Recent Results in Cancer Research 93

Leukemia

Recent Developments in Diagnosis and Therapy

Edited by E. Thiel and S. Thierfelder

With 36 Figures and 63 Tables

Springer-Verlag
Berlin Heidelberg New York Tokyo 1984

Priv.-Doz. Dr. Eckhard Thiel
Professor Dr. Stephan Thierfelder

Gesellschaft für Strahlen- und Umweltforschung mbH
Institut für Hämatologie, Abteilung für Immunologie
Landwehrstrasse 61, 8000 München 2, FRG

Sponsored by the Swiss League against Cancer

ISBN 3-540-13289-9 Springer-Verlag Berlin Heidelberg New York Tokyo
ISBN 0-387-13289-9 Springer-Verlag New York Heidelberg Berlin Tokyo

Library of Congress Cataloging in Publication Data. Main entry under title: Leukemia: recent developments in diagnosis and therapy. (Recent results in cancer research; 93) "Sponsored by the Swiss League against Cancer" – T.p. verso. Includes bibliographies and index. 1. Leukemia-Congresses. I. Thiel, Eckhard, 1944– . II. Thierfelder, Stefan, 1933– . III. Schweizerische Krebsliga. IV. Series: Recent results in cancer research; v. 93. [DNLM: 1. Leukemia-diagnosis. 2. Leukemia-therapy. W1 RE106P v.93./WH 250 L6556] RC261.R35 vol. 93 616.99'4 s [616.99'419] 84-10510 [RC643].

Typesetting and printing: v. Starck'sche Druckereigesellschaft m.b.H., Wiesbaden
Binding: J. Schäffer OHG, Grünstadt
2125/3140–543210

Preface

Much of the attention presently paid to leukemia is the result of recent progress in understanding and treatment. Chemotherapy of leukemia started in the late 1940s, and combination therapy evolved in the late 1950s. It was at that time that the clonality of leukemia was realized, after the discovery of chromosomal and then biochemical and immunological markers. And now we have the new data on retroviral and cellular oncogenes and the reports on human T-cell lymphoma/leukemia viruses. Many more steps forward could be enumerated in a field which is so rapidly making the hematological textbooks outdated.

In this volume, thirteen in-depth reviews from large multicenter trials in the Federal Republic of Germany summarize the current state of diagnosis and management of leukemias. Childhood ALL and AML adult ALL and AUL were investigated. While cure appears to be achievable for more and more patients with acute leukemia, we still pursue the aim of optimal palliation in chronic leukemias. The management of patients with leukemia therefore varies to a large extent in aggressiveness of therapy. In some situations, rescue from an otherwise lethal disease is provided by bone marrow transplantation, which is discussed in two chapters.

Propertailoring of therapy depends from the beginning of the disease on accurate and complete diagnosis. Classification of leukemias according to immunological markers and to cytochemical/ultrastructural criteria is dealt with comprehensively in two reviews. There is even a chapter on atypical leukemias, comprising preleukemia, smoldering leukemia, and hypoplastic leukemia. Extensive up-to-date bibliographies and tabulations of published data will help the reader find the original references.

It is hoped that this volume will orient clinicians, hematologists, and researchers in their quest for valuable new insights into leukemia.

February 1984 The Editors

Contents

*List of Contributors**

* The address of the principal author is given on the first page of each contribution
1 Page, on which contribution commences

Current Understanding of Virus Etiology in Leukemia

R. Hehlmann, H. Schetters, C. Leib-Mösch, and V. Erfle

Medizinische Poliklinik, Universität München, Pettenkoferstrasse 8a, 8000 München 2, FRG

Introduction

Epidemiological studies demonstrate that irradiation, genetic factors, immunological deficiencies, drugs, and environmental agents represent risk factors for the development of human leukemia, but cannot be considered common causes of this disease [1]. The same studies show that human leukemias are clearly not acute infectious diseases in the usual sense. In fact, tumor viruses or their footprints have been found only in a minority of human leukemias and lymphomas in spite of considerable efforts, and their role as possible etiological agents or cofactors remains uncertain. These observations and the recognition of certain preleukemic states which are not neoplastic in themselves but can convert to overt leukemia support the concept of a multifactorial etiology and/or multistep development of human leukemias. Why then pursue the concept of a *viral* etiology in human leukemias? There are four main reasons why the virus approach to leukemia remains an important issue: (a) Viruses are the cause of naturally occurring leukemias in several animal species including primates; (b) viruses have been associated regularly and repeatedly with certain forms of human leukemias and lymphomas; (c) a viral etiology may be obscured in human leukemias by several factors, such as long latency period, requirement for unknown cofactors, vertical transmission of the agent, congenital infection of the embryo, etc., all of which are known to occur in virus-induced leukemias in animals; and (d) the study of oncogenesis by viruses has contributed and continues to contribute a great deal to our knowledge of the molecular events and basic mechanisms involved in carcinogenesis in general.

Two groups of viruses are known to cause leukemias and lymphomas in animals and are suspected of being etiologically involved in some forms of human leukemias: members of the herpesvirus group and certain retroviruses. Herpesviruses contain DNA as genetic material and possess a complex genetic structure. *Herpesvirus saimiri* and *herpesvirus ateles* cause rapidly fatal leukemias and lymphomas in susceptible monkeys. Marek's disease virus (MDV) has been recognized as the etiological agent of one form of lymphomatosis in chickens. And the Epstein-Barr virus (EBV), which causes infectious mononucleosis, is implicated in the etiology of African Burkitt's lymphoma and some forms of nasopharyngeal carcinoma in man. Since the herpesviruses have been reviewed recently and extensively in several series of articles by workers in the field [2, 3], this review will concentrate on leukemogenesis by retroviruses. Retroviruses (or RNA tumor viruses) are RNA-containing viruses and the etiological agents of leukemias and lymphomas in chickens, mice, rats, guinea pigs, cats, cattle, and gibbon apes.

This article will briefly summarize the basic properties of retroviruses, present the new data on retroviral and cellular oncogenes, and discuss evidence for and against various models of

Recent Results in Cancer Research. Vol. 93

retroviral leukemogenesis. Furthermore, it will give a broad overview over the virus-induced leukemias in animals and finally review the recent developments in virus association with human leukemias and lymphomas, including the recently discovered human T cell lymphoma/leukemia viruses HTLV and ATLV.

Basic Properties of Retroviruses

Basic features of retroviruses and retroviral replication have been the subjects of many recent review articles [4–8] and will therefore be only summarized here.

Modes of Transmission

Retroviruses may exist either as so-called endogenous viruses integrated in the genomes of their host cells, or as exogenous viruses infecting their host cells from outside. Endogenous viruses are replicated as parts of their host cell DNAs and are transmitted vertically through the germ line from one generation to the next. They can be activated by several chemical and physical agents to form infectious retroviral particles. Most endogenous retroviruses are not pathogenic for their respective hosts and are usually xenotropic, i.e., they have lost their capability to infect cells of their hosts of origin. Most vertebrate species appear to harbor endogenous viruses.
Exogenous retroviruses are transmitted horizontally, either from one individual to another, in utero, or through mother's milk by means of an infectious process. The complete genetic information of these viruses is not found as a part of the genome of the species in which they cause disease. Most oncogenic retroviruses are exogenous.

Structure of Retroviruses

All retroviruses share common morphological and structural features. The genetic information is contained in a 70S RNA that consists of two identical 35S RNA subunits held together by hydrogen bonds at their 5′ ends [9]. The viral RNA is similar to messenger RNA in that it has a cap structure of 5′-methyl-GpppG at its 5′ end [10] and a poly(A) sequence of about 200 nucleotides at its 3′ end. An RNA dependent DNA polymerase, the reverse transcriptase, is associated with the 70S RNA; this enzyme is responsible for transcription of the viral RNA into DNA during virus replication.
Furthermore, virus particles contain structural proteins which represent about 95% of the total retroviral weight. The structural proteins consist of the inner core proteins and the envelope proteins which are in most cases glycoproteins. They are designated by a small p or gp (for protein or glycoprotein) and a number which specifies their molecular weights in thousands, e.g., p30, gp70 etc. All replication-competent retroviruses harbor at least three viral genes that are necessary for their replication: the *gag* gene coding for the internal or core proteins of the viral particles; the *pol* gene coding for the viral RNA-dependent DNA polymerase or reverse transcriptase; and the *env* gene coding for the envelope glycoproteins and proteins. The gene sequence has been determined as 5′-*cap-gag-pol-env*-poly(A) 3′.
In addition, all retroviral genomes carry noncoding terminal sequences: the terminally redundant *R* regions, and the unique regions at the 5′ and 3′ ends next to the *R* regions,

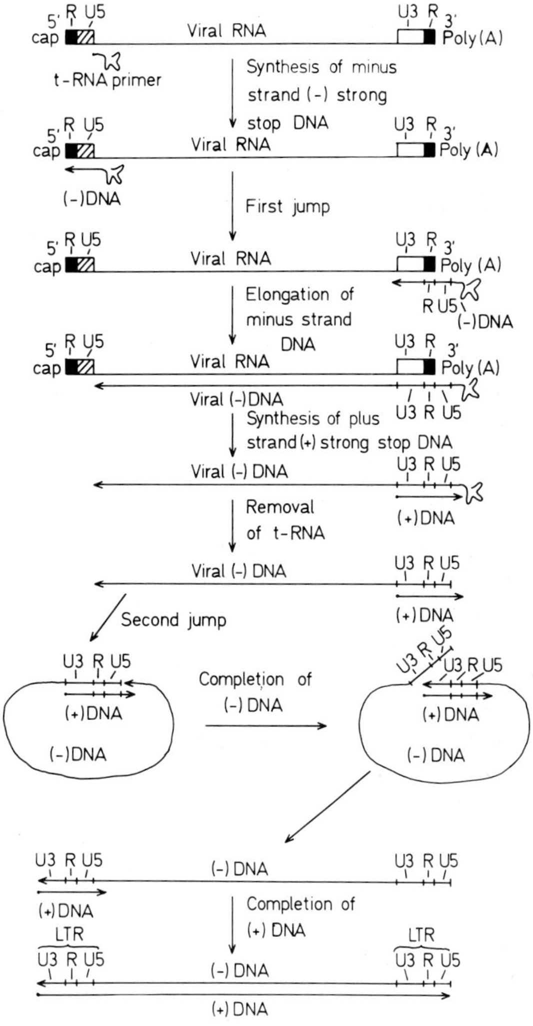

Fig. 1. Reverse transcription. For explanation see text

called *U5* and *U3* (Fig. 1). These noncoding regions are duplicated during the formation of the DNA provirus in a complex process and form the domains called long terminal repeats (LTRs) at either end of the provirus [11] in the sequence *U3-R-U5*. On the basis of nucleotide sequencing data [12–19], the LTRs appear to provide basic functions for regulation and expression of proviral genes [20]. The *U3* regions of all LTRs contain a sequence closely related to the so-called TATAA box, which is thought to promote initiation of transcription of eukaryotic genes [21]. Another common eukaryotic signal contained in the LTR is the AATAAA sequence for polyadenylation.

Replication of Retroviruses

RNA tumorviruses infect cells by adhesion to the cellular membrane at specific receptors. After penetration, the uncoated RNA is transcribed into DNA (reverse transcription) as summarized in Fig. 1. This step is initiated by a host cell transfer-RNA primer.

Transcription of retroviral RNA into DNA starts close to the 5′ terminus of the viral RNA molecule resulting in a short piece of complementary DNA also called "strong stop" DNA and then "jumps" to the 3′ terminus of the same, if circularized, or of another RNA molecule. The viral RNA is then transcribed into a "minus"-strand DNA beginning with the *U3* region. Synthesis of complementary or "plus"-strand DNA is initiated at the 5′ boundary of *U3*. Extension of the plus-strand DNA occurs in a similar fashion to that of the minus-strand DNA. Transcription results in a double-stranded proviral DNA with the terminally redundant *U3, R,* and *U5* regions on either side of the provirus forming the LTRs.

The proviral DNA is covalently incorporated into the host cellular genome by a mechanism that is not yet understood. It is not clear whether linear provirus DNA or circular DNA forms are required for integration. The integration sites seem to be multiple and not dependent on particular host cell DNA sequences. The proviral DNA is then replicated with the cellular DNA as part of the host cell genome. Viral RNA synthesis is mediated by host RNA polymerase II [4], probably under the influence of the promotor region of the LTR.

Viral RNA has to fulfill the twofold function of providing (a) mRNA for viral protein synthesis and (b) genomic RNA for the synthesis of progeny virus. Assembly of RNA and viral proteins occurs in the cytoplasm near the cellular membrane. The details of the formation of complete viral particles that bud from the cell surface are largely unknown.

Oncogenicity

The remarkable property of retroviruses which has given this virus group the name RNA tumorviruses is the capability of some retroviruses to cause tumors (leukemias, sarcomas, lymphomas, carcinomas) in various animal species (chickens, mice, rats, guinea pigs, cats, cattle, monkeys) and to mediate neoplastic transformation of cultured cells (for review see 106). The oncogenicity of retroviruses follows two patterns: 1. Some viruses induce tumors rapidly, i.e., in two to four weeks and possess a gene called "oncogene" which is responsible for their capacity to induce tumors. 2. Other viruses do not possess oncogenes and induce tumors by other not yet fully recognized pathways. Oncogenesis by the second category of viruses is much slower and requires long latent periods (i.e., several months) for tumor induction.

In most rapidly oncogenic viruses the oncogenes are present at the expense of replication genes. These viruses are therefore defective and need for their replication the presence of a replication competent helper virus. The exception is the avian Rous sarcoma virus (RSV) which possesses an oncogene in addition to a complete set of replication genes. Most remarkably, however, the 5′ and the 3′ ends of all defective viruses have been conserved and result in proviruses carrying complete LTR regions as determined by nucleotide sequence analysis [16, 18, 22–24].

Several general structures of oncogene products of the acutely transforming retroviruses have been recognized (Table 1). Some viruses, including most of the acute avian leukemia viruses, Abelson murine leukemia virus, and feline sarcoma viruses, have retained part of their *gag* genes (*Δgag*) immediately preceding the *onc*-specific information (X), and therefore synthesize a *Δgag*-X transformation polyprotein. Other viruses with different genomic locations of their oncogenes synthesize oncogene products without portions of viral structural proteins; examples of such viruses are RSV, avian myeloblastosis virus (AMV), the murine sarcoma viruses, and possibly also simian sarcoma virus (SiSV) [25].

Table 1. Structures of acutely transforming viruses

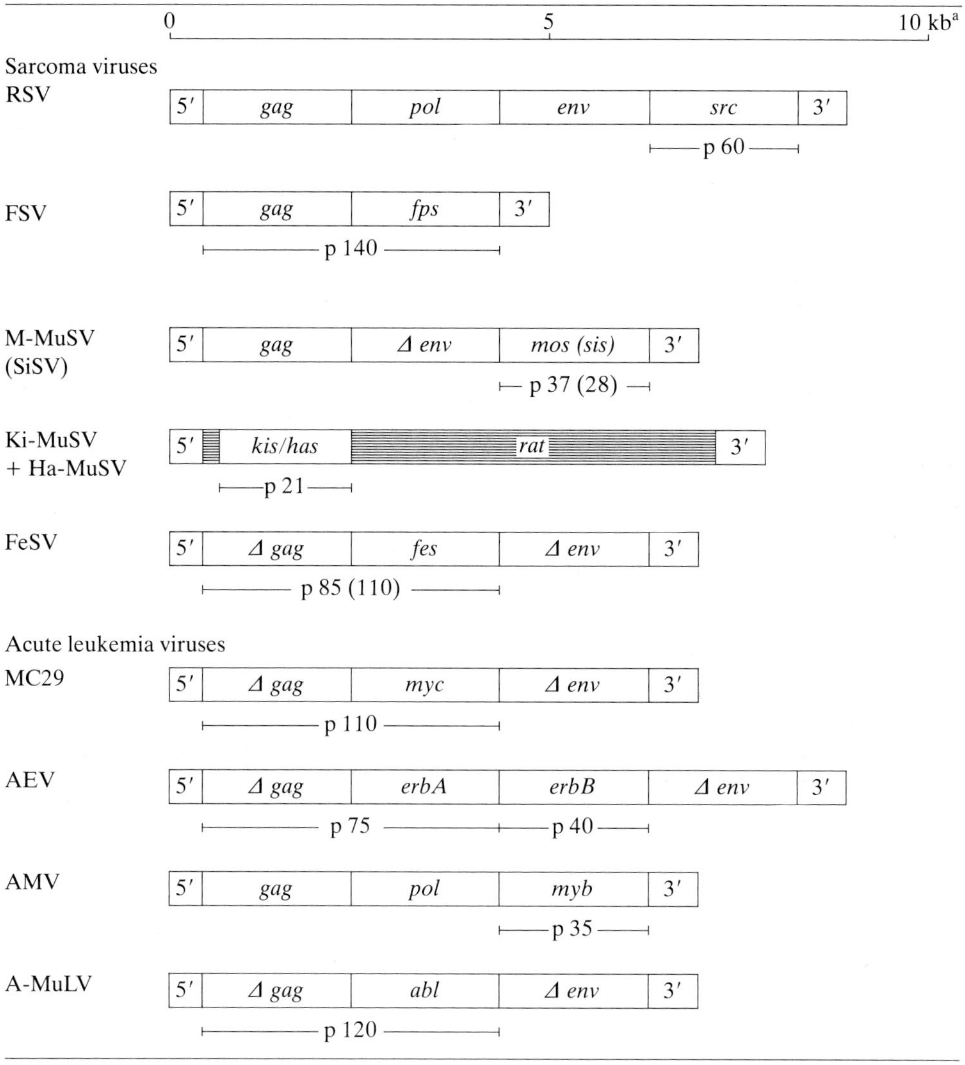

[a] Number of kb approximate values

The structures deduced for several defective viruses have now been confirmed by the determination of the complete nucleotide sequences of one murine and two avian sarcoma viruses [22–24, 26].

Oncogenes

Oncogenes are retroviral or cellular genes that have been shown to induce tumors or transform tissue culture cells under certain defined conditions.

Table 2. Onc genes of acutely transforming retroviruses

Onc gene	Virus of origin	Human chromosome	Neoplasias induced
A) Acute leukemia viruses			
myc	MC29 avian myelocytomatosis virus	8	Leukemias, sarcomas, carcinomas
myc, mil	MH2 avian leukemia virus		Leukemias, sarcomas, carcinomas
myb	Avian myeloblastosis virus (AMV)	6	Myeloblastosis
myb, ets	E26 myeloblastosis virus		Erythroblastosis, Myeloblastosis
erb B, erb A	Avian erythroblastosis virus (AEV)		Leukemias
rel	Avian reticuloendotheliosis virus T (REV)		Reticuloendotheliosis
abl	Abelson murine leukemia virus (A-MuLV)	9	Leukemias
B) Sarcoma viruses			
src	Rous avian sarcoma virus (RSV)	20	Sarcomas
fps	Fujinami avian sarcoma virus (FSV)	15	Sarcomas
yes	Yamaguchi avian sarcoma virus (Y73)		Sarcomas
ros	UR2 avian sarcoma virus		Sarcomas
ski	Avian SkV 770 virus	1	Sarcomas
mos	Moloney murine sarcoma virus (M-MuSV)	8	Sarcomas
raf	3611 MuSV	3	Sarcomas
ras	Rasheed rat sarcoma virus (RaSV)		Sarcomas
has	Harvey MuSV	11	Sarcomas
kis	Kirsten MuSV	12	Sarcomas
bas	Balb MuSV		Sarcomas
fos	FBJ MuSV	2	Osteosarcomas
fes	Feline sarcoma virus (FeSV) (strains Gardner-Arnstein and Snyder-Theilen)	15	Sarcomas
fms	FeSV (strain McDonough-Sarma)	5	Sarcomas
fgr	FeSV (strain Gardner-Rasheed)		Sarcomas
sis	Simian sarcoma virus (SiSV)	22	Sarcomas

Retroviral Oncogenes

Oncogenes have been detected in most acutely transforming retroviruses (leukemia- and sarcoma viruses) and are responsible for tumor induction by these viruses [4, 27, 30, 32]. Oncogenesis via viral oncogenes is rapid and predominates over all other cellular genes. The best studied of these oncogenes is the *src* gene of Rous sarcoma virus (RSV). The knowledge that a separate gene is involved in neoplastic transformation was originally derived from observations with transformation-defective (td) and with temperature-sensitive (ts) conditional mutants of RSV [27, 28]. When ts mutant RSV-transformed cells were maintained at a permissive temperature they remained transformed. When the temperature was made higher and nonpermissive the transformed cells regained normal morphology. By additional work with td mutants it was possible to assign the transforming property to a fragment of RNA contained in wild-type RSV-RNA, but missing from td RSV-RNA [29].

After detection of the *src* gene further *onc* genes were identified in other oncogenic retroviruses [25, 30]. More than 20 different viral oncogenes have so far been detected [31, 32, 199, 202] (Table 2). The complete nucleotide sequence of several of these retroviral oncogenes, e.g., of *src, mos, kis, has, sis,* has been determined [12, 16, 18, 19, 23], and it has confirmed that most *onc* genes are not related to each other. Homology, however, found between *fps* from Fujinami avian sarcoma virus (FSV) and *fes* from the Gardner-Arnstein and Snyder Theilen strains of feline sarcoma virus (FeSV) [33] and between *src* from RSV and *mos* from Moloney-murine sarcoma virus, for example, indicates that the number of oncogenes probably may be limited [34].

Transformation Proteins

The translation products of the *onc* genes which mediate cellular transformation are the so-called transformation or onc proteins. Molecular weights and approximate viral coding domains of some of these proteins are depicted in Table 1. Many of these proteins still lack functional definition. The best characterized transformation protein is that of RSV, a 60,000 dalton phosphoprotein called $pp60^{src}$ [35]. $pp60^{src}$ possesses protein kinase activity, and specifically phosphorylates tyrosine, an uncommon aminoacid, to be phosphorylated under normal conditions [36]. $pp60^{src}$ was shown to be present in RSV-transformed cells and absent in normal cells and is thought to be responsible for cellular transformation. The transformation process at the translational level is still not well understood, but appears to be associated with the cytoskeleton. $pp60^{src}$ has been found associated with the inner plasmalemma of the cell membrane and in close proximity to the cytoskeleton component vinculin [37, 38], which is responsible, among other proteins, for adhesion of cells to surfaces. Phosphorylation of vinculin and breakdown of the cytoskeleton appear to be interrelated processes during transformation. By work with ts transformation-defective RSV mutants and with antibodies against synthetic oligopeptides, a multifunctional and/or pleiotropic effect of $pp60^{src}$ has been suggested [39].
Several other transformation proteins also possess kinase activities. In contrast, the *onc* product of *myc*, the oncogene of the avian acute leukemia virus MC 29, has been shown to possess DNA-binding capacity and seems to be localized in the nucleus [40], and the transformation protein of simian sarcoma virus, $p28^{sis}$, is structurally related to a cellular growth factor, the platelet-derived growth factor (PDGF) [41, 42].

Origin of Oncogenes

Retroviral oncogenes designated *v-onc* are derived from cellular progenitor DNA sequences designated *c-onc*. These sequences are thought to have been acquired by replication of retroviruses upon passage through rodents, cats, chickens, and primates. The source of these new sequences has been traced, in most cases, to the genomes of the host animal through which the original virus was passed. This was first shown for *src* of RSV [43] by the hybridization of ^{3}H-*src* DNA with nuclear DNA of normal uninfected chickens.
The cellular progenitors of retroviral *onc* genes appear to be highly conserved from the evolutionary aspect. This is concluded from the observation that sequences homologous to *src* are not only found in DNAs of vertebrate species as diverse as chicken, calf, mouse, man, and salmon [44], but also in the DNA of *Drosophila melanogaster* [45]. Similar observations have been made with sequences homologous to the *onc* gene of SiSV (*v-sis*), which have been found in the DNAs of gibbon apes, marmosets, rats, cats, and man [46]. There is accumulating evidence that human DNA and the DNAs of all other vertebrate species contain progenitors of most *onc* genes analysed. Sequences related to the following viral *onc* genes have been detected in human DNA: *v-myc* of avian myelocytomatosis virus

MC 29, *v-myb* of avian myeloblastosis virus (AMV), *v-mos* of Moloney murine sarcoma virus (M-MuSV), *v-has* of Harvey murine sarcoma virus (Ha-MuSV), *v-kis* of Kirsten murine sarcoma virus (Ki-MuSV), *v-bas* of Balb murine sarcoma virus (Balb-MuSV), *v-abl* of Abelson murine leukemia virus (A-MuLV), and *v-fes* of feline sarcoma virus (FeSV) [47–50]. Expression of some of these sequences has been observed in human cells and tissues [51, 52, 201].

Chromosomal Assignment of Human Oncogene Homologs

Chromosomal assignment has been possible for several human oncogene homologs by means of the somatic cell hybrid technique. The human homologs of the transforming sequence of A-MuLV, *c-abl,* of the transforming sequences of FeSV, *c-fes,* of Ha-MuSV, *c-has,* of Ki-MuSV, *c-kis,* of myelocytomatosis virus MC 29, *c-myc,* of M-MuSV, *c-mos,* of AMV, *c-myb,* and of SiSV, *c-sis,* have been assigned to the human chromosomes 9, 15, 11, 12, 8, 8, 6, and 22, (Table 2) [53–62, 64]. Aberrations and translocations of several of these chromosomes (numbers 6, 8, 9, 15, 22) have been observed in chronic myelogenous leukemia, in Burkitt's lymphomas, and in acute leukemias. The location of some human oncogene homologs (*c-abl, c-myc, c-mos, c-myb*) at the breakpoints involved in these chromosome translocations [53, 55, 59, 61] suggest a causal relationship between chromosomal aberrations and oncogene activity in these human neoplasms. Most remarkably, the human oncogene homolog *c-sis* of SiSV, the only known transforming primate retrovirus, which has been assigned to human chromosome 22 [62, 63], is translocated to chromosome 9 in chronic myelogenous leukemia [63a] in exchange for the human oncogene homolog of A-MuLV, *c-abl,* which is translocated from chromosome 9 to chromosome 22, the so-called Philadelphia chromosome [53].

Oncogenes Isolated by Transfection

There is evidence that the detection of oncogenes through retroviruses was fortuitous and that oncogenes do exist and transform cells quite independently of retroviruses. This evidence has been obtained by transfection studies with isolated DNA from various normal, chemically transformed, and tumor-derived cell lines. DNAs from chemically transformed and from normal rodent and avian cells not associated with retroviruses were found to transform contact-inhibited NIH/3T3-mouse fibroblasts [65, 66]. Transforming activity has also been reported for DNA of cell lines from human tumors, including bladder, lung, colon, and mammary carcinomas, and from lymphoid and myeloid neoplasias, neuroblastomas, and sarcomas [67–73]. In several cases, the transforming sequences have been isolated from the NIH/3T3 cells by molecular cloning and characterized by hybridization studies. These studies showed that (a) human (tumor) DNA contains transforming sequences; (b) different tumor types tend to be associated with distinct oncogenes; and (c) some of these cellular transforming sequences are closely related to known retroviral oncogenes.

The transforming sequences isolated from the human bladder carcinoma lines EJ and T24 are homologs of *v-has,* the *onc* gene of Harvey murine sarcoma virus (74–76], and the transforming sequences from lung and colon carcinomas are homologs of *v-kis,* the *onc* gene of Kirsten MuSV [76]. No homology to retroviral oncogenes could be detected in transformation sequences from other human tumors [73]. Sequence analyses have revealed that the transforming sequences isolated from the EJ and T24 lines differ from the homologous sequences in normal human DNA by a single base exchange [77, 78]. It appears from these observations that oncogenes can act independently of retroviruses and that retroviruses function rather as vehicles for the transduction of cellular oncogenes. Possibly oncogenes represent a final common pathway for carcinogenesis by various carcinogenic agents.

Possible Mechanisms of Viral Leukemogenesis

Leukemogenesis mediated by viruses appears to follow several pathways. Experimental support exists for several distinct theories of viral leukemogenesis. Clearly, the rapid induction of leukemia by the acute leukemia viruses which possess oncogenes is quite different from the slow leukemia induction by the chronic leukemia viruses which do not possess oncogenes but might utilize cellular oncogenes. And leukemogenesis by certain recombinant retroviruses, or via chronic mitogenic stimulation as a consequence of virus infection, appears, thus far, not to be associated with oncogenes at all.

Leukemogenesis by Oncogene-Virogene Recombinants (Acute Leukemia Viruses)

Oncogenes have been found in almost all acutely transforming sarcoma and leukemia viruses [25, 79, 80] with few exceptions, e.g., some strains of MuLV and the spleen focus-forming virus (SFFV) of the murine Friend virus complex [81]. The only known function of the oncogenes is malignant transformation. The sporadic isolation of oncogene-carrying viruses and the absence of horizontal spread of retroviruses with oncogenes, however, lead to the question as to whether retroviral oncogenes are relevant to the majority of natural cancers. The acutely transforming oncogene-carrying retroviruses do, in any case, represent excellent models for the study of carcinogenesis.

The transforming property of oncogenes was established by the use of ts conditional mutants [28, 83] and td deletion mutants [27] (see above), and by transfection studies with *onc* genes isolated from a murine sarcoma virus [84] and from normal cellular, including human, DNA [87]. The transforming efficiency of the oncogenes could be markedly increased if they were ligated to LTR sequences [85, 86, 88].

Transformation by oncogenes is probably mediated by the protein products (= transformation proteins) of the oncogenes, since presence and absence of transformation proteins correlate with transformed and nontransformed states of the cells. The mechanism(s) of action of the transformation proteins is unclear.

Since the cellular progenitor oncogenes present in normal cells are usually not detectably expressed, or expressed at low levels, transformation has been assumed to be a *quantitative* problem due to an enhanced production of transformation proteins. If correct, this hypothesis assumes that cells normally control cellular oncogenes to prevent expression above a certain critical level. Expression of transformation proteins above this critical level would lead to transformation or carcinogenesis. This assumption is supported by the observation that expression of oncogenes may be greatly enhanced in transformed cells and after infection by acutely transforming retroviruses [25].

Alternatively, it has been suggested that *qualitative* differences may exist between retroviral oncogenes and their cellular progenitors. Evidence for this alternative comes from the observation that most cellular *onc* sequences are interrupted by several stretches of unrelated DNA (introns). Also, biological activity does not occur following transfection with cellular DNA related to avian oncogenes (*src* or *myc*), even on ligation to LTR sequences [25]. And the discovery of point mutations as critical events for the acquisition of transforming properties in the case of the EJ and T24 bladder carcinoma oncogenes further argues for a mechanism of carcinogenesis by qualitative changes of cellular oncogenes [77, 78]. Qualitative (sequence) differences have also been observed between viral oncogenes and cellular progenitor sequences of Moloney murine sarcoma virus *(mos)*, avian myeloblastosis virus *(myb)* [89], and others [200].

The sporadic isolation of oncogene carrying viruses and the absence of horizontal spread of retroviruses with oncogenes argue against *retroviral* oncogenes being a major cause of natural cancers. The location of oncogenes at critical points of chromosomal translocations associated with cancer (see above) suggests that this conclusion is not valid for *cellular* oncogenes.

Leukemogenesis by Promotor Insertion and Activation of Oncogenes (Chronic Leukemia Viruses)

An enhanced production of transformation proteins might also be the mechanism of leukemogenesis by chronic leukemia viruses which do not carry oncogenes. This hypothesis assumes the insertion of the promotor sequences of retroviral LTR DNA adjacent to a cellular oncogene and subsequent promotion of expression of this oncogene. A promotor insertion next to a cellular oncogene would be a rare recombinational event and would be consistent with a long latency period prior to tumor development. Evidence for this model has been obtained in avian leukosis virus (ALV)-induced leukemia of chickens by Hayward et al. [90], who showed the ALV proviral DNA is inserted adjacent to the cellular oncogene *c-myc,* and that as a consequence expression of *c-myc* is stimulated 30- to 100-fold. Hayward's observation was extended by Payne et al. [91] who found that enhanced expression of *c-myc* occurs with proviruses in any of three configurations: (a) on the 5′ side ('upstream') of *c-myc* in the same transcriptional orientation; (b) on the 3′ side ('downstream') of *c-myc* in the same orientation; (c) upstream, in the opposite orientation. The implication of these findings is that for the validity of the promotor insertion model several modes of transcriptional promotion would have to be postulated.

Leukemogenesis by Recombination Among Non-oncogenic Retroviruses

A possibly entirely different mechanism of leukemogenesis has been concluded from observations on the creation of highly leukemogenic retroviruses in mice by recombinational events in the *env* gene region of the viruses [92, 93]. The molecular events underlying leukemogenesis by these recombinant viruses are far from clear. It has been suggested, however, that the recombination in *env* might alter the antigenicity of the envelope glycoprotein (see below) and/or that the recombination includes part of the regulating sequences in the adjacent 3′ terminal region. These alterations of antigenicity and/or regulating capacity are assumed to be responsible for leukemogenesis.

Leukemogenesis by Chronic Mitogenic Stimulation

This hypothesis proposes the involvement of retroviruses in leukemogenesis not by genetic mechanisms, as discussed above, but by cell surface signals mediated by retroviral antigens and antibodies. The expression of retroviral antigens on the surface of lymphocytes is postulated as signal for some steps of differentiation. These antigens can be activated by certain mitogenic substances, and the proliferation of these activated cells can be stimulated or blocked by specific antiviral antibodies [94]. The induction of a potent and specific antiviral antibody response could lead to a block of differentiation, to stimulation of proliferation, and to an accumulation of undifferentiated cells.

Alternatively, it is assumed that the viral glycoprotein may act as a specific mitogen for certain hematopoietic target cells. Such a model has been put forward for the formation of murine T cell lymphomas [95, 96]. This model proposes a mitogenic effect of retroviruses on target cells via cell surface receptors for retroviral envelope glycoproteins with the consequence that the target cells may produce blastogenic factors (lymphokines) which induce proliferation of another cell population [96, 97]. Experimental support for this model stems from characterization of surface phenotypes of retrovirus-induced leukemias [98], blocking of virus binding sites with monoclonal antibodies [99], and demonstration of lymphokines in supernatants of gp70-induced lymphocytes [96].

The mitogenic stimulation model could also explain leukemia and lymphoma induction by chronic leukemia viruses.

Transition to Irreversible State of Transformation

In the last model, as in the other hypotheses discussed above, a hypothetical second step would be required for transition from the reversible polyclonal transformed or preleukemic state of tumorvirus-infected cells to the state of irreversible, mostly monoclonal growth characteristics of malignant tumors. This second step has been suggested by Klein [100] to be permanent DNA or chromosomal rearrangement.

Indeed, characteristic chromosomal aberrations have been correlated with distinct malignant tumors of several species, and specific translocations (for example, the trisomy of chromosome 15 in MuLV-induced T cell leukemias and the 8; 14 translocation in Burkitt's lymphoma) have been found in several virus-associated neoplasias [100, 101].

The mechanisms by which permanent chromosomal changes are induced are unknown. But retroviruses, for instance, possess structural properties of transposable elements of bacteria, yeast, maize, and *drosophila* which can induce transposition of genetic material. These structural features, in essence, are short inverted repeats at the ends of the transposable DNA molecule (as contained in the LTRs of the retroviral provirus) and short sequences of duplication at the insertion site flanking the inserted DNA segment. Integration of these elements has been shown to create recombinations between inserting elements and flanking DNA and, probably as a consequence of this recombination, chromosomal deletions, inversions, and translocations [102]. The inverted repeats seem to be the hot-spots for the initiation of the recombination event.

The location of oncogenes at the breakpoints involved in chromosomal translocations, e.g., the location of *c-myc* at the break point of chromosome 8 in the 8; 14 translocation in Burkitt's lymphoma [53, 59, 60] and of *c-abl* at the breakpoint of chromosome 9 in the 9; 22 translocation in CML, suggests a critical role of oncogenes at this step.

Retroviruses with their structural similarities to transposable elements would be suitable entities to provide the necessary basis for the initiation of recombination and for the stable inheritance of the resulting DNA reorganization in subsequent cell generations [14, 103].

Virus Etiology of Leukemia in Animal Systems

Avian Leukemia

Avian leukemia was the first neoplasia that was shown to be caused by a virus [104]. On the basis of their biological properties and genetic structures two main groups of avian leukemia viruses are distinguished: the chronic lymphoid leukosis viruses (LLV or ALV), which cause lymphoid leukemia and lymphomatosis in chickens after long latency periods, and the replication-defective acute leukemia viruses, which carry oncogenes and rapidly induce various leukemias, sarcomas and carcinomas [106, 107].

Spontaneous ALV-induced leukemia of chickens in the form of a lymphoproliferative disease of the visceral organs is a major natural cause of death in chicken flocks. Transmission of ALV can be horizontal but appears to be mostly through the egg. In contrast, the isolation of an acute leukemia virus is a rare event and the significance of these viruses for naturally occurring disease is questionable.

A separate form of lymphomatosis of chicken affecting T lymphocytes is Marek's disease. This disease is caused by a member of the herpesvirus group, the Marek's disease virus (MDV) [108].

Murine Leukemia

The first murine leukemia virus was isolated by Gross in 1951 [105]. A series of murine leukemia viruses (MuLV) have been isolated since then. Further in vivo passage of these isolates gave rise to a number of prototype leukemia virus strains, which allowed an insight into basic processes of virus-cell interactions leading to malignant transformation of hematopoietic cells. These viruses are exogenous; their only mode of transmission is by injection; and the course and the picture of the diseases induced are not necessarily those of naturally occurring leukemias.

Several different types of leukemias can be induced with exogenous MuLV in mice. These are T cell leukemias (with Gross, Moloney, radiation MuLV), B cell leukemias (with Abelson MuLV), myeloid leukemias (with Graffi MuLV), or erythroleukemias and polycythemia (with Rauscher and Friend MuLV). The development of the leukemias is rapid, with latent periods of only 1–3 weeks. In most instances the viruses seem to transform stem cells committed to specific differentiation pathways, but under certain conditions infection of pluripotent stem cells may occur [109]. The question of target cells was investigated essentially with in vitro long-term bone marrow cultures [110].

In vivo inoculation of the viruses is followed by a viremic state, marked immunosuppression, and later the production of virus-neutralizing and cytotoxic antibodies. The viral genomes can be found integrated as proviruses in the genomes of leukemic cells [111], and from these proviruses leukemic viruses can again be isolated. Horizontal transmission of these viruses from leukemic to healthy animals has not been observed. Prevention of virus spread and of the onset of leukemia was achieved by preimmunization of the animals with a viral vaccine or with anti-MuLV gp70 antibodies [112, 113].

The best-studied example of the association of endogenous retroviruses with naturally occurring murine leukemias is the spontaneous T cell leukemia of AKR mice. In AKR leukemia, which develops within 5–6 months after birth, a high amount of infectious, nonleukemogenic viruses can be isolated from the thymus and other lymphoreticular organs during the entire lifetime of the animals. In the preleukemic phase biologically different, leukemogenic viruses are found in the thymus [92]. After leukemia induction with these viruses the same types of viruses can be recovered from the resulting thymic lymphomas. Protein and genome analyses indicate that the leukemogenic isolates have arisen by a recombination event between different proviruses present in the mouse genome. The newly created leukemia viruses can be found integrated in the DNA of the leukemic cells at varying locations. For possible molecular pathways leading to the transformed state of the cells see above.
Besides spontaneous AKR leukemia, radiation-induced leukemia in mice has also been discussed with reference to causation by the activation of endogenous retroviruses. The isolation of leukemogenic recombinant viruses from these leukemias supports the hypothesis of a possible role of endogenous retroviruses in carcinogenesis [114].

Feline Leukemia

A leukemogenic virus was first isolated from leukemic cats in 1964 [115]. The virus has been identified as retrovirus (FeLV), and has been shown to transmit the disease. Subsequent epidemiological and biochemical studies by Jarrett, Essex, Hardy, and others [79] established FeLV as the major cause of naturally occurring leukemia and lymphoma in domestic cats. Feline leukemia and lymphoma occur in several forms. Acute lymphoblastic leukemia, thymic lymphoma, and multicentric lymphoma appear to be T cell malignancies. In the alimentary form of lymphoma, the B cell appears to be the target cell. Most field isolates of FeLV cause neoplastic disease only after long latency periods. Viremia precedes the outbreak of overt leukemia, and therefore viremia may be present in apparently healthy cats. High titers of infectious virus are present in the saliva of infected cats, and this presumably is the main route of infection. FeLV is transmitted horizontally and is not an endogenous virus of the cat [116]. Virus-induced feline leukemias and sarcomas can be prevented by vaccination with antiviral antibodies [79, 118].
Analysis of viral antigen expression in leukemic cats provided evidence not only for expression of viral structural proteins (gp70, p30), but also for an antigen originally found in cell clones nonproductively transformed by feline sarcoma virus (FeSV). The antigen was termed FOCMA (feline oncornavirus-associated cell membrane antigen) [117]. Even leukemic cells negative for FeLV and FeLV structural proteins were regularly positive for FOCMA. Recent evidence indicates that FOCMA and the gene product of the feline oncogene *fes* share antigenic determinants and may be identical [119]. The role of FOCMA in FeLV-transformed cells is not yet clear, but it probably represents expression of an activated cellular oncogene.

Bovine Leukemia

Bovine leukemia virus (BLV) is the causative agent of the enzootic form of bovine leukemia (EBL) and of persistent lymphocytosis (PL) in cattle [120]. EBL is a herd disease and is clearly distinguished from sporadic bovine leukosis (SBL), which is not associated

with BLV or any other known virus. BLV infection and development of disease appear to depend on genetic and environmental factors, since certain herds have a much higher incidence of leukemia than others and since not all infected animals of a given herd develop disease (for review see [121]). BLV is transmitted horizontally and is exogenous to cattle, i.e., the BLV genome is not present in the DNA of normal uninfected animals [122]. BLV appears to infect only B lymphocytes. Virus cannot be isolated from diseased animals, probably due to the good humoral antibody response elicited. In fact, this virus has only been obtained after in vitro culture of leukemic cells from cattle with EBL [120].
The origin of BLV is unclear. Epidemiological studies indicate that BLV probably originates from Eastern Prussia and Poland at the southern Baltic seacoast [121]. From there it spread by export of cattle to North America, and by movement of cattle during and after World War I to Russia and Western Europe. Diagnosis was originally made by hematological criteria. Now the application of very sensitive serological assays for the detection of viral antigens or antibodies allows the recognition of disease-free virus-carrier cattle and provides the possibility of designing eradication programs by eliminating seropositive animals [121].

Primate Leukemia

Leukemia viruses have been isolated from naturally occurring leukemias in gibbon apes. The isolated retroviruses have been designated gibbon ape leukemia viruses (GaLV). They induce myelogenous or lymphoblastic leukemias in gibbons in captivity [123]. The virus is present in saliva of infected animals in high levels. An efficient immune response apparently prevents most of the exposed animals from developing leukemia. GaLV is not endogenous to gibbon apes or any other primates, including man, and is presumed to originate from an endogenous virus of wild mice from Asia [124].
Two primate herpesviruses, *herpesvirus saimiri* and *herpesvirus ateles,* which are not oncogenic in their natural hosts, induce rapidly fatal lymphoma and lymphatic leukemia in several monkey species under laboratory conditions [3, 125, 126]. Transmission can occur horizontally [127]. *Herpesvirus saimiri* is unlike EBV and similar to MDV in that the target cells for this virus appear to be T cells [128].

Virus Association with Human Leukemias and Lymphomas

Epstein-Barr Virus

Epstein-Barr virus (EBV) will not be reviewed here in detail since reviews by workers in the field are available [2, 3].
EBV causes infectious mononucleosis [129] in man. After inoculation into primates EBV also caused malignant lymphomas [130–132]. EBV is etiologically implicated in African Burkitt's lymphomas and some nasopharnygeal carcinomas [3]. Recent observations suggest that it may cause fatal lymphoproliferation in immune-deficient children and in the elderly [133, 134, 136, 137]. The molecular events by which EBV induces malignant growth are not fully understood, but it appears that the initial events are mitogenic stimulation of B cells leading to a profound T cell response. Mitogenic stimulation of human B lymphocytes by EBV has been shown in vitro. Other factors are assumed to convert the mitogen-stimulated growth to overt malignancy. These factors may be immune

incompetence, which may be inherited or caused by disease (e.g., malaria), or chromosomal aberrations such as the 8; 14 translocation observed in Burkitt's lymphoma [100].

Animal Retroviruses (SiSV, GaLV, BaEV)

The similarity of some malignancies in man (e.g., leukemias, lymphomas, sarcomas, breast cancer) with certain tumors in animals for which an etiology by retroviruses has been demonstrated has stimulated an intensive search for analogous viruses in human cancer. The leukemias are, without doubt, the human neoplasia studied most extensively for its possible association with retroviruses [137, 138, 140, 142]. Research has included the search for complete viral particles by electron microscopy and by cultivation attempts in tissue culture, and that for structural components such as viral RNA, reverse transcriptase, viral proteins, and antiviral antibodies.

The presence of a reverse transcriptase in at least some of the human leukemias has been demonstrated by several independent studies [137, 139]. The reverse transcriptase purified from human leukemic cells and tissues [139, 144, 145] has a molecular weight of 70,000 daltons, which is characteristic of the reverse transcriptase of mammalian leukemia viruses. It shows a serological relationship with the reverse transcriptase of SiSV and of the murine leukemia viruses and prefers the synthetic templates dT : rA and dG : rC (dG : rCm), which are diagnostic for reverse transcriptases. In some instances the polymerase was found associated with 70S RNA and/or virus-like particles [135].

The existence of retrovirus-specific cytoplasmic RNA in at least some human leukemias has been confirmed by several laboratories [135, 139]. The RNA detected shows homology with the RNAs of MuLV, MuSV, and SiSV. The RNA has a high molecular weight and possesses poly-A sequences like retroviral RNA.

Good evidence also exists for the presence in some human leukemias of proteins cross-reacting with structural proteins of the primate retroviruses SiSV and babbon endogenous virus (BaEV) [146, 148, 149]. Proteins cross-reacting with the p30 proteins of SiSV and BaEV were detected in 35%–40% of the sera from patients with acute leukemias. The purified proteins showed a molecular weight of approximately 70,000 daltons and competed with SiSV p30 in competition assays. Peptide mapping experiments with proteins isolated from sera of two different leukemic patients showed that the two proteins were virtually identical. Major peptides from the human proteins possessed significant similarity with peptides from SiSV p30 and BaEV p30. A protein of similar molecular weight with antigenic determinants of retroviral reverse transcriptases has been reported in one case of chronic myelogenous leukemia in blast crisis [150].

Antigens cross-reacting with SiSV gp70 have been detected in a variety of human leukemic and nonleukemic sera, and a correlation of presence of antigens with shorter survival has been obtained in patients with acute leukemias and chronic myelogenous leukemia in blast crisis [147, 149]. In none of these studies has the retroviral nature of the cross-reacting antigens yet been established with certainty.

Corresponding human antibodies to the internal core proteins p30 of SiSV, BaEV, and MuLV, and to the envelope glycoprotein gp70 of SiSV have been reported in several instances [151, 152]. Antibodies to retroviral p30 were reported in various human sera and exudate fluids from leukemic and nonleukemic patients [153, 154]. Antibodies occurring in human sera and reactive with the envelope glycoprotein of SiSV [155, 157], however, were shown to be heterophilic and directed against the sugar moieties of the glycoproteins [156,

Table 3. Retroviral isolates from human leukemic and embryonic tissue

Origin	Reference	Related viruses
Acute myelogenous leukemia	Gallagher and Gallo [161]	SiSV, BaEV
Acute lymphoblastic leukemia	Nooter et al. [162]	SiSV
Acute lymphatic leukemia	Gabelman et al. [164]	SiSV
Embryonic tissue	Panem et al. [163]	SiSV, BaEV
Diffuse histiocytic lymphoma	Kaplan et al. [165]	SiSV
Testicular carcinoma	Bronson et al. [166]	BaEV (?)
Cutaneous T cell lymphoma and leukemia	Poiesz et al. [170, 171]	None
Adult T cell leukemia	Hinuma et al. [173]	None

158, 159]. Antibody molecules reactive with reverse transcriptase of FeLV and of SiSV have been detected on the surface of leukocytes of patients with acute myelogenous leukemia and chronic myelogenous leukemia in blast crisis [160].

Most attempts to isolate viral particles from cultivated human leukemic cells have been without success. Several successful isolations of retroviruses from cultured leukemic and embryonic cells, however, have been reported since 1975 (Table 3) [161–166]. All these presumably human isolates showed RNA and antigenic similarity or identity with SiSV and/or BaEV, thus leaving the question of contamination with animal retroviruses unsettled.

The application of modern gene technology has also allowed the detection of retrovirus-related sequences in normal human nuclear DNA [82, 167]. The sequences are related to structural genes of MuLV and BaEV.

Overall, it is concluded that some human leukemias contain nucleic acids, proteins, and/or viral particles related to known animal retroviruses, in particular to SiSV and BaEV. Retroviruses related to SiSV and BaEV probably do occur in man, but complete particles appear to be infrequent. No epidemiological or causal relationship has yet been shown between these viruses, or viral components, and the development of human leukemia.

HTLV/ATLV

An entirely new approach to the question of human leukemia viruses was made possible by research on cellular growth factors and by the successful propagation of human T lymphocytes with the help of a factor, the so-called T cell growth factor (TCGF) or interleukin 2 [168, 169]. Long-term cultivation of T lymphocytes from patients with T cell neoplasias (mycosis fungoides, Sézary syndrome) yielded retroviruses of C-type morphology, which were unrelated to all other known retroviruses [170–172]. Similar viruses were isolated from adult T cell leukemias (ATL) endemic in Japan [173, 175, 177], and comparative studies of the different isolates showed that they represented similar, if not identical viruses [143, 178]. The viruses were designated human T cell lymphoma virus (HTLV) and adult T cell leukemia virus (ATLV).

HTLV has a density of 1.16 g/cm^3 in sucrose, has C-type morphology, and possesses a 70S RNA consisting of two identical 35S RNA subunits, a reverse transcriptase, and structural proteins, like all other replication competent C-type retroviruses [171]. The six major structural proteins are designated p10, p13, p19, p24, p42, and p52, and have molecular weights of approximately 10,000, 13,000, 19,000, 24,000, 42,000, and 52,000 daltons, respectively. The sizes of some of these proteins (p24, p42) are distinct from those of most other retroviruses. The major HTLV core protein (p24) was shown to be serologically distinct from the core proteins of all previously described viruses [179]. Its aminoacid sequence is in part homologous to that of the major core protein p24 of bovine leukemia virus [181]. This relationship is not detectable by conventional serological assays. The complete nucleotide sequence of the proviral genome of ATLV (9,032 bases) has been determined [182].

Cocultivation of HTLV (ATLV)-producing cell lines with leukocytes from adult peripheral blood and umbilical cord blood resulted in transformation of the leukocytes and expression of HTLV (ATLV) antigens by these cells [176, 183, 184]. The transformed cell lines exhibited T cell and non-T, non-B cell surface properties.

HTLV is not an endogenous human virus and was not transmitted through the germ line of the patient from whom HTLV was first isolated, since HTLV sequences were present in the DNA of T cells and absent from B cells of the same patient [141].

Antibodies to HTLV/ATLV p24 and/or p19 have been detected both in the sera of patients with HTLV-positive T cell neoplasias and in the sera of normal contact persons of these patients [174, 179, 180, 185].

Antibodies to HTLV have also been detected in apparently healthy individuals both in endemic areas and, to a lesser extent, in a random population [186, 174].

Most T cell leukemia cases positive for HTLV are identifiable by common clinical features: adult onset, a rapid disease course, often hepatosplenomegaly, hypercalcemia, lymphadenopathy, large and pleomorphic lymphocytes with lobulated nuclei, and mature T cell surface phenotype markers (OKT4 +) [142].

A seroepidemiological survey of patients with adult T cell leukemia (ATL) from the region in Southwestern Japan that is endemic for ATL showed that almost all patients with ATL and 26% of normal persons from the endemic region had specific antibodies to HTLV p19 and p24 [173]. A survey of black patients with ATL and of healthy blacks from the West Indies gave similar results [187, 188]. Asymptomatic carriers of HTLV have been found in a family of a patient with ATL [189].

In Japan, a nationwide seroepidemiological study showed that 140 of 142 patients with ATL, mainly from the endemic area in Southwestern Japan, were positive for HTLV/ATLV and that 6%–37% of 473 healthy individuals from various regions were positive for HTLV antibodies [174]. Worldwide epidemiological studies revealed HTLV or HTLV antibodies in various areas of the United States (southeast, Boston, Seattle), among the eskimo populations of Alaska and Greenland, in South America (Venezuela, Brazil, Guyana, Ecuador), in Israel, and particularly in the West Indies [142, 187, 188, 190]. Most of the HTLV isolates are very similar, but some differences in serological reactivity have been noted [191].

At the time of writing (August 1982) it has been estimated from the data presently available that the prevalence of T cell malignancies in HTLV-positive reactors is about 1 in 2,000. No definite information exists, at present, on the transmission or the etiological relevance of HTLV. Possibly, HTLV has been acquired from monkeys; HTLV was isolated from some Japanese macaques [192] and HTLV antibodies were found in African green monkeys [193]. But from observations with cell cultures it seems that HTLV is not readily infectious, because it requires prolonged intimate contact for the infection of target cells. Therefore the transmission of the virus among individuals may occur by sexual contact, breast-milk, blood transfusion, or insect vectors.

Similar to the T cell tropic feline leukemia virus (FeLV), which induces immune deficiency in addition to leukemia in cats [194] HTLV has recently been associated with acquired immune deficiency syndrome (AIDS) in man [195–198].

Conclusion

Considerable progress has been made concerning the elucidation of viral leukemogenesis by the detection and characterization of retroviral and cellular oncogenes and by the isolation of a first unambiguously human retrovirus. Oncogenes can induce malignant transformation, as observed in vivo and in vitro under experimental conditions, although it remains unclear whether oncogenes are a common cause of naturally occurring neoplasias. A role of retroviruses in human leukemogenesis becomes more likely in consideration of the recent human retroviral isolates and the accumulating evidence implicating primate retroviruses. But in view of the well known role of many factors in carcinogenesis and the probable multifactorial etiology of human cancer, the concept of cocarcinogenesis and the role of cofactors other than viruses, such as radiation and chemicals, aging, hormones, graft-vs-host reaction, environmental factors, etc., as well as carcinogenesis as a multistep process, will have to be carefully considered. Finally, recent advances concerning retroviruses and oncogenes probably will be of no immediate clinical relevance either for diagnosis or for prognosis and therapy. Rather they will help to improve our understanding of the events leading up to leukemogenesis on a molecular basis, which might indicate some practical implications. Possibly epidemiological data on HTLV/ATLV will allow etiological conclusions with subsequent inference of prophylactic measures for human T cell malignancies.

References

1. Alderson M (1980) The epidemiology of leukemia. Adv Cancer Res 31: 167
2. In: Klein G (ed) (1980) Viral oncology. Raven, New York, pp 665–832
3. zur Hausen H (1981) Oncogenic herpesviruses. In: Tooze J (ed) DNA tumorviruses. Cold Spring Harbor Laboratory, Cold Spring Harbor, pp 747–795
4. Bishop JM (1978) Retroviruses. Annu Rev Biochem 47: 35–88
5. Bishop JM (1980) The molecular biology of RNA tumor viruses: a physician's guide. N Engl J Med 303: 675–692
6. Erikson RL (1980) Avian sarcoma viruses: molecular biology. In: Klein G (ed) Viral oncology. Raven, New York, pp 39–54
7. Varmus HE (1982) Form and function of retroviral proviruses. Science 216: 812–820
8. Weiss RA, Teich N, Varmus HE, Coffin JM (eds) (1982) The molecular biology of tumor viruses, part III. RNA tumor viruses. Cold Spring Harbor Laboratory, Cold Spring Harbor
9. Bender W, Davidson N (1976) Mapping of poly(A) sequences on the electron microscope reveals unusual structure of type-C oncornavirus RNA molecules. Cell 7: 595–599
10. Furuichi Y, Shatkin AJ, Stravenzer E, Bishop JM (1975) Blocked methylated 5′-terminal sequences in avian sarcoma virus RNA. Nature 257: 618–621
11. Hsu TW, Sabran JL, Mark GE, Guntaka RV, Taylor JW (1978) Analysis of unintegrated avian RNA tumorvirus double-stranded DNA intermediates. J Virol 28: 810–818
12. Czernilofsky AP, Levinson AD, Varmus HE, Bishop JM, Tischer E, Goodman HM (1980) Nucleotide sequence of an sarcoma virus oncogene (src) and proposed amino acid sequence for gene product. Nature 287: 198–203

13. Yamamoto T, de Crombrugghe B, Pastan J (1980) Identification of a functinal promotor in the long terminal repeat of Rous sarcoma virus. Cell 22: 787–797
14. Shimotohno K, Mizutani S, Termin HM (1980) Sequence of retrovirus resembles that of bacterial transposable elements. Nature 285: 550–554
15. Dhar R, McClements WL, Enquist LW, van de Woude GF (1980) Nucleotide sequences of integrated Moloney sarcoma provirus long terminal repeats and their host and viral junctions. Proc Natl Acad Sci USA 77: 3937–3941
16. Dhar R, Ellis RW, Shih TY, Oroszlan S, Shapiro B, Maizel J, Lowy D, Scolnick E (1982) Nucleotide sequence of the p21 transforming protein of Harvey murine sarcoma virus. Science 217: 934–937
17. Shinnick TM, Lerner RA, Sutcliff JG (1981) Nucleotide sequence of Moloney murine leukemia virus. Nature 293: 543–548
18. Tsuchida N, Ryder T, Ohtsubo E (1982) Nucleotide sequence of the oncogene encoding the p21 transforming of Kirsten murine sarcoma virus. Science 217: 937–939
19. Devare SG, Reddy EP, Robbins KC, Andersen PR, Tronick SR, Aaronson SA (1982) Nucleotide sequence of the transforming gene of simian sarcoma virus. Proc Natl Acad Sci USA 79: 3179–3182
20. Temin HM (1982) Function of the retrovirus long terminal repeat. Cell 28: 3–5
21. Breathnach R, Chambon P (1981) Organization and expression of eukaryotic split genes coding for proteins. Annu Rev Biochem 50: 349–383
22. Reddy EP, Smith MJ, Aaronson SA (1981) Complete nucleotide sequence and organization of the Moloney sarcoma virus genome. Science 214: 445–450
23. van Beveren C, van Straaten F, Galleshaw JA, Verma IM (1981) Nucleotide sequence of the genome of a murine sarcoma virus. Cell 27: 97–108
24. Kitamura N, Kitamura A, Toyoshima K, Hirayama Y, Yoshida M (1982) Avian sarcoma virus Y73 genome sequence and structural similarity of its transforming gene product to that of Rous sarcoma virus. Nature 297: 205–208
25. Bister K, Duesberg PH (1982) Genetic structure and transforming genes of avian retroviruses. Adv Viral Res Therapy 1: 3–42
26. Schwartz D, Tizard R, Gilbert W (1983) The nucleotide sequence of Prague Rous sarcoma virus. Cell 32: 853–869
27. Duesberg PH, Vogt PK (1970) Differences between the ribonucleic acids of transforming and nontransforming avian tumor viruses. Proc Natl Acad Sci USA 67: 1673–1680
28. Martin GS (1970) Rous sacroma virus: a function required for the maintenance of the transformed state. Nature 227: 1021–1023
29. Wang L-H (1978) The gene order of avian RNA tumor viruses derived from biochemical analyses of deletion mutants and viral recombinants. Annu Rev Microbiol 32: 561–593
30. Graf T, Stéhelin D (1982) Avian leukemia viruses. Oncogenes and genome structure. Biochim Biophys Acta 651: 245–271
31. Coffin JM, Varmus HE, Bishop JM, Essex M, Hardy WD, Martin GS, Rosenberg NE, Scolnick EM, Weinberg RA, Vogt PK (1981) A proposal for naming host cell derived inserts in retrovirus genomes. J Virol 40: 953–957
32. Cooper GM (1982) Cellular transforming genes. Science 218: 801–806
33. Shibuya M, Hanafusa T, Hanafusa H, Stephenson JR (1980) Homology exists among the transforming sequences of avian and feline sarcoma viruses. Proc Natl Acad Sci USA 77: 6536–6540
34. Weinberg RA (1982) Fewer and fewer oncogenes. Cell 30: 3–4
35. Brugge JS, Erikson RL (1977) Identification of a transformation-specific antigen induced by an avian sarcoma virus. Nature 269: 1673–1680
36. Hunter T, Sefton BM (1980) Transforming gene product of Rous sarcoma virus phosphorylates tyrosine. Proc Natl Acad Sci USA 77: 1311–1315
37. Rohrschneider LR (1980) Adhesion plaques of Rous sarcoma virus-transformed cells contain the src gene product. Proc Natl Acad Sci USA 77: 3514–3518

38. Nigg EA, Sefton BM, Hunter T, Walter G, Singer J (1982) Immunofluorescent localization of the transforming protein of Rous sarcoma virus with antibodies against a synthetic src peptide. Proc Natl Acad Sci USA 79: 5322–5326
39. Tamura T, Bauer H, Birr C, Pipkorn R (1983) Antibodies against synthetic peptides as a tool for functional analysis of the transforming protein pp60^{src}. Cell 34: 587–596
40. Donner P, Greiser-Wilcke J, Moelling K (1982) Nuclear localization and DNA binding of the transforming gene product of myelocytomatosis virus. Nature 296: 262–266
41. Waterfield MD, Scrace GT, Whittle N, Stroobant P, Johnsson A, Wasteson A, Westermark B, Heldin CH, Huang JS, Deuel TF (1983) Platelet-derived growth factor is structurally related to the putative transforming protein p28^{sis} of simian sarcoma virus. Nature 304: 35–39
42. Doolittle RF, Hunkapiller MW, Hood LE, Devare SG, Robbins KC, Aaronson SA, Antoniades HN (1983) Simian sarcoma virus onc gene, v-sis, is derived from the gene (or genes) encoding a platelet-derived growth factor. Science 221: 275–277
43. Stéhelin D, Varmus HE, Bishop JM, Vogt PK (1976) DNA related to the transforming gene(s) of avian sarcoma viruses is present in normal DNA. Nature 260: 170–173
44. Spector DH, Varmus HE, Bishop JM (1978) Nucleotide sequences related to the transforming gene of avian sarcoma virus are present in DNA of uninfected vertebrates. Proc Natl Acad Sci USA 75: 4102–4106
45. Shilo BZ, Weinberg RA (1981) DNA sequences homologous to vertebrate oncogenes are conserved in Drosophila melanogaster. Proc Natl Acad Sci USA 78: 6789–6792
46. Dalla-Favera R, Gelman EP, Gallo RC, Wong-Staal F (1981) A human onc gene homologous to the transforming gene (v-sis) of simian sarcoma virus. Nature 292: 31–35
47. Groffen J, Heisterkamp N, Grosveld F, van de Ven W, Stephenson JR (1982) Isolation of human oncogene sequences (v-fes homolog) from a cosmid library. Science 216: 1136–1138
48. Watson R, Oskarsson M, van de Woude GF (1982) Human DNA sequence homologous to the transformation gene (mos) of Moloney murine sarcoma virus. Proc Natl Acad Sci USA 79: 4078–4082
49. Bergmann DG, Sonza LM, Baluda MA (1981) Vertebrate DNAs contain nucleotide sequences related to the transforming gene of avian myeloblastosis virus. J Virol 40: 450–455
50. Wong-Staal F, Gallo RC (1982) The transforming genes of primate and other retroviruses and their human homologs. In: Klein G (ed) Advance in viral oncology. Raven, New York, pp 159–171
51. Eva A, Robbins KC, Andersen PR, Srinivasan A, Tronick SR, Reddy RP, Ellmore NW, Galen AT, Lautenberger JA, Papas TS, Westin EH, Wong-Staal F, Gallo RC, Aaronson SA (1982) Cellular genes analogous to retroviral onc genes are transcribed in human tumor cells. Nature 295: 116–119
52. Westin EH, Wong-Staal F, Gelmann EP, Dalla Favera R, Papas TS, Lautenberger JA, Eva A, Reddy EP, Tronick SR, Aaronson SA, Gallo RC (1982) Expression of cellular homologues of retroviral onc genes in human hematopoietic cells. Proc Natl Acad Sci USA 79: 2490–2494
53. deKlein A, van Kessel AG, Grosveld G, Bartram CR, Hagemeijer A, Bootsma D, Spurr NK, Heisterkamp N, Groffn J, Stephenson JR (1982) A cellular oncogene is translocated to the Philadelphia chromosome in chronic myelocytic leukemia. Nature 300: 765–767
54. Heisterkamp N, Groffen J, Stephenson JR, Spurr NK, Goodfellow PN, Solomon E, Carritt B, Bodmer WF (1982) Chromosomal localization of human cellular homologues of two viral oncogenes. Nature 299: 747–749
55. Dalla-Favera R, Franchini G, Martinotti S, Wong-Staal F, Gallo RC, Croce CM (1982) Chromosomal assignment of the human homologues of feline sarcoma virus and avian myeloblastosis virus onc genes. Proc Natl Acad Sci USA 79: 4714–4717
56. McBride OW, Swan DC, Santos E, Barbacid M, Tronick SR, Aaronson SA (1982) Localization of the normal allele of T24 human bladder carcinoma oncogene to chromosome 11. Nature 300: 773–774

57. Sakaguchi AY, Naylor SL, Shows TB, Toole JJ, McCoy M, Weinberg RA (1983) Human c-Ki-ras2 proto-oncogene on chromosome 12. Science 219: 1081–1083
58. Ryan J, Barker PE, Shimizu K, Wigler M, Ruddle FH (1983) Chromosomal assignment of a family of human oncogenes. Proc Natl Acad Sci USA 80: 4460–4463
59. Dalla Favera R, Bregni M, Erikson J, Patterson D, Gallo RC, Croce CM (1982) Human c-myc onc gene is located on the region of chromosome 8 that is translocated in Burkitt lymphoma cells. Proc Nat Acad Sci USA 79: 7824–7828
60. Taub R, Kirsch L, Morton C, Lenoir G, Swan D, Tronick S, Aaronson S, Leder P (1982) Translocation of the c-myc gene into the immuno-globulin heavy chain locus in human Burkitt lymphoma and murine plasmacytoma cells. Proc Natl Acad Sci USA 79: 7837–7841
61. Neel BG, Jhanwar SC, Chaganti RSK, Hayward WS (1982) Two human c-onc genes are located on the long arm of chromosome 8. Proc Natl Acad Sci USA 79: 7842–7846
62. Swan DC, McBride OW, Robbins KC, Keithley DA, Reddy EP, Aaronson SA (1982) Chromosomal mapping of the simian sarcoma virus onc gene analogue in human cells. Proc Natl Acad Sci USA 79: 4691–4695
63. Dalla Favera R, Gallo RC, Giallongo A, Croce CM (1982) Chromosomal localization of the human homolog (c-sis) of the simian sarcoma virus onc gene. Science 218: 686–688
63a. Groffen J, Heisterkamp N, Stephenson JR, van Kessel AG, deKlein A, Grosveld G, Bootsma D (1983) c-sis is translocated from chromosome 22 to chromosome 9 in chronic myelocytic leukemia. J Exp Med 158: 9–15
64. Prakash K, McBride OW, Swan DC, Devare SG, Tronick SR, Aaronson SA (1982) Molecular cloning and chromosomal mapping of a human locus related to the transforming gene of Moloney murine sarcoma virus. Proc Natl Acad Sci USA 79: 5210–5214
65. Shih C, Shilo BU, Goldfarb HP, Dannenberg A, Weinberg RA (1979) Passage of phenotypes of chemically transformed cells via transfection of DNA and chromatin. Proc Natl Acad Sci USA 76: 5714–5718
66. Cooper GM, Okenquist S, Silverman L (1980) Transforming activity of DNA of chemically transformed and normal cells. Nature 284: 418–421
67. Murray MJ, Shilo BZ, Shih C, Cowing D, Hsu H, Weinberg RA (1981) Three different human tumor cell lines contain different oncogenes. Cell 25: 355–361
68. Perucho M, Goldfarb M, Shimizu K, Lama C, Fogh J, Wigler M (1981) Human tumor-derived cell lines contain common and different transforming genes. Cell 27: 467–476
69. Lane M-A, Sainten A, Cooper GM (1981) Activation of related transforming genes in mouse and human mammary carcinomas. Proc Natl Acad Sci USA 78: 5185–5189
70. Goldfarb M, Shimizu K, Perucho M, Wigler M (1982) Isolation and preliminary characterization of a human transforming gene from T24 bladder carcinoma cells. Nature 296: 404–409
71. Shih C, Weinberg RA (1982) Isolation of a transforming sequence from a human bladder carcinoma cell line. Cell 29: 161–169
72. Pulciani S, Santos E, Lauver AV, Longi LK, Robbins KC, Barbacid M (1982) Oncogenes in human tumor cell lines: Molecular cloning of a transforming gene from human bladder carcinoma cells. Proc Natl Acad Sci USA 79: 2845–2849
73. Marshall CJ, Hall A, Weiss RA (1982) A transforming gene present in human sarcoma cell lines. Nature 299: 171–173
74. Parada LF, Tabin CJ, Shih C, Weinberg RA (1982) Human EJ bladder carcinoma oncogene is homologue of Harvey sarcoma virus has gene. Nature 297: 474–478
75. Santos E, Tronick SR, Aaronson SA, Pulciani S, Barbacid M (1982) T24 human bladder carcinoma oncogene is an activated form of the normal human homologue of Balb- and Harvey-MSV transforming genes. Nature 298: 343–347
76. Der CJ, Krontiris TG, Cooper GM (1982) Transforming genes of human bladder and lung carcinoma cell lines are homologous to the ras genes of Harvey and Kirsten sarcoma viruses. Proc Natl Acad Sci USA 79: 3637–3640

77. Tabin CJ, Bradley SM, Bargmann CI, Weinberg RA, Papageorge AG, Scolnick EM, Dhar R, Lowy DR, Chang EH (1982) Mechanism of activation of a human oncogene. Nature 300: 143–149
78. Reddy EP, Reynolds RK, Santos E, Barbacid M (1982) A point mutation is responsible for the acquisition of transforming properties by the T24 human bladder carcinoma oncogene. Nature 300: 149–152
79. Essex M (1980) Feline leukemia and sarcoma viruses. In: Klein G (ed) Viral oncology. Raven, New York, pp 205–230
80. Risser R (1982) The pathogenesis of Abelson virus lymphomas of the mouse. Biochim Biophys Acta 651: 213–244
81. Troxler DH, Ruscetti SK, Scolnick EM (1980) Molecular biology of Friend-virus. Biochim Biophys Acta 605: 305–324
82. Martin MA, Bryan T, Rasheed S, Khan AS (1981) Identification and cloning of endogenous retroviral sequences present in human DNA. Proc Natl Acad Sci USA 78: 4892–4896
83. Graf T, Ade N, Beug H (1978) Temperature-sensitive mutant of avian erythroblastosis virus suggests a block of differentiation as mechanism of leukemogenesis. Nature 257: 496–501
84. Blair DG, McClements WL, Oskarsson MK, Fischinger PJ, Van de Woude GF (1980) Biological activity of cloned Moloney sarcoma DNA: terminally redundant sequences may enhance transformation efficiency. Proc Natl Acad Sci USA 77: 3504–3508
85. Blair DG, Oskarson M, Wood TG, McClement WL, Fischinger PJ, Van de Woude G (1981) Activation of the transforming potential of a normal cell sequence: a molecular model for oncogenesis. Science 212: 941–943
86. Chang EH, Ellis RW, Scolnick EM, Lowy DR (1980) Transformation by cloned Harvey sarcoma virus DNA: Efficiency increased by long terminal repeat DNA. Science 210: 1249–1251
87. Chang EH, Furth ME, Scolnick EM, Lowy DR (1982) Tumorigenic transformation of mammalian cells induced by a normal human gene homologous to the oncogene of Harvey murine sarcoma virus. Nature 297: 479–483
88. De Feo D, Gonda MA, Young HA, Chang EH, Lowy DR, Scolnick EM, Ellis RW (1981) Analysis of two divergent rat genomic clones homologous to the transforming gene of Harvey murine sarcoma virus. Proc Natl Acad Sci USA 78: 3328–3332
89. Klempnauer KH, Gonda TJ, Bishop JM (1982) Nucleotide sequence of the retroviral leukemia gene v-myb and its cellular progenitor c-myb: the architecture of a transduced oncogene. Cell 31: 453–463
90. Hayward WS, Neel BG, Astrin SM (1981) Activation of a cellular onc gene by promotor insertion in ALV-induced lymphoid leukosis. Nature 290: 475–480
91. Payne GS, Bishop JM, Varmus HE (1982) Multiple arrangements of viral DNA and an activated host oncogene in bursal lymphomas. Nature 295: 209–214
92. Hartley JW, Wolford NK, Old LJ, Rowe WP (1977) A new class of murine leukemia virus associated with development of spontaneous lymphomas. Proc Natl Acad Sci USA 74: 789–792
93. Chattopadhyay SK, Lander MR, Gupta S, Rands E, Lowy DR (1981) Origin of mink cytopathic focus-forming (MCF) viruses: comparison with ecotropic and xenotropic murine leukemia virus genomes. Virology 113: 465–483
94. Moroni C, Forni L, Hunsmann G, Schumann G (1980) Antibody directed against Friend leukemia virus stimulates DNA synthesis in a subpopulation of mouse B lymphocytes. Proc Natl Acad Sci USA 77: 1486–1490
95. McGrath MS, Weissman IL (1979) AKR leukemogenesis: identification and biological significance of thymic lymphoma receptors for AKR retroviruses. Cell 17: 65–75
96. Ihle JN, Enjuanes L, Lee JC, Keller J (1982) The immune response to C-type viruses and its potential role in leukemogenesis. Curr Top Microbiol Immunol 101: 31–49
97. Lee JC, Ihle JN (1979) Mechanisms of C-type viral leukemogenesis: Correlation of in vitro lymphocyte blastogenesis to viremia and leukemia. J Immunol 123: 2351–2358

98. Zielinski CC, Waksal SD, Tempelis LD, Khiroya RH, Schwartz RS (1980) Surface phenotypes in T-cell leukemia are determined by oncogenic retroviruses. Nature 288:489–491
99. McGrath MS, Pillemer E, Weissman IL (1980) Murine leukaemogenesis: monoclonal antibodies to T-cell determinants arrest T-lymphoma cell proliferation. Nature 285:259–261
100. Klein G (1981) The role of gene dosage and genetic transpositions in carcinogenesis. Nature 294:313–318
101. Wiener F, Ohno S, Spira J, Haran-Ghera N, Klein G (1978) Cytogenetic mapping of the trisomic segment of chromosome 15 in murine T-cell leukemia. Nature 285:658–660
102. Shapiro JA, Cordell B (1982) Eukaryotic mobile and repeated genetic elements. Biol Cell 43:31–54
103. Temin HM (1980) Origin of retroviruses from cellular moveable genetic elements. Cell 21:599–600
104. Ellermann V, Bang O (1908) Experimentelle Leukämie bei Hühnern. Zentralbl Bakteriol 46:595
105. Gross L (1951) "Spontaneous" leukemia developing in C3H mice following inoculation in infancy, with AK leukemic extracts, or AK embryos. Proc Soc Exp Biol Med 76:27
106. Gross L (1983) Oncogenic viruses, 3rd ed. Pergamon, Oxford
107. Beard JW (1980) Avian oncorna viruses: biology. In: Klein G (ed) Viral oncology. Raven, New York, pp 55–87
108. Biggs PM (1968) Marek's disease – current state of knowledge. Curr Top Microbiol Immunol 43:91
109. Seidel HJ (1982) Hemopoietic stem cells and target cells in murine virus induced leukemias. J Cancer Res Clin Oncol (to be published)
110. Dexter TM, Testa NG (1976) Differentiation and proliferation of hemopoietic cells in culture. In: Prescott DM (ed) Methods in cell biology, vol. 14, pp 387–405
111. Sweet RW, Goodman NC, Cho J-R, Ruprecht RM, Redfield RR, Spiegelman S (1974) The presence of unique DNA sequences after viral induction of leukemia in mice. Proc Natl Acad Sci USA 71:1705–1709
112. Schäfer W, Claviez M, Frank H, Hunsmann G, Moennig V, Schwarz H, Thiel HJ, Bolognesi DP, Green RW, Langlois AJ, Fischinger PJ, deNoronha F (1976) Mammalian C-type oncorna viruses: relationship between structural virus and cell surface antigens and their possible significance in immunological defense mechanisms. Proceedings of the VIIth international symposium on comparative leukemia research, Copenhagen 1975. Karger, Basel, pp 88–96
113. Hunsmann G, Moennig V, Schäfer W (1975) Properties of mouse leukemia viruses IX. Active and passive immunization of mice against Friend leukemia with isolated viral gp71 glycoprotein and its corresponding antiserum. Virology 66:327–329
114. Declève A, Lieberman M, Ihle IN, Kaplan HS (1977) Biological and serological characterization of the C-type RNA viruses isolated from the C57 BL/Ka strain of mice. III. Characterization of the isolates and their interactions in vitro and in vivo. In: Duplan JF (ed) Radiation-induced leukemogenesis and related viruses. Elsevier, Amsterdam, pp 247–264
115. Jarrett WFH, Martin WB, Crighton GW, Dalton RG, Steward MF (1964) Leukemia in the cat: transmission experiments with leukemia (Lymphosarcoma). Nature 202:566–568
116. Hardy WD Jr, Old LJ, Hess PW, Essex M, Cotter S (1973) Horizontal transmission of feline leukemia virus. Nature 244:266–269
117. Essex M, Klein G, Deinhardt F, Wolfe LG, Hardy WD Jr, Theilen GH, Pearson LD (1972) Induction of the feline oncornavirus associated cell membrane antigen in human cells. Nature 238:187–189
118. deNoronha F, Baggs R, Schäfer W, Bolognesi DP (1977) Prevention of oncornavirus-induced sarcomas in cats by treatment with antiviral antibodies. Nature 267:54–56
119. Chen AP, Essex M, Shadduck JA, Niederkorn JY, Albert D (1981) Retrovirus-encoded transformation-specific polyproteins: expression coordinated with malignant phenotype in cells from different germ layers. Proc Natl Acad Sci USA 78:3915–3919

120. Miller JM, Miller LD, Olson C, Gilette KG (1969) Virus-like particles in phythemagglutinin-stimulated lymphocyte cultures with reference to bovine lymphosarcoma. JNCI 43: 1297–1305
121. Burny A, Bex F, Chantrenne H, Cleuter Y, Dekege D, Ghysdael J, Kettman R, Leclercq M, Leunen J, Mammerickx M, Portetelle D (1978) Bovine leukemia virus involvement in enzootic bovine leukosis. Adv Cancer Res 28: 251–311
122. Kettmann R, Portetelle D, Mammerickx M, Dekegel Y, Galoux M, Ghysdael J, Burny A, Chantrenne H (1976) Bovine leukemia virus: an exogenous RNA oncogenic virus. Proc. Natl. Acad. Sci. USA 73: 1014–1018
123. Kawakami TG, Huff SD, Buckley PM, Dungworth DL, Snyder SP, Gilden RV (1972) C-type virus associated with gibbon lymphosarcoma. Nature 235: 170–171
124. Kawakami TG, Sun L, McDowell TS (1978) Distribution and transmission of primate type-C virus. In: Yohn P (ed) Advances in comparative leukemia research 1977. Elsevier, Amsterdam, pp 33–36
125. Meléndez LV, Hunt RD, Daniel MD, Blake BJ, Garcia FG (1971) Acute lymphatic leukemia in owl monkeys (Aotus trivirgatus) inoculated with herpesvirus saimiri. Science 171: 1161–1163
126. Meléndez LV, Hunt RD, Kind NW, Barahona HH, Daniel MD, Fraser CEO, Garcia FG (1972) Herpesvirus ateles, a new virus of monkeys. Nature 235: 182
127. Deinhardt F, Falk L, Wolfe LG (1973) Simian herpesviruses. Cancer Res 33: 1424
128. Wallen W, Neubauer RH, Rabin H, Cicmanec HL (1973) Nonimmune rosette formation by lymphoma and leukemia cells from herpesvirus saimiri-infected owl monkeys. J. Natl. Cancer Inst. 51: 967
129. Henle G, Henle W, Diehl V (1968) Relation of Burkitt's tumor-associated herpes-type virus to infectious mononucleosis. Proc Natl Acad Sci USA 59: 94–101
130. Shope T, Dechairo D, Miller G (1973) Malignant lymphoma in cottontop marmosets after inoculation with Epstein-Barr virus. Proc Natl Acad Sci USA 70: 2487–2491
131. Epstein MA, Hunt RD, Rabin H (1973) Pilot experiments with EB virus in owl monkeys (Aotus trivirgatus) I. Reticuloproliferative disease in an inoculated animal. Int J Cancer 12: 309–318
132. Epstein MA, Rabin H, Ball G, Rickinson AB, Jarvis J, Melendez LV (1973) Pilot experiments with EB virus in owl monkeys (Aotus trivirgatus) II. EB virus in a cell line from an animal with reticuloproliferative disease. Int J Cancer 12: 319–332
133. Purtilo DT, Cassel C, Yang JP (1974) Fatal infectious mononucleosis in familial lymphohistiocytosis. N Engl J Med 291: 736
134. Purtilo DT (1980) Epstein-Barr-Virus-induced oncogenesis in immune-deficient individuals. Lancet 2: 300–303
135. Hehlmann R (1976) RNA tumorviruses and human cancer. In: Current topics in microbiology and immunology. Springer, Berlin Heidelberg New York, pp 141–215
136. Hehlmann R, Walther B, Zöllner N, Wolf H, Deinhardt F (1980) Infectious mononucleosis and acute monocytic leukemia. Lancet 2: 652–653
137. Hehlmann R, Walther B, Zöllner N, Wolf H, Deinhardt F, Schmid M (1981) Fatal lymphoproliferation and acute monocytic leukemia-like disease following infectious mononucleosis in the elderly. Klin Wochenschr 59: 477–483
138. Pimentel E (1979) Human oncovirology. Biochim Biophys Acta 560: 169–216
139. Gallo RC, Gallagher RE, Miller NR, Mondal H, Saxinger WC, Mayer RJ, Smith RG, Gillespie DH (1975) Relationships between components in primate RNA tumor viruses and in the cytoplasm of human leukemic cells: implications to leukemogenesis. Cold Spring Harbor Symp Quant Biol 39: 933–961
140. Gallo RC (1979) Cellular and virological studies directed to the pathogenesis of the human myelogenous leukemias. In: Neth R, Gallo RC, Hofschneider P-H, Mannweiler K (eds) Modern trends in human leukemia 3. Springer, Berlin Heidelberg New York, pp 7–24 (Hämatologie und Bluttransfusion, vol 23)

141. Gallo RC, Mann D, Broder S, Ruscetti FW, Maeda M, Kalyanaraman VS, Robert-Guroff M, Reitz MS Jr (1982) Human T-cell leukemia-lymphoma virus (HTLV) is in T but not B lymphocytes from a patient with cutaneous T-cell lymphoma. Proc Natl Acad Sci USA 79: 5680–5683
142. Gallo RC, Wong-Staal F, Ruscetti F (1982) Viruses and adult leukemia-lymphoma of man and relevant animal models. In: Bloomfield CD (ed) Adult leukemias. pp 1–41
143. Gallo RC, Reitz MS (1982) Human retroviruses and adult T-cell leukemia-lymphoma. J. Natl. Cancer Inst. 69: 1209–1214
144. Chandra P, Steel LK (1977) Purification, biochemical characterization and serological analysis of cellular deoxyribonucleic acid polymerases and a reverse transcriptase from spleen of a patient with myelofibrotic syndrome. Biochem J 167: 513–524
145. Witkin SS, Ohno T, Spiegelman S (1975) Purification of RNA-instructed DNA polymerase from human leukemic spleens. Proc Natl Acad Sci USA 72: 4133–4136
146. Hehlmann R, Schetters H, Erfle V, Leib-Mösch C (1983) Detection and biochemical characterization of antigens in human leukemic sera that crossreact with primate C-type viral p30 proteins. Cancer Res 43: 392–399
147. Hehlmann R, Schetters H, Erfle V (1981) ELISA for the detection of antigens crossreacting with primate C-type viral proteins (p30, gp70) in human leukemic sera. In: Neth R, Gallo RC, Graf I, Mannweiler K, Winkler K (eds) Modern trends in human leukemia 4. Springer, Berlin Heidelberg New York, pp 530–536 (Hämatologie und Bluttransfusion, vol 26)
148. Hehlmann R, Schetters H, Leib C, Erfle V (1982) Antigens crossreacting with primate C-type viral p30 proteins in human leukemic sera. In: Advances in comparative leukemia research 1981. Elsevier Biomedical, Amsterdam, pp 387–388
149. Hehlmann R, Erfle V, Schetters H, Luz A, Rohmer H, Schreiber MA, Essers U, Pralle H, Weber W (1984) Antigens and circulating immune complexes related to the primate retroviral glycoprotein SiSVgp70: indicators of early mortality in human acute leukemias and chronic myelogenous leukemias in blast crisis. Cancer (to be published)
150. Jaquemin PC (1983) Purification of a reverse transcriptase-like protein from the plasma of a chronic myelogenous leukemia patient and production of monoclonal antibodies. In: Modern trends in human leukemia 5. Springer, Berlin Heidelberg New York, pp 282–283 (Hämatologie und Bluttransfusion, vol 28)
151. Aoki R, Walling MJ, Bushar GS, Liu M, Hsu KC (1976) Natural antibodies in sera from healthy humans to antigens on surfaces of type C RNA viruses and cells from primates. Proc Natl Acad Sci USA 73: 2492–2495
152. Kurth R, Teich NM, Weiss R, Oliver RT (1977) Natural human antibodies reactive with primate type-C viral antigens. Proc Natl Acad Sci USA 74: 1237–1241
153. Herbrink P, Moen JET, Brouwer J, Warnaar SO (1980) Detection of antibodies cross-reactive with type C RNA tumor viral p30 protein in human sera and exudate fluids. Cancer Res 40: 166–173
154. Mellors RC, Mellors JW (1978) Type C RNA virus-specific antibody in human systemic lupus erythematosus demonstrated by enzymoimmunoassay. Proc Natl Acad Sci USA 75: 2463–2467
155. Snyder HW, Pincus T, Fleissner E (1976) Specificities of human immunoglobulins reactive with antigens in preparations of several mammalian type C viruses. Virology 75: 60–73
156. Snyder HW, Fleissner E (1980) Specificity of human antibodies to oncovirus glycoproteins: Recognition of antigen by natural antibodies directed against carbohydrate structures. Proc Natl Acad Sci USA 77: 1622–1626
157. Kurth R, Mikschy U (1978) Human antibodies reactive with purified envelope antigens of primate type-C tumor viruses. Proc Natl Acad Sci USA 75: 5692–5696
158. Barbacid M, Bolognesi D, Aaronson SA (1980) Humans have antibodies capable of recognizing oncoviral glycoproteins: demonstration that these antibodies are formed in response to cellular modification of glycoproteins rather than as consequence of exposure to virus. Proc Natl Acad Sci USA 77: 1617–1621

159. Löwer J, Davidson EA, Teich NM, Weiss RA, Joseph AP, Kurth R (1981) Heterophil antibodies recognize oncornavirus envelope antigens: epidemiological parameters and immunological specificity of the reaction. Virology 109: 409–417
160. Jacquemin PC, Saxinger C, Gallo RC (1978) Surface antibodies of human myelogenous leukemia leukocytes reactive with specific type-C viral reverse transcriptases. Nature 276: 230–236
161. Gallagher RE, Gallo RC (1975) Type-C RNA tumor virus isolated from cultured human acute myelogenous leukemia cells. Science 187: 350–353
162. Nooter K, Aarson AM, Bentvelzen P, deGroor FG, van Pelt FG (1975) Isolation of infectious C-type oncornavirus from human leukemic bone marrow cells. Nature 256: 595–597
163. Panem S, Prochownik EV, Reale FR, Kirsten WH (1975) Isolation of type C virions from a normal human fibroblast strain. Science 189: 297–299
164. Gabelman N, Waxman S, Smith W, Douglas SD (1975) Appearance of C-type viruslike particles after co-cultivation of a human tumor cell line with rat (XC) cells. Int J Cancer 16: 355–356
165. Kaplan HS, Goodenow RS, Epstein AL, Gartner S, Decleve A, Rosenthal PN (1977) Isolation of a type C RNA virus from an established human histiocytic lymphoma cell line. Proc Natl Acad Sci USA 74: 2564–2568
166. Bronson DL, Ritzi DM, Fraley EE, Dalton AJ (1978) Morphologie evidence for retrovirus production by epithelial cells derived from a human testicular tumor metastasis – brief communication. J. Natl. Cancer Inst 60: 1305–1308
167. Bonner TI, O'Connell C, Cohen M (1982) Cloned endogenous retroviral sequences from human DNA. Proc Natl Acad Sci USA 79: 4709–4713
168. Morgan DA, Ruscetti FW, Gallo RC (1976) Selective in vitro growth of T lymphocytes from normal human bone marrows. Science 193: 1007–1008
169. Mier JW, Gallo RC (1980) Purification and some characteristics of human T-cell growth factor from phytohemagglutinin-stimulated lymphocyte-conditioned media. Proc Natl Acad Sci USA 77: 6134–6138
170. Poiesz BJ, Ruscetti FW, Mier JW, Woods AM, Gallo RC (1980) T-cell lines established from human T-lymphocytic neoplasias by direct response to T-cell growth factor. Proc Natl Acad Sci USA 77: 6815–6819
171. Poiesz BJ, Ruscetti FW, Gazdar AF, Bunn PA, Minna JD, Gallo RC (1980) Detection and isolation of type C retrovirus particles from fresh and cultured lymphocytes of a patient with cutaneous T-cell lymphoma. Proc Natl Acad Sci USA 77: 7415–7419
172. Poiesz BH, Ruscetti FW, Reitz MS, Kalyanaraman VS, Gallo RC (1981) Isolation of a new type C retrovirus (HTLV) in primary uncultured cells of a patient with Sézary T-cell leukemia. Nature 294: 268–271
173. Hinuma Y, Nagata K, Hanaoka M, Nakai M, Matsumoto T, Knishita K, Shirakawa S, Miyoshi I (1981) Adult T-cell leukemia: Antigen in an ATL cell line and detection of antibodies to the antigen in human sera. Proc Natl Acad Sci USA 78: 6476–6480
174. Hinuma Y, Komoda H, Chosa T, Kondo T, Kohakura M, Takenaka T, Kikuchi M, Ichimaru M, Yunoki K, Sato I, Matsuo R, Takiuchi Y, Uchino H, Hanaoka M (1982) Antibodies to adult T-cell leukemia-virus-associated antigen (ATLA) in sera from patients with ATL and controls in Japan: a nation-wide sero-epidemiologic study. Int J Cancer 29: 631–635
175. Miyoshi I, Kubonishi I, Yoshimoto S, Akagi T, Ohtsuki Y, Shiraishi Y, Nagata K, Hinuma Y (1981) Type C virus particles in a cord T-cell line derived by co-cultivating normal human cord leukocytes and human leukemic T cells. Nature 294: 770–771
176. Miyoshi I, Yoshimoto S, Kubonishi I, Taguchi H, Shiraishi Y, Ohtsuki Y, Akagi T (1981) Transformation of normal human cord lymphocytes by co-cultivation with a lethally irradiated human T-cell line carrying type C virus particles. Gan 72: 997–998
177. Yoshida M, Miyoshi I, Hinuma Y (1982) Isolation and characterization of retrovirus from cell lines of human adult T-cell leukemia and its implication in the disease. Proc Natl Acad Sci USA 79: 2031–2035

178. Popovic M, Reitz MS, Sarngadharan MG, Robert-Guroff M, Kalyanaraman VS, Nakao Y, Miyoshi I, Minowada J, Yoshida M, Ito Y, Gallo RC (1982) The virus of Japanese adult T cell leukemia is member of the human T-cell leukemia virus group. Nature 300: 63–66

179. Kalyanaraman VS, Sarngadharan MG, Poiesz B, Ruscetti FW, Gallo RC (1981) Immunological properties of a type C retrovirus isolated from cultured human T-lymphoma cells and comparison to other mammalian retroviruses. J Virol 38: 906–915

180. Kalyanaraman VS, Sarngadharan MG, Nakao Y, Ito T, Aoki T, Gallo RC (1982) Natural antibodies to the structural core protein (p24) of the human T-cell leukemia (lymphoma) retrovirus found in sera of leukemia patients in Japan. Proc Natl Acad Sci USA 79: 1653–1657

181. Oroszlan S, Sarngadharan MG, Copeland TD, Kalyanaraman VS, Gilden RV, Gallo RC (1982) Primary structure analysis of the major internal protein p24 of human type C T-cell leukemia virus. Proc Natl Acad Sci USA 79: 1291–1294

182. Seiki M, Hattori S, Hirayama Y, Yoshida M (1983) Human adult T-cell leukemia virus: Complete nucleotide sequence of the provirus genome integrated in leukemia cell DNA. Proc Natl Acad Sci USA 80: 3618–3622

183. Yamamoto N, Okada M, Koyanagi Y, Kannagi M, Hinuma Y (1982) Transformation of human leukocytes by cocultivation with an adult T-cell leukemia virus producer cell line. Science 217: 737–739

184. Popovic M, Lange-Wantzin G, Sarin PS, Mann D, Gallo RC (1983) Transformation of human umbilical cord blood T cells by human T-cell leukemia/lymphoma virus. Proc. Natl. Acad. Sci. USA 80: 5402–5406

185. Robert-Guroff M, Nakao Y, Notake K, Ito Y, Sliski A, Gallo RC (1982) Natural antibodies to human retrovirus HTLV in a cluster of Japanese patients with adult T-cell leukemia. Science 215: 975–978

186. Gotoh Y-I, Sugamura K, Hinuma Y (1982) Healthy carriers of a human retrovirus, adult T-cell leukemia virus (ATLV): demonstration by clonal culture of ATLV-carrying T-cells from peripheral blood. Proc Natl Acad Sci USA 79: 4780–4782

187. Catovsky D, Rose M, Goolden AWG, White JM, Bourikas G, Brownell AI, Blattner WA, Greaves MF, Galton DA, McCluskey DR, Lampert I, Ireland R, Bridges JM, Gallo RC (1982) Adult T cell lymphoma-leukemia in blacks from the West Indies. Lancet 1: 639–643

188. Schüpbach J, Kalyanaraman VS, Sarngadharan MG, Blattner WA, Gallo RC (1983) Antibodies against 3 purified proteins of the human type C retrovirus, HTLV, in adult T-cell leukemia/lymphoma patients and healthy blacks from the Caribbean. Cancer Res 43: 886–891

189. Miyoshi I, Taguchi H, Fujishita M, Niiya K, Kitagawa T, Ohtsuki Y, Akagai T (1982) Asymptomatic type C virus carriers in the family of an adult T-cell leukemic patient. Gan 73: 339–340

190. Blattner WA, Saxinger C, Clark J, Hanchard B, Gibbs, W, Robert-Guroff M, Lofters W, Campbell M, Gallo RC (1983) Human T-cell leukemia/lymphoma virus-associated lymphoreticular neoplasia in Jamaica. Lancet 2: 61–64

191. Kalyanaraman VS, Sarngadharan MG, Robert-Guroff M, Miyoshi I, Blayney D, Golde D, Gallo RC (1982) A new subtype of human T-cell leukemia virus (HTLV-II) associated with a T-cell variant of hairy cell leukemia. Science 218: 571–573

192. Miyoshi I, Fujishita M, Taguchi H, Niiya K, Kobayashi M, Matsubayashi K, Miwa N (1983) Horizontal transmission of adult T-cell leukemia virus from male to female Japanese monkey. Lancet 1: 241

193. Yamamoto N, Hinuma Y, zur Hausen H, Schneider J, Hunsmann G (1983) African green monkeys are infected with adult T-cell leukemia virus or a closely related agent. Lancet 1: 240–241

194. Trainin Z, Wernicke D, Unga-Waron H, Essex M (1983) Suppression of the humoral antibody response in natural retrovirus infections. Science 220: 858–859

195. Essex M, McLane MF, Lee TH, Falk L, Howe CWS, Mullins JI, Cabradilla C, Francis DP (1983) Antibodies to cell membrane antigens associated with human T-cell leukemia virus in patients with AIDS. Science 220: 859–862
196. Gallo RC, Sarin PS, Gelmann EP, Robert-Guroff M, Richardson E, Kalyanaraman VS, Mann D, Sidhu GD, Stahl RE, Zolla-Pazner S, Leibowitch J, Popovic M (1983) Isolation of human T-cell leukemia virus in acquired immune deficiency syndrome (AIDS). Science 220: 865–867
197. Gelmann EP, Popovic M, Blayney D, Masur H, Sidhu G, Stahl RE, Gallo RC (1983) Proviral DNA of a retrovirus, a human T-cell leukemia virus, in two patients with AIDS. Science 220: 862–865
198. Barré-Sinoussi F, Chermann JC, Rey F, Nugeyre MT, Chamaret S, Gruest J, Dauguet C, Axler-Blin C, Vézinet-Brun F, Rouzioux C, Rozenbaum W, Montagnier L (1983) Isolation of a T-lymphotropic retrovirus from a patient at risk for acquired immune deficiency syndrome (AIDS). Science 220: 868–871
199. Land H, Parada LF, Weinberg RA (1983) Cellular oncogenes and multistep carcinogenesis. Science 222: 771–778
200. Duesberg PH (1983) Retroviral transforming genes in normal cells? Nature 304: 219–226
201. Müller R, Tremblay JM, Adamson ED, Verma IM (1983) Tissue and cell type-specific expression of two human c-onc genes. Nature 304: 454–456
202. Jansen HW, Lurz RL, Bister K, Bonner TI, Mark GE, Rapp UR (1984) Homologous cell-derived oncogenes in avian carcinoma virus MH2 and murine sarcoma virus 3611. Nature 307: 281–284

Cytogenetics in Leukemia: Implications for Pathogenesis and Prognosis*

D. K. Hossfeld and H.-J. Weh

Abteilung für Onkologie und Hämatologie, Medizinische Universitätsklinik,
Martinistrasse 52, 2000 Hamburg 20, FRG

Introduction

Since the first description of the chromosome constitution of leukemic cells by Ford et al. in 1958 [1], leukemia cytogenetics has become a valuable tool for both researchers and practicing physicians. It has revived the stem cell concept, contributed to our understanding of clonal evolution and progression, and climaxed recently in the localization of "cancer genes" on certain chromosome segments. For the physician, chromosome analysis of leukemic cells gained an important role in diagnosis and differential diagnosis, and also in the follow-up of patients with preleukemic and leukemic disorders; in addition, in a number of diseases chromosomal findings were shown to be an independent prognostic factor which should be considered in the planning of therapeutic strategies. In this article we will concentrate on what cytogenetics can tell us about the pathogenesis of leukemias, leukemogenesis, and the role of chromosomes in the prognosis of patients with leukemic conditions. Diagnostic chromosomal findings will be described only briefly in the context of the aforementioned topics.

Some Remarks on Chromosome Techniques

For readers who are not acquainted with the techniques of leukemia cytogenetics some introductory remarks seem to be appropriate not only to improve their understanding of the following text but also to help them realize the limitations and drawbacks of such techniques.

Chromosome analysis requires a sufficient number of well spread metaphases with slim chromosomes. Usually, leukemia tissue – be it bone marrow, peripheral blood, lymph node or spleen – does not fill any of these requirements when investigated shortly after it has been obtained from the patient (direct preparation). Instead, the number of metaphases is small, overlapping of chromosomes occurs frequently, and the chromosomes are dull and fuzzy. The reasons for the fuzzy morphology of leukemic chromosomes compared with chromosomes of normal cells are unknown, but appear to be intimately related to the leukemic process. Metaphases with such fuzzy chromosomes are likely to be overlooked, resulting either in a false-normal report (when only the well-defined metaphases of normal cells have been analysed) or in a report claiming technical failure.

* Cytogenetic studies in the Department of Oncology and Hematology were supported by the Hamburger Krebsgesellschaft

The low number of metaphases is a reflection of the low proliferation rate of leukemic cells, which can, however, be enhanced under in vitro conditions. Recent reports even suggest that short-term culture conditions may provide a selective growth advantage for leukemic cells, and that some specific chromosomal changes cannot be detected unless the leukemic cells are cultured [2–5]. Also, the morphology of leukemic chromosomes can be improved by culturing the cells for 24–48 h. Thus, short-term culture appears to be the method of choice in leukemia cytogenetics. Yet this is only partly true, since we have shown that in (exceptional?) cases culture conditions may also obscure the leukemic karyotype [6]. It is therefore essential to use both direct and culture methods to reveal the total spectrum of chromosomal changes in leukemia, and the report must indicate which results have been obtained with what method to allow comparison of the results from different laboratories.

Another limitation of chromosome analysis is that the techniques used to obtain chromosome preparations destroy the cytological and cytochemical characteristics of the cell. This is of no importance when the tissue to be examined is uniformly infiltrated by just one cell type. However, particularly in bone marrow one is quite often confronted not only with both presumably leukemic and normal blasts, but also with granulocytic, erythrocytic and megakaryocytic cells. If chromosome analysis in such a bone marrow were to reveal a mixture of normal and abnormal metaphases, the conclusion would be that the abnormal metaphases were derived from leukemic blasts and the normal ones from normal precursor cells and their derivatives. However, such a conclusion may be questionable, since it is known that chromosomally abnormal cells can mature up to the stage of neutrophils [7] and that chromosomally normal leukemic blasts can coexist with abnormal ones. Thus, as long as no technique is available to allow identification of the cellular derivation of a given metaphase the correlations of cytogenetic findings with cytology remain indirect, resting largely on the observation of which cells enter mitosis in cytologic smears. The demonstration of radioactive iron in a metaphase is a more direct indication that such a metaphase is derived from an erythropoietic cell.

Results of chromosome analysis and the conclusions based upon them will be influenced not only by the quality and quantity of metaphases, but also by the number of metaphases studied under the microscope, photographed, and karyotyped. Most cytogeneticists agree that the analysis of 20 metaphases affords a representative picture of the actual chromosome constitution of a given tissue provided that the analysis is not restricted to "nice" metaphases (see above).

Considering the enormous leukemic mass at the time of diagnosis one wonders whether this is sufficient. It has been shown that when a much larger number of metaphases is counted a higher percentage of abnormal cells is in fact found [8]. Yet at present it appears that with regard to diagnosis and prognosis the amount of information gained by analysing such large numbers of metaphases is small. If more refined and specific modalities for the treatment of patients with leukemia should become available in the future this situation may change. For the elucidation of the pathogenesis of leukemias the evaluation of only a small number of metaphases is certainly insufficient, as will be discussed below.

To sum up this section, the reader should keep in mind that due to the paucity of metaphases and their poor chromosome morphology, leukemia cytogenetics (and cancer cytogenetics in general) is a tedious and time-consuming business, particularly when banding techniques are applied, which is a prerequisite nowadays. The cytogeneticist must withstand the temptation to analyse only nicely spread metaphases, since this may lead to false-normal results. Because chromosome preparation destroys cellular characteristics the relationship of normal or abnormal metaphases and the cellular composition can only be estimated. The notion that a chromosome analysis should be based on the analysis of 20 metaphases is a compromise enforced by technical difficulties rather than biologically well founded.

Finally, for those not acquainted with cytogenetics some definitious and symbols should be explained: The term "clone" is used when two or more metaphases share an identical structural or supernumerary chromosomal anomaly or when three metaphases have an identical chromosome loss [9]. The system of terminology and notation used for the description of chromosomal findings was defined at the Paris Chromosome Conference [10]. According to this system the chromosome number is indicated first, followed by the sex chromosomes, and then by gains, losses, or rearrangements of autosomes. Autosomes are identified by a number in the series 1–22. The symbols "+" and "−" before a chromosome number indicate gain or loss of such a chromosome, e.g., +8 means gain of one chromosome No. 8. The letters "p" and "q" stand for the short and long arms of a chromosome, respectively; for example, 5q− refers to loss (deletion) of a part of the long arms of chromosome No. 5. Translocations are described by the letter "t" followed by the chromosomes involved in the first set of parentheses and the location of breaks in the second set of parentheses; for example t (8; 21) (q22; q22) means a translocation between band 22 on the long arms of chromosome 8 and band 22 on the long arms of chromosome 21. Further symbols are explained below and in the report published following the Paris Conference [10].

Implications for Pathogenesis

Chronic Myelocytic Leukemia (CML)

CML was the first neoplastic disease shown to be associated with an acquired, specific chromosome anomaly in the leukemic cells [11]. The anomaly became known as the Philadelphia (Ph^1) chromosome, and it was later identified as a translocation of a part of 22q to another chromosome, most frequently 9q, i.e., t(9; 22) (q34; q11) [12]. There is now morphological [13] and molecular [14] evidence to show that the translocation is reciprocal, which means that the exchange does not lead to loss of genetic material.

The observation that the translocation always involved a No. 22, while the recipient chromosome of the deleted material varied in 8% of the cases, led to the opinion that the decisive event in the genesis of the Ph^1 (and of CML?) must be the alteration of chromosome 22. Recently, however, it has been demonstrated that chromosome 9 is at least as important as No. 22. The human oncogene *c-abl* is normally localized on chromosome 9q. In CML, with the typical translocation (9; 22), even in patients with variant translocation (without cytological involvement of No. 9), *c-abl* is translocated to 22q- [14, 15]. On the basis of these data, therefore, the critical event appears to be the transposition of genes from chromosome No. 9 to No. 22. It is known that most of the oncogene-coded proteins phosphorylate tyrosine, and that tyrosine phosphorylation has a central role in cell proliferation [16]. From this one could conclude that the uncontrolled proliferation of hematopoietic cells in patients with CML is the result of altered gene function due to the transposition of the *c-abl* gene on chromosome 9 to an hypothetical promotor region on chromosome 22. It is conceivable that the same mechanism applies to Ph^1-negative, but otherwise typical CML, in which the reciprocal exchange between chromosomes 9 and 22 might be too small to be detected.

This new look at the nature of the Ph^1 chromosome does not detract from its importance as an easily identifiable cell marker. Study of the Ph^1 anomaly has considerably deepened our knowledge of CML in particular and of leukemia in general.

In patients with CML the Ph^1 chromosome can be found not only in cells of myeloid lineage (granulocytes, erythrocytic cells, megakaryocytes, monocytes-macrophages), but also in lymphoid cells. The involvement of B lymphoid cells has been demonstrated convincingly, while for T cells such evidence is so far restricted to some rare case reports [17–19]. Occurrence of the Ph^1 in B cells is based indirectly on the observation of patients with Ph^1-positive blastic phase, in whom the apparently lymphoid blasts had pre-B cell characteristics, e.g., intracytoplasmatic IgM [20, 21], and more directly by analyses of continuous B cell lines established from Epstein-Barr virus-infected blood cells from patients with CML [22]. In the latter study it was shown that the B lymphoid cells had in common with myeloid cells not only the Ph^1 but also the same type of the X-linked enzyme glucose-6-phosphate dehydrogenase (G6PD). The participation of the B cell was finally proven by an elegant combined study of surface immunoglobulins on Ph^1-positive metaphases [23].

Thus there is now ample cytogenetic, enzymatic, and immunologic evidence that CML arises in a pluripotent stem cell which has the ability to differentiate into myeloid cells, including cells of the monocytic/macrophage series, and into B cells.

On the basis of G6PD studies it is apparent that the enormous mass of leukemic cells at the time of diagnosis of CML is derived from a single clone [24]. This is also suggested by chromosomal findings in CML patients with constitutional chromosome anomalies (either mosaicism or heteromorphism) in whom the Ph^1 occurs strictly in only a single cell type [25, 26]. Obviously, the Ph^1 endows the affected cell with a very powerful growth advantage, resulting in a more or less complete outgrowth and/or suppression of normal hematopoiesis. This is evidenced by findings that in about 95% of the patients with Ph^1-positive CML exclusively Ph^1-positive metaphases will be detected, and by the impossibility of detecting the nonclonal cell in vitro by the G6PD method [27, 28]. However, in roughly 5% of patients with Ph^1-positive CML a varying proportion (4%–40%) of bone marrow-derived metaphases is normal. The nature of such normal cells was, until recently, beyond doubt. It was believed that they represented the normal residual hematopoiesis. A number of observations favor this interpretation: first, in the majority of patients such "normal" metaphases will be replaced by Ph^1-positive ones as the disease progresses [27, 29, 30]; second, after chemotherapy-induced marrow hypoplasia a partial or complete reversion of a previously Ph^1-positive to a Ph^1-negative state can be obtained in about 40% of patients, and this conversion correlates with the hematological status of complete remission [31, 32] and the restoration of nonclonal hematopoiesis [33].

Recently, however, the hypothesis was advanced that at least in untreated patients the Ph^1-negative cells may also belong to the leukemic clone. This hypothesis, too, can be supported by several findings: first, there are papers claiming that the prognosis of patients with a mixture of Ph^1-positive and Ph^1-negative cells is no different from that of patients with 100% Ph^1-positive cells [34, 35; for an opposite view see 36]; second, some patients were observed to remain in the mosaic (Ph^1-positive/Ph^1-negative) state or to become Ph^1-negative when a monomorphic blastic phase developed [29, 37, 38], and others, who were Ph^1-negative at the time of diagnosis, not to become Ph^1-positive until later [39]; third, Fialkow et al. provided evidence that some (but not all) B lymphocytes which are Ph^1-negative arise from the CML clone [40]; finally it must be mentioned that about 5% of the patients with classic CML are and remain Ph^1-negative.

Thus, the possibility must be seriously considered that in CML Ph^1-positive and Ph^1-negative leukemic cells derived from the same clone coexist. If this turns out to be correct then the causative role of the Ph^1 chromosome as such in the genesis of CML must be questioned, as it has been by Fialkow, who proposed that the formation of the Ph^1 is the second step in the evolution of CML [40]. Direct proof of the leukemic nature of Ph^1-negative bone marrow cells in patients with Ph^1-positive CML would be provided by demonstration of the transposition of the *c-abl* gene to chromosome 22.

With or without the formation of the Ph^1, the leukemic CML stem cell is characterized by an exceptional karyotypic instability. During the course of the disease, particularly upon entering the blastic phase, 80%–85% of the patients are found to have new or additional numerical and/or structural abnormalities [30, 41]. There is good reason to believe that the blastic phase is not a de novo event but the consequence of an additional mutation in a CML stem cell. Accordingly, the blasts retain the Ph^1 (if it was present in the chronic phase), and the population of blasts is monoclonal [42]. Again, however, exceptions to this rule have been described. In these cases a loss of the Ph^1 or the presence of cytogenetically and/or morphologically different population has been noted and taken as an indication for multiclonality [29, 37, 41, 43, 44].

The enormous variety of morphological and immunological phenotypes of blasts in the blastic phase of CML (M1–M6 and L1-L2 morphology according to the FAB classification [45]; myeloid, B and T lymphoid, erythroid, megakaryocytic and undifferentiated as determined by monoclonal antibodies) suggests the possibility that the additional mutation affects stem cells at different stages of maturation. It is also conceivable that the type of genetic alteration determines the differentiation pattern of the cells. This notion is corroborated by the fact that the isochromosome 17q, which is a very reliable marker of impending or overt blastic phase, is always associated with the myeloid type, and has never yet been seen in the lymphoid type of the blastic phase [46, 47].

Serial chromosomal analyses have demonstrated continuous genetic instability of blasts throughout the disease, which is reflected in a remarkably predictable pattern of increasing chromosomal anomalies. Most commonly the transition into the blastic phase begins with addition of a chromosome No. 8, followed by an extra Ph^1, followed by an extra 19. Trisomies 6 and 4 and the duplication of a sex chromosome are the final events. This chain of events is a classic demonstration of clonal evolution. It reflects increasing anarchy of the cells. There is no indication that these progressive genetic changes are related to therapy during the chronic phase, since identical chromosomal changes have been observed in patients with so-called primary blastic phase.

Acute Leukemias (AL)

Before the introduction of banding techniques cytogenetics of acute leukemias lacked the fascination which it had in CML. No chromosome marker comparable to the Ph^1 had been found, an association between morphology and chromosomal pattern was not evident, and at least 50% of the cases exhibited an apparently normal karyotype. At that time most chromosome workers considered chromosomal changes in AL as epiphenomena [48]. Today the situation is quite different. Although, with conventional banding techniques [49], the percentage of cases with karyotypic anomalies did not change substantially (between 40% and 70%, mean 53%), a number of anomalies specific for certain types of leukemia have been detected, and the role of chromosomes as independent prognostic factors has been established; moreover, it appears that the karyotypic pattern may allow conclusions as to the etiology of AL [50–57].

As in CML, chromosomal and G6PD studies support the view that AL (both myeloid and lymphoid) is usually a monoclonal disease, i.e., the leukemic cells present at diagnosis are derived from a single cell [58–60]. In a given patient the cells share the same G6PD type and an identical karyotype. If different karyotypes are found a closer look will demonstrate a relationship among them in most cases. Some rare cases with apparently strictly unrelated clones have been reported, suggesting bi- or multiclonality [61, 62]. At this juncture it should be added that the demonstration of monoclonality at *diagnosis* does not imply single-cell origin at the time of *induction* of leukemia. What is seen at diagnosis represents the result of a more or less protracted selection process during which a number of genetic changes occur in a number of cells before a certain genetic constellation (e.g., Ph^1) provides one clone with a growth advantage [60].

During complete remission, chromosomal findings in an initially abnormal marrow will become normal, which is in striking contrast to busulfan-induced remission in CML [48]. This observation strongly suggests that the marrow is repopulated by normal cells. G6PD analysis supports such an interpretation [58] as do long-term observations of AL patients in continuous remission. However, one problem remains, which is whether all normal metaphases are indeed derived from normal cells, or whether some are also derived from leukemic ones. Theoretically this possibility has to be considered, unless one denies the above-mentioned concept of clonal selection and implicates visible chromosomal changes as very early events in leukemogenesis [63].

This theory is undermined by reports that upon relapse a change from an initially abnormal to a normal karyotype has been observed only very rarely [54, 59, 64]. The rule is that in relapse the same clone that dominated at diagnosis reappears. During recent years we have learnt that karyotypic progression is not limited to CML, but also occurs in AL. Karyotypic progression preceding or going along with relapse was seen in 10%–40% of AML patients [51, 54, 64–66] and even more often (20%–60%) in ALL patients [59, 67–69]. In AML, the additional changes superimposed on the initial karyotype are mostly numerical in nature, e.g., +8, and thus resemble the blastic phase, while in ALL structural anomalies are more common. The emergence of one or more new clone(s) seemingly unrelated to the original one does occur but is exceptional. Thus, cytogenetics of acute leukemia in relapse indicates that relapse represents the re-emergence of the original leukemic clone which treatment had failed to eradicate; that genetic instability is a continuous feature, particularly in ALL; and that new clones with normal or abnormal karyotype may arise, which either had already been present at diagnosis as a minor subclone or represent a secondary leukemia.

The contribution of cytogenetics to determination of the stem cell category from which acute leukemias may arise is limited, mainly because we do not know from which cell types which karyotypes are derived. It is very likely that in different types of leukemia different stem cell maturation stages are affected. It is probably quite safe to postulate that the translocations 8; 21 and 15; 17, which are diagnostic for M2 and M3 leukemias, respectively, are limited to granulopoietic cells and their progeny. The 11q− appears to arise in stem cells that are in an earlier stage of the differention pathway of myeloid cells, e.g., mainly committed to monocytoid differentiation; at the Fourth International Workshop on Chromosomes in Leukemia [107] it was reported that 60% of patients with 11q− (with and without translocation of the deleted segment) had M5 leukemia, 15% had M4 leukemia, and 7% had M2 leukemia. The translocation 4; 11 is considered to be specific for lymphoid leukemias [71, 72]; on the basis of ultrastructural and immunological findings [73], it now seems that it affects a pluripotential stem cell close to the differentiation stage of cells in which the Ph^1 is commonly induced.

The involvement of different stem cell categories in acute leukemias can also be deduced from other observations: Inoue et al. [74] and Fialkow et al. [58] described children in whom the leukemic karyotypic and enzymatic phenotypes were restricted to the granulocytic-monocytic pathway while erythropoiesis was unaffected; in other patients with myeloid leukemia it has been demonstrated directly [75] and indirectly [76] that the leukemic karyotype involves *both* myeloid and erythroid cells.

Secondary Acute Leukemias

Among the more important contributions of cytogeneticists to leukemia research are findings in so-called secondary acute leukemias. By definition, secondary leukemia is a disease developing in a patient with a previous neoplasm in his history, which may or may not have been treated by radio- and/or chemotherapy. Such findings have led to a number of other observations which are likely to assist in the elucidation of leukemogenesis and the modification of the present treatment strategies applied in malignant diseases.

The story began with the realization that particularly patients with Hodgkin's disease and plasmocytoma who had been treated with cytostatic drugs had a greatly increased risk of developing acute leukemia [77] and that such leukemias were almost invariably accomparied by a strikingly abnormal karyotype [78]. The application of banding techniques then revealed a highly typical chromosome pattern, characterized by partial deletion or loss of chromosomes 5, 7, 17, and possibly 3 [56, 79, 80]. In addition, in more than half the cases a hypodiplid clone was detected, and karyotypic instability was rather frequent. Such findings are in contrast to those in de novo acute leukemia (without a known prior exposure to cytostatic drugs and/or radiation), in which particularly the constellation −5/5q− and −7/7q− occurs in less than 10% of cases and the chromosome modes are evenly distributed among hypo-, pseudo-, and hyperdiploidy. Although most of the secondary leukemias fall into the M2 category, it is extremely striking that the translocation 8; 21 has not yet been observed. This is also true for t (15; 17), t (9; 22=Ph^1), and 11q−, which allows the conclusion that the causation of acute leukemias characterized by these specific structural chromosome anomalies is different from that of those with −5/5q−, −7/7q−, and −17 [56, 78].

In this context, important aspects have been emphasized by Pedersen-Bjeergaard et al. [81]. They pointed out that the typical karyotype occurred mainly in patients who became leukemic 30−60 months after the start of therapy of the preceding disease, who had a preleukemic phase, and who had received chemotherapy. Of patients who developed secondary leukemia earlier or later, only one-third had the typical karyotype, half had a preleukemic phase, and three-quarters had received radiotherapiy exclusively. These workers concluded that the last group of patients represented mostly de novo leukemias rather than therapy-related secondary leukemias. Yet the fact remained that the karyotype typical for chemotherapy-related leukemia could also be demonstrated in about a third of the patients without a corresponding history. There could be a connection between these observations and those reported by Mitelman et al. [82], which were later confirmed [83] but also contradicted [84]. They discovered that most patients with de novo leukemia and a −5/5q−; −7/7q− chromosome constitution in their leukemic cells had had occupational exposure to agents known to be mutagenic and/or carcinogenic, such as insecticides, petroleum products, and various chemicals and solvents. Again, among the leukemias with the "iatrogenic" chromosome pattern, the M1−M2 types predominated heavily. Not surprisingly, females are underrepresented in this group and its incidence increased with

increasing age of the patients. These last observations could be related to the duration of exposure [57, 66, 85, 86]. In children and young adults (less than 20 years of age) the iatrogenic karyotype has not yet been described [57], while de novo karyotypes [t (8; 21); 11q−] account for the majority of anomalies.
It thus appears that chromosome analysis has allowed important insights into the etiology of acute leukemias. The differentiation between patients with iatrogenic and those with de novo leukemias, which cannot be accomplished cytologically, also has considerable clinical relevance, since the former group of patients is unlikely to respond to the chemotherapeutic measures currently in use [81].

Implications for Prognosis

Chronic Myelocytic Leukemia

For years the prognostic value of chromosome analysis in CML was considered to be clear: patients with Ph^1-positive CML live almost 4 times as long as patients with Ph^1-negative CML [87]. However, the situation turned out not to be so simple: in the first place, it was realized that Ph^1-negative CML represents a highly heterogeneous group of diseases, which renders a comparison with well defined Ph^1-positive CML questionable; secondly, apart from the presence or absence of the Ph^1 a number of other chromosomal aspects appeared to have prognostic significance.
In evaluation of the influence of the Ph^1 on the course of CML, care must be taken that both the Ph^1-positive and the Ph^1-negative groups include only patients with typical CML (which is not always an easy task). No such study has been reported as yet. From our own experience [88] we would expect that about a third of Ph^1-negative patients will have a similar prognosis to Ph^1-positive CML patients, and that for the other patients with Ph^1-negative disease the role of Ph^1-negativity as an independent prognostic factor will be difficult to prove. Admittedly, this interpretation is at variance with most reports devoted to this subject [89, 90].
Within the Ph^1-positive group of patients, loss of the Y chromosome, the presence of normal metaphases, and the absence of additional chromosome anomalies have been as factors with a favorable effect on prognosis. The first two aspects are controversial. Some authors insist on the missing Y as a positive prognostic factor [35], while others deny it [91]. We analysed seven such patients and suggested that CML patients do not live particularly long because they have lost the Y, but rather lose the Y because they survive longer [92]. The finding that patients with a mixture of Ph^1-positive and Ph^1-negative (normal?) metaphases have a better prognosis was theoretically attractive and plausible, especially in the light of a similar observation in AML [36]. However, this was not corroborated in larger series of patients [34, 35]. There is general agreement (with one exception [93]) that the translocation type involved in formation of the Ph^1 does not alter the course of CML [94]. The detection of new clones during the chronic phase is an ominous sign if the clone is characterized by an additional Ph^1, or +19, or isochromosome 17q. Most of such patients are in a transitional phase of the disease, and many of them, particularly those with an isochromosome 17q, are about to enter the blastic phase. Since isochromosome 17 is restricted to the myeloid type, the outlook for such patients is very poor [30, 41, 47]. With regard to manifest blastic phase most cytogeneticists agree that an inverse correlation exists between length of survival and proportion of metaphases with additional anomalies, as well

as extent of anomalies [27, 46, 47, 95, 96]. Apart from isochromosome 17q there is only one other undisputed karyotypic pattern that is related to a particular morphologic type; this is near-haploidy in the lymphoid blastic phase.

Acute Myeloid Leukemia

Role of Normal Metaphases

In 1973 Sakurai and Sandberg [97] reported that the demonstration of normal metaphases in the bone marrow of patients with AML means a favorable prognosis. In subsequent years many authors have addressed themselves to this finding; most of them confirmed it, while some did not (Table 1).

Sakurai and Sandberg divided the patients into three groups, those without chromosomal abnormalities (NN), those with a mixture of normal and abnormal metaphases (AN), and those with exclusively abnormal metaphases (AA). Their interpretation of the findings was that normal metaphases reflect the presence of a residual normal population which is of vital importance for repopulation of the marrow after chemotherapy-induced aplasia. This view was generally adopted. Nilsson et al. [98] offered an alternative explanation, proposing that all acute leukemias start with a normal (NN) and end up with an exclusively (AA) abnormal karyotype; thus, AA patients are those diagnosed in a more advanced stage of the disease than NN patients.

The results of Sakurai and Sandberg were based on unbanded chromosome preparations. Banding studies [64, 66, 98, 99, 102] did not reveal any fundamentally different data, but did contribute a number of important subgroups, which will be discussed below.

In any attempt at critical review, in the studies mentioned in Table 1, of the role of normal and abnormal metaphases in the prognosis of patients with AML the following facets will have to be considered: patient selection; type of treatment; type of supportive care; material used for chromosome analysis; chromosome techniques; and number of metaphases studied.

Obviously, if one believes that normal metaphases represent, at least in part, a normal residual hematopoiesis, studies carried out in peripheral blood cells [53] are not relevant. The situation would be quite different if leukemic cells with a normal karyotype were considered less aggressive or more responsive to chemotherapy than karyotypically abnormal cells. Data available (remission rate, survival rate) do not reveal which of these premises is correct.

It has already been stated that the results of chromosome analysis are greatly influenced by whether the cells are prepared directly or after short-term culture [2–6]. Usually the latter method provides leukemic cells with a growth advantage, with the consequence that an NN status may become AN and an AN status may convert to AA (2–5, 104]. In some of the studies listed in Table 1 only direct preparations were used [52, 97, 101, 105], in some only 24-hour cultures [66, 100], and in others both methods, including culture times up to 48 hours [51, 64, 102]. This situation makes a comparative evaluation of the results difficult, even though no clear-cut evidence emerges for the proposition that the proportions of patients within the three chromosome groups are substantially changed by the method applied. Particularly with regard to the AA group, which is of major interest since the NN and NA groups do not have different prognoses, the proportion of patients is remarkably similar, ranging from 11% to 30% in nine studies evaluable; in six of them the proportion was 15%–20%.

Table 1. Remission rate and median survival of AML patients classified according to normal and abnormal karyotype

Authors[a]	Culture time[b]	No. of metaphases counted	Remission rate (%)			Median survival (months)		
			NN	AN	AA	NN	AN	AA
Sakurai and Sandberg [97]	d	25	–	–	–	12.5	7.4	3.6
Nilson et al. [98]	d	> 30	–	–	–	8.0	2.5	1.0
Alimena et al. [101]	d	13–30	–	–	–	7.0	2.0	
Fitzgerald et al. [103]	d	5–33	–	–	–	3.0	2.7	2.5
Golomb et al. [99]	d, 24	> 20	50	33	8	8.0	6.5	2.0
Prigogina et al. [53]	d, 24		15	20		5.4	6.2	
Hossfeld et al. [100]	24	> 25	73	60	36	12.5	8.5	4.0
Lawler et al. [64]	d, 24	3–30	74	57	66	12.0	11.2	3.5
Takeuchi et al. [52]	d	> 25	59	58		6.4	8.2	
Hagemeijer et al. [51]	d, 24, 48	> 32	13	19		3.0	5.0	3.0
Bernard et al. [102]	d, 48	20–30	78	77	80	25.0	20.0	1.0
Li et al. [66]	24	10–30	59	54	50	15.0	12.5	2.0
Brodeur et al. [105]	d	10–25	78	77	80	14.0	14.8	18.3

[a] Numbers in parenthesis refer to list of references
[b] *d*, direct preparation; 24, 48 h of culture time

The effect of patient- and treatment-related factors is borne out by findings reported by Hagemeijer et al. [51] who analyzed a rather unfavorable group of patients with advanced disease, one-fourth of whom did not receive cytostatic treatment. The median survival of all patients (including untreated patients) was 3 months for NN patients, 5 months for NA patients, and 3 months for AA patients. On the other hand, if results of "modern" chemotherapy (Ara-C plus daunomycin ± 6-thioguanin) are compared with results of "older" chemotherapy (Ara-C+thioguanin) the impression emerges that, particularly in AA patients, remission rates have improved, which has not, however, led to a marked improvement in survival [64, 66]. This interpretation contrasts with results published by Brodeur et al. [105] who observed a high remission rate and prolonged survival in *children* with AA leukemia. It should also be added that the data published do not allow analysis of the possible impact of maintenance therapy on survival in different studies.

The definition of the chromosome group also depends on the total number of metaphases analyzed per patient. It is quite likely that the analysis of 50 metaphases instead of 20 will move a patient from a NN status to AN or from AA to AN. But again, the studies referred to in Table 1 do not allow the conclusion that the proportions of patients in the different groups are significantly altered by the number of metaphases analysed. In the majority of studies more than 20 metaphases were investigated.

Admittedly, despite this rather lengthy discussion the reader is left in the dark concerning the nature and significance of normal metaphases in the prognosis of patients with AML. It is hoped that the results of the Fourth Chromosome Workshop [107] can give answers to at least some of the questions raised.

Specific Chromosome Anomalies

t(8; 21). This translocation is closely correlated with M_2 leukemia. The morphological changes associated with t(8; 21) are believed to be so distinct that this particular subtype of M2 can be predicted by means of cytology alone [104]; cytochemically it is characterized by a low activity of alkaline phosphatase [106]. The t (8; 21) is not absolutely specific for M2: at the Fourth International Workshop on Chromosomes in Leukemia [107], 4 of 45 cases were classified as M4, and in the literature we found two cases with M1 morphology [104, 105]. The overall incidence of t(8; 21) among M2 leukemias was reported as 15% at the Fourth Workshop. However, there is a peculiar geographic distribution, hitherto unexplained, with a low incidence of about 5% in Europe and a high incidence of about 30% in Japan [108], which may relate to genetic and/or carcinogenic factors. The t(8; 21) anomaly is rare in patients older than 50 years, and it occurs more frequently in males than in females [57].

Patients with t(8; 21) are considered to have a favorable prognosis [108, 109]. This statement needs specification and modification. If all patients with t(8; 21) are considered together it can be seen that 70%–80% will enter a complete remission, but survival is unlikely to exceed 12 months [108, 110, 111]. Longer survival occurs only in patients with a mixture of normal and abnormal (AN) metaphases. For patients in whom loss of a sex chromosome is detected in addition to t(8; 21) survival time is short, being less than 4 months [108]. Roughly half the patients belong to the group with poor prognosis. What is not yet known is whether t(8; 21) represents an independent prognostic factor. There are no larger series comparing the clinical course of M2 patients with and without t(8; 21).

t(15; 17). Among the characteristic chromosome anomalies associated with myeloid leukemias the translocation (15; 17) is the most specific. It has not been found in any other leukemia but M3. However, not all M3 leukemias have the t(15; 17). In two large collaborative studies [107, 108] 61% and 41% of cases, respectively, had the translocation. Chromosomal findings in APL are remarkable for another reason, in that anomalies other than t(15; 17) can be seen in less than 10% of the cases only.
Remission rates and survival appear to be somewhat more favorable in patients with karyotypically normal M3 than in those with the translocation [108]. Among the patients with t(15; 17) those with a mixture of normal and abnormal metaphases do better than those with exclusively abnormal metaphases [108, 112].
The variant form of M3 leukemia [113] is almost invariably linked with t(15; 17) [108, 114].

del 11q. The deletion 11q is the most recent discovery of a specific structural anomaly associated with a particular type of leukemia, i.e., M5. The frequent involvement of the long arm of chromosome 11 in monoblastic (M5) and myelomonocytic (M4) leukemias was not recognized until 1980 [115]. Among 118 cases of M5 leukemia submitted to the Fourth Chromosome Workshop [107] del 11q was present in 23% of the cases. The breakpoint was band q23 in 80% of cases. Recently, evidence was provided that in a significant proportion of M5 leukemias the deleted material is translocated to the short arm of chromosome No. 9, resulting, for example, in t(9; 11) [116, 117]. The anomaly occurs more often in the poorly differentiated subtype of monoblastic leukemia, e.g., M5a.
Deletions of 11q have also been detected in other types of AML, particularly in M4. The incidence, however, is much lower, the breakpoints are located in different bands, and t(9; 11) appears to be restricted to M5 [54].
It is not yet known whether del 11q correlates with a particular clinical course and prognosis.

−5/5q−; −7/7q−. Pathogenetic and clinical aspects of AML related to the −5/5q−; −7/7q− chromosome constitution have been discussed previously. It was stressed that most of the patients affected have a preleukemic phase preceding the development of M1, M2, or M6 leukemia, that elderly males predominate, and that a history of a previously treated neoplasm or occupational exposure to carcinogenic substances is common. In at least 70% of the patients no normal metaphases can be found once they have entered an overt leukemic phase [57, 59, 80]. Response to chemotherapy in such patients is very poor, and a complete remission exceptional. The mean survival, accordingly, is less than 5 months from diagnosis of frank leukemia. In our recent series of 42 unselected AML patients three of 42 had secondary leukemia, and 2 of them presented with the −5/5q−, −7/7q− chromosome constitution. None of them entered a complete remission [119].

Acute Lymphoid Leukemia

Role of Chromosome Number

Only 20 years after the introduction of chromosome analysis into leukemia research the relationship of chromosome anomalies to prognosis in ALL was recognized. Secker-Walker et al. [119] classified patients, according to the chromosomal characteristics of the major proportion of their leukemic cells, into five categories: hyperdiploid (more than 46 chromosomes), pseudodiploid, normodiploid, hypodiploid (less than 46 chromosomes), and mixed. They found that patients in the hyperdiploid group had significantly longer first remissions than those in the other groups, and that those in the pseudodiploid group had the shortest. These findings were substantiated and extended by a collaborative study [70] and a large single-institution study [120].

At the Third International Workshop of Chromosomes in Leukemia [7] and in the Memphis study [120] patients were divided into five categories according to modal numbers: hyperdiploid (more than 50 chromosomes), hyperdiploid (47–50 chromosomes), pseudodiploid, normodiploid, and hypodiploid. The Workshop series consisted of 330 newly diagnosed patients, 157 of whom were children and 173 adults. The Memphis study was concerned with children only. Treatment was more heterogeneous in the Workshop series than in the Memphis series, but type of treatment did not appear to influence the relationship of chromosome findings to prognosis.

Both studies showed that in *children,* achievement of complete remission, duration of first complete remission, and survival were highly significantly different in the > 50 category versus the pseudodiploid category. After a follow-up period of up to 35 months (median follow-up period not given), in the Memphis study only two of 41 patients in the > 50 category had failed, but 19 of 28 pseudodiploid patients. An updating of the Workshop results after a median follow-up of 40 months demonstrated that 70% of the children in the > 50 category remained alive in their first complete remission, while in the pseudodiploid group median survival was 5–22 months, depending on the type of chromosomal anomaly [121]. Patients with normodiploid and hyperdiploid (47–50 chromosomes) karyotypes had an intermediate prognosis. Remission rates and survival in *adults* were comparably poor in all chromosome groups; however, in the > 50 group only, a median duration of first complete remission of more than 1 year was observed.

Most importantly, the karyotype was revealed to be an independent prognostic factor not related to leukocyte count, age, surface markers, FAB morphology, etc. The prognostic power of the karyotype was at least as strong as that of the leukocyte number.

Role of Specific Anomalies

In addition to modal numbers the type of karyotypic anomaly within the pseudodiploid category and its relationship to prognosis were analysed at the Third International Workshop on Chromosomes in Leukemia [70]. Particular attention was paid to the translocation 4; 11, 8; 14, and the Ph^1. Interestingly, the prognosis of *both* adults and children with such anomalies was very poor. Since these translocations have been shown to be associated with certain clinical and hematological characteristics, some details will be provided (Table 2).

The Ph^1 Chromosome. It was many years before the existence of Ph^1-positive ALL was accepted. We now know that the Ph^1 occurs in 15%–20% of cases of adult ALL and in about 5% of cases of childhood ALL. There is no ready explanation for this peculiar age distribution. It is possible that it may be related to the age distribution of CML, which is also much more frequent in adults than in children. At the Third International Workshop the data relating to 39 cases of Ph^1-positive ALL had been collected. All these cases had a non-T, non-B phenotype. L2 morphology (FAB) predominated. Median WBC and the percentage of circulating blasts were somewhat higher than in ALL patients with a normal karyotype. After a median follow-up of 40 months only three patients are known to be alive

Table 2. Clinical and hematological characteristics of ALL patients according to karyotype[a]

	> 50	47–50	46N	46A	< 46	Ph^1	t (4; 11)	t (8; 14)
Number of patients	31	28	112	41	17	39	18	16
Sex: % male	48	54	62	56	65	54	50	81
Median age (years)	5	16	15	18	19	30	14	22
Signs at diagnosis (%)								
Lymphadenopathy	42	63	51	66	65	44	50	38
Splenomegaly	74	56	53	71	59	49	78	60
CNS leukemia	3	8	6	5	0	3	22	33
Hematological findings at diagnosis								
Hgb (g/dl, median)	8	9	10	10	8	10	8	10
WBC (10^9/l, median)	6	9	12	28	36	34	183	12
FAB								
%L1	48	46	52	32	29	39	43	6
%L2	48	55	47	68	71	61	50	ß
%L3	4	0	1	0	0	0	7	94
LSM								
% Non-T, non-B	100	87	67	74	80	100	88	0
% T	0	13	33	26	20	0	12	0
% B	0	0	0	0	0	0	0	100
% Complete remission (CR)								
Children	95	86	97	100	100	78	88	83
Adults	78	67	87	61	50	46	50	44
Median duration of CR (months)								
Children	60+	49	27	17	13	15	3	4
Adults	17	10	0	11	5	7	–	–
Median survival (months)								
Children	58	81	50	26	21	15	9	5
Adults	21	8	24	10	7	11	7	5

[a] Results collected for the Third Workshop on Chromosomes in Leukemia [70, 121]

[121]. The median survival was 15 months for children and 11 months for adults, figures which resemble our own experience [122].

t(8; 14). The Third International Workshop confirmed the invariable association of t(8; 14) and L3 morphology (FAB) which had been described before [123, 124]. All cases were found to have B cell characteristics. CNS leukemia was diagnosed in a third of the patients, more frequently than in any other of the various chromosome groups. WBC tended to be low (median 12×10^9/l). In all, 80% of the patients were males. Although a complete remission was obtained in 60% of the patients, median survival was only 5 months.

t(4; 11). The most typical feature of patients with the t(4; 11) translocation is a very high tumor load, as evidenced by a greatly increased WBC (median 183×10^9/l), splenohepatomegaly, and lymphadenopathy. The median age of the patients considered at the Workshop was 14 years; a literature survey reveals that more than half the patients were children below 1 year. Of the 18 patients collected by the Workshop only three survived beyond 16 months, the longest survivor living 32 months. Median survival was 7 months. Both the patients with t(4; 11) whom we have observed recently developed diffuse intravascular coagulopathy and died within 6 days after diagnosis [125].
The possibility has been discussed that the cells affected by t(4; 11) are not lymphoid but early myeloid [73].

Conclusion

In this paper we have tried to give a brief review of the implications of chromosomal findings in the pathogenesis and prognosis of leukemia. Fortunately the editors did not ask us to write about the role of chromosomes in the causation of leukemia, which would have been an extremely difficult task. We believe that it is still too early for an unambiguous definition of the place of chromosomal changes in the multistep process that eventually leads to leukemia. However, some recent, exciting developments should be touched upon, which may lead the protagonists of chromosomes' identity as epiphenomena to reconsider their dogma. The developments relate to cellular genes which have come to be called oncogenes. What must be considered a major step forward in the appreciation of chromosomal anomalies in carcinogenesis is the demonstration that a number of such oncogenes are located in chromosome regions which are involved in specific translocations. Thus, *c-mos* has been mapped to 8q22, which is precisely the region participating in the translocation 8; 21 in M2 leukemia [126], and *c-myc* is located in band q24 of chromosome 8, the region involved in the translocation 8; 14 in L3 leukemia and Burkitt's lymphoma [127, 128]. The location of *c-abl* on 9q34 and its translocation to 22q11 in CML [14] has already been mentioned. The significance of these findings is not yet clear. However, they will unquestionably throw new light on the significance of chromosome anomalies in oncogenesis.

References

1. Ford CE, Jacobs PA, Lajtha LG (1958) Human somatic chromosomes. Nature 181: 1565–1568
2. Berger R, Bernheim A, Flandrin G (1980) Absence d'anomalie chromosomique et leucémie aigue: Relation avec les cellules médullaires normales. C R Acad Sci [D] (Paris) 290: 1557–1559
3. Carbonell F, Grilli G, Fliedner TM (1981) Cytogenetic evidence for a clonal selection of leukemic cells in culture. Leuk Res 5: 395–398
4. Knuutila S, Vuopio P, Elonen E, Siimes M, Kovanen R, Borgström GH, de la Chapelle A (1981) Culture of bone marrow reveals more cells with chromosomal abnormalities than the direct method in patients with hematologic disorders. Blood 58: 369–375
5. Yunis JJ (1982) Comparative analysis of high-resolution chromosome technique for leukemic bone marrows. Cancer Genet Cytogenet 7: 43–50
6. Weh HJ, von Paleske A, Hossfeld DK (to be published) Disappearance of hypotetraploid clones after short term culture of leukemic cells. A case report. Cancer Genet Cytogenet
7. Pedersen-Bjergaard J, Vindeløv L, Philip P, Ruutu P, Elmgreen J, Repo H, Christensen IJ, Killmann S-A, Jensen G (1982) Varying involvement of peripheral granulocytes in the clonal abnormality – 7 in bone marrow cells in preleukemia secondary to treatment of other malignant tumors: cytogenetic results compared with results of flow cytometric DNA analysis and neutrophil chemotaxis. Blood 60: 172–179
8. Sonta SI, Sandberg AA (1977) Chromosomes and causation of human cancer and leukemia. XXVIII. Value of detailed chromosome studies on large numbers of cells in CML. Am J Hematol 3: 121–126
9. First International Workshop on Chromosomes in Leukemia (1978) Cancer Res 38: 867–868
10. ISCN (1978) An international system for human cytogenetic nomenclature, 1978. Birth defects: original article series, vol 14, no 8. The National Foundation, New York
11. Nowell PC, Hungerford DA (1960) A minute chromosome in human chronic granulocytic leukemia. Science 132: 1497
12. Rowley JD (1973) A new consistent chromosomal abnormality in chronic myelogenous leukemia identified by quinacrine fluorescence and Giemsa staining. Nature 243: 290–293
13. Wayne AW, Sharp JC (1982) A photometric study of the standard Philadelphia (Ph^1) translocation of chronic myeloid leukemia (CML). Cancer Genet Cytogenet 5: 253–256
14. De Klein A, van Kessel AG, Grosveld G, Bartram CR, Hagemeijer A, Bootsma D, Spurr NK, Heisterkamp N, Groffen J, Stephenson JR (1982) A cellular oncogene is translocated to the Philadelphia chromosome in chronic myelocytic leukemia. Nature 300: 765–767
15. Bartam CR, de Klein A, Hagemeier A, Agthoven T, van Kessel AG, Bootsma D, Grosveld G, Ferguson-Smith MA, Davies T, Stone M, Heisterkamp N, Stephenson JR, Groffen J (1983) Translocation of *c-abl* oncogene correlates with the presence of a Philadelphia chromosome in chronic myelocytic leukemia. Nature 306: 277–280
16. Bishop JM (1982) Oncogenes. Sci Am 3: 69–78
17. Roozendaal KJ, van der Reijden HJ, Geraedts JPM (1981) Philadelphia chromosome positive acute lymphoblastic leukemia with T-cell characteristics. Br J Haematol 47: 145–147
18. Dankbaar H, Willemze R, Spaander PJ, Geraedts JPM (1982) Philadelphia chromosome positive T-ALL. Br J Haematol 50: 543–546
19. Hernandez P, Carhot J, Cruz C (1982) Chronic myeloid leukemia blast crisis with T-cell features. Br J Haematol 51: 175–180
20. Greaves MF, Verbi W, Reeves R, Hoffbrand A, Drysdale HC, Jones L, Sacker LS, Samaratunga J (1979) "Pre-B" phenotypes in blast crisis of Ph^1-positive CML: evidence for a pluripotential stem cell "target". Leuk Res 3: 181–186
21. LeBien TW, Hozier J, Minowada J, Kersey JH (1979) Origin of chronic myelocytic leukemia in a precursor of pre-B lymphocytes. N Engl J Med 301: 144–147

22. Martin PJ, Majfeld V, Fialkow PJ (1982) B-lymphoid cell involvement in chronic myelogenous leukemia: implications for the pathogenesis of the disease. Cancer Genet Cytogenet 6: 359–368
23. Bernheim A, Berger R, Preud'homme JL, Labaume S, Bussel A, Barot-Ciorbaru R (1981) Philadelphia chromosome positive blood B lymphocytes in chronic myelocytic leukemia. Leuk Res 5: 331–339
24. Fialkow PJ, Jacobson RJ, Papayannopoulou T (1977) Chronic myelocytic leukemia: clonal origin in a stem cell common to the granulocyte, erythrocyte, platelet and monocyte/macrophage. Am J Med 63: 125–130
25. Hossfeld DK (1975) Additional chromosomal indication for the unicellular origin of chronic myelocytic leukemia. Z Krebsforsch 83: 269–273
26. Chaganti RSK, Bailey RB, Jhanwar SC, Arlin ZA, Clarkson BD (1982) Chronic myelogenous leukemia in the monosomic cell line of a fertile Turner syndrome mosaic (45, X/46, XX). Cancer Genet Cytogenet 5: 215–221
27. Hossfeld DK (1975) Chronic myelocytic leukemia: Cytogenetic findings and their relations to pathogenesis and clinic. Ser Haemat 8: 53–72
28. Singer JW, Pialkow PJ, Steinmann L, Najfeld V, Stein SJ, Robinson WA (1979) Chronic myelocytic leukemia (CML): Failure to detect residual normal committed stem cells in vitro. Blood 53: 264–268
29. Wayne AW, Sharp JC, Joyner MV, Sterndale H, Pulford KAF (1979) The significance of Ph^1 mosaicism: A report of six cases of chronic granulocytic leukaemia and two cases of acute myeloid leukaemia. Br J. Haematol 43: 353–360
30. Carbonell E, Benitez J, Prieto F, Badia L, Sánchez-Payos J (1982) Chromosome banding patterns in patients with chronic myelocytic leukemia. Cancer Genet Cytogenet 7: 287–297
31. Cunningham I, Gee T, Dowling M, Chaganti R, Bailey R, Hopfan S, Bowden L, Turnbull A, Knapper W, Clarkson B (1979) Results of treatment of Ph^1 – chronic myelogenous leukemia with an intensive treatment regimen (L-5 protocol). Blood 53: 375–395
32. Sharp JC, Joyner MV, Wayne AW, Kemp J, Crofts M, Birch A, McArthur G, Lai S, Sterndale H, Williams Y (1979) Karyotypic conversion in Ph^1-positive CML with combination chemotherapy. Lancet 1: 1370–1372
33. Singer JW, Clarkson BD, Fialkow PJ (1980) Restoration of nonclonal hematopoiesis in chronic myelogenous leukemia (CML) following a chemotherapy-induced loss of the Ph^1 chromosome. Blood 56: 356–360
34. Sokal J (1980) Significance of Ph^1-negative marrow cells in Ph^1-positive chronic granulocytic leukemia. Blood 56: 1072–1076
35. Oguma S, Takatsuki K, Uchino H, Kamada N, Oguma N, Kuramoto A (1982) Factors influencing survival in Philadelphia chromosome positive chronic myelocytic leukemia. Cancer 50: 2928–2934
36. Sakurai M, Hayata I, Sandberg AA (1976) Prognostic value of chromosomal findings in Ph^1-positive chronic myelocytic leukemia. Cancer Res 36: 313–318
37. Hagemeijer A, Smit EME, Löwenberg B, Abels J (1979) Chronic myeloid leukemia with permanent disappearance of the Ph^1 chromosome and development of new clonal subpopulations. Blood 53: 1–14
38. Appelbaum FR, Najfeld V, Singer JW (1983) Chronic myelogenous leukemia. Prolonged survival with spontaneous decline in the frequency of Ph^1-positive cells and subsequent development of mixed Ph^1-positive and Ph^1-negative blast crisis. Cancer 51: 149–153
39. Lisker R, Casas L, Mutchinick O, Pérez-Chávez F, Labardini J (1980) Late-appearing Philadelphia chromosome in two patients with chronic myelogenous leukemia. Blood 56: 812–814
40. Fialkow PJ, Martin PJ, Najfeld V, Penfold GK, Jacobson RJ, Hansen JA (1981) Evidence for a multistep of chronic myelogenous leukemia. Blood 58: 158–163

41. Hagemeijer A, Stenfert Kroeze WF, Abels J (1980) Cytogenetic follow-up of patients with nonlymphocytic leukemia. I. Philadelphia chromosome-positive chronic myeloid leukemia. Cancer Genet Cytogenet 2: 317–326
42. Motomura S, Ogi K, Horie M (1973) Monoclonal origin of acute transformation of chronic myelogenous leukemia. Acta Haematol (Basel) 49: 300–305
43. Janossy G, Woodruff RK, Paxton A, Greaves MF, Capellaro D, Kirk B, Innes EM, Lewis C, Eden OB, Catovsky D, Hoffbrand AV (1978) Membrane marker and cell separation studies in Ph[1]-positive leukemia. Blood 51: 861–877
44. Griffin JD, Todd RF III, Ritz J, Nadler LM, Canellos GP, Rosenthal D, Gallivan M, Beveridge RP, Weinstein H, Karp D, Schlossman F (1983) Differentiation patterns in the blastic phase of chronic myeloid leukemia. Blood 61: 85–91
45. Bennett JM, Catovsky D, Daniel M-T, Flandrin G, Galton DAG, Gralnick HR, Sultan C (1976) Proposals for the classification of the acute leukaemias. Br J Haematol 33: 451–458
46. Alimena G, Dallapiccola B, Gastaldi R, Mandelli F, Brandt L, Mitelman F, Nilsson PG (1982) Chromosomal, morphological and clinical correlations in blastic crisis of chronic myeloid leukaemia. A study of 69 cases. Scand J Haematol 28: 103–117
47. Fleischman EW, Prigogina EL, Volkova MA, Frenkel MA, Zakhartchenko NA, Konstantinova LN, Puchkova GP, Balakirev SA (1981) Correlations between the clinical course, characteristics of blast cells, and karyotype patterns in chronic myeloid leukemia. Hum Genet 58: 285–293
48. Sandberg AA, Hossfeld DK (1970) Chromosomal abnormalities in human neoplasia. Annu Rev Med 21: 379–408
49. Garson OM (1979) Chromosome-banding techniques and their implication in hematology. Prog Hematol 21: 83–114
50. First International Workshop in Chromosomes in Leukemia (1978) Chromosomes in acute non-lymphocytic leukaemia. Br J Haematol 39: 311–316
51. Hagemeijer A, Hählen K, Abels J (1981) Cytogenetic follow-up of patients with nonlymphocytic leukemia. II. Acute nonlymphocytic leukemia. Cancer Genet Cytogenet 3: 109–124
52. Takeuchi J, Ohshima T, Amaki I (1981) Cytogenetic studies in adult acute leukemias. Cancer Genet Cytogenet 4: 293–302
53. Prigogina EL, Fleischman EW, Puchkova GP, Kulagina OE, Majakova SA, Balakirev SA, Prenkel MA, Khvatova NV, Peterson IS (1979) Chromosomes in acute leukemia. Hum Genet 53: 5–16
54. Fitzgerald PH, Morris CM, Fraser GJ, Giles LM, Hamer JW, Heaton DC, Beard MEJ (1983) Nonrandom cytogenetic changes in New Zealand patients with acute myeloid leukemia. Cancer Genet Cytogenet 8: 51–66
55. Mitelman F, Nilsson PG, Brandt L, Alimena G, Gastaldi R, Dallapiccola B (1981) Chromosome pattern, occupation, and clinical features in patients with acute nonlymphocytic leukemia. Cancer Genet Cytogenet 4: 197–214
56. Rowley JD, Golomb HM, Vardiman JW (1981) Nonrandom chromosome abnormalities in acute leukemia and dysmyelopoietic syndromes in patients with previously treated malignant disease. Blood 58: 759–767
57. Rowley JD, Alimena G, Garson OM, Hagemeijer A, Mitelman F, Prigogina EL (1982) A collaborative study of the relationship of the morphological type of acute nonlymphocytic leukemia with patient age and karyotype. Blood 59: 1013–1021
58. Fialkow PJ, Singer JW, Adamson JW, Vaidya K, Dow LW, Ochs J, Moohr JW (1981) Acute nonlymphocytic leukemia: heterogeneity of stem cell origin. Blood 57: 1068–1073
59. Zuelzer WW, Inoue S, Thompson RI, Ottenbreit MJ (1976) Long-term cytogenetic studies in acute leukemia of children; the nature of relapse. Am J Hematol 1: 143–190
60. Nowell PC (1978) Tumors as clonal proliferation. Virchows Arch [Cell Pathol] 29: 145–150
61. Morse HG, Ducore JM, Hays T, Peakman D, Robinson A (1978) Multiple leukemic clones in acute leukemia of childhood. Hum Genet 40: 269–278

62. Testa JR, Kanofsky JR, Rowley JD, Baron JM (1981) Multiple cytogenetically abnormal clones in two polycythemia vera patients. Hum Genet 57: 165–168
63. McCulloch EA, Howatson AF, Buick RN, Minden MD, Izaguirre CA (1979) Acute myeloblastic leukemia considered as a clonal hemopathy. Blood Cells 5: 261–282
64. Lawler SD, Summersgill B, Clink HM, McElwain TJ (1980) Cytogenetic follow-up study of acute non-lymphocytic leukaemia. Br J Haematol 44: 395–405
65. Testa JR, Mintz U, Rowley JD, Vardiman JW, Golomb HM (1979) Evolution of karyotypes in acute nonlymphocytic leukemia. Cancer Res 39: 3619–3627
66. Li YS, Khalid G, Hayhoe FGJ (1983) Correlation between chromosomal pattern, cytological subtypes, response to therapy, and survival in acute myeloid leukaemia. Scand J Haematol 30: 265–277
67. Kaneko Y, Rowley JD, Variakojis D, Chilcote RR, Check I, Sakurai M (1982) Correlation of karyotype with clinical features in acute lymphoblastic leukemia. Cancer Res 42: 2918–2929
68. Whang-Peng J, Knutsen T, Ziegler J, Leventhal B (1976) Cytogenetic studies in acute lymphocytic leukemia: special emphasis in long-term survival. Med Pediat Oncol 2: 333–351
69. Secker-Walker LM, Swansbury GJ, Lawler SD, Hardisty RM (1979) Bone marrow chromosomes in acute lymphoblastic leukaemia: a long- term study. Med Pediat Oncol 7: 371–385
70. Third International Workshop on Chromosomes in Leukemia (1981) Chromosomes in acute lymphoblastic leukemia. Cancer Genet Cytogenet 4: 101–137
71. Van den Berghe H, David G, Broeckaert-van Orshoven A, Louwagie A, Verwilghen R, Casteels-van Daele M, Eggermont E, Eeckels R (1979) A new chromosome anomaly in acute lymphoblastic leukemia (ALL). Hum Genet 46: 173–180
72. Arthur DC, Bloomfield CD, Lindquist LL, Nesbit ME Jr (1982) Translocation 4; 11 in acute lymphoblastic leukemia: clinical characteristics and prognostic significance. Blood 59: 96–99
73. Parkin JL, Arthur DC, Abramson CS, McKenna RW, Kersey JH, Heideman RL, Brunning RD (1982) Acute leukemia associated with the t (4; 11) chromosome rearrangement: Ultrastructural and immunologic characteristics. Blood 60: 1321–1331
74. Inoue S, Ravindranath Y, Zuelzer WW (1975) Cytogenetic analysis of erythroleukaemia in two children – Evidence of nonmalignant nature of erythron. Scand J Haematol 14: 129–139
75. Blackstock AM, Garson OM (1974) Direct evidence for involvement of erythroid cells in acute myeloblastic leukaemia. Lancet II: 1178–1182
76. Brandt L, Mitelman F, Sjögren U (1975) Megaloblastic changes and chromosome abnormalities of erythropoietic cells in acute myeloid leukaemia. Acta Haematol 54: 280–283
77. Holland JF (1970) Epidemic acute leukemia. N Engl J Med 283: 1165–1166
78. Hossfeld DK, Holland JF, Cooper RG, Ellison RR (1975) Chromosome studies in acute leukemias developing in patients with multiple myeloma. Cancer Res 35: 2808–2813
79. Rowley JD, Golomb HM, Vardiman J (1977) Nonrandom chromosomal abnormalities in acute nonlymphocytic leukemia in patients treated for Hodgkin disease and non-Hodgkin lymphomas. Blood 50: 759–769
80. Sandberg AA, Abe S, Kowalczyk JR, Zedgenidze A, Takeuchi J, Kakati S (1982) Chromosomes and causation of human cancer and leukemia. L Cytogenetics of leukemias complication other diseases. Cancer Genet Cytogenet 7: 95–136
81. Pedersen-Bjergaard J, Philip P, Mortensen BT, Ersbøll J, Jensen G, Panduro J, Thomsen M (1981) Acute nonlymphocytic leukemia. Preleukemia, and acute myeloproliferative syndrome secondary to treatment of other malignant diseases. Clinical and cytogenetic characteristics and results of in vitro culture of bone marrow and HLA typing. Blood 57: 712–723
82. Mitelman F, Brandt L, Nilsson PG (1978) Relation among occupational exposure to potential mutagenic/carcinogenic agents, clinical findings, and bone marrow chromosomes in acute nonlymphocytic leukemia. Blood 52: 1229–1237

83. Golomb HM, Alimena G, Rowley JD, Vardiman JW, Testa JR, Sovik C (1982) Correlation of occupation and karyotype in adult with acute nonlymphocytic leukemia. Blood 60: 404–411
84. Lawler SD, Summersgill BM, Clink HMcD, McElwain TJ (1979) Chromosomes, leukaemia, and occupational exposure to leukaemogenic agents. Lancet 2: 853–854
85. Rowley JD (1981) Association of specific chromosome abnormalities with type of acute leukemia and with patient age. Cancer Res 41: 3407–3410
86. Brandt L, Mitelman F, Nilsson PG (1983) Chromosome pattern and survival in acute non-lymphocytic leukaemia in relation to age and occupational exposure to potential mutagenic/carcinogenic agents. Scand J Haematol 30: 227–231
87. Ezdinli EZ, Sokal JE, Crosswhite L, Sandberg AA (1970) Philadelphia-chromosome-positive and – negative chronic myelocytic leukemia. Ann Intern Med 72: 175–182
88. Hossfeld DK (to be published) Die chronische myeloische Leukämie. In: Gross R, Schmidt CG (Hrsg) Klinische Onkologie. Thieme, Stuttgart
89. Lawler SD (1982) Significance of chromosome abnormalities in leukemia. Semin Hematol 19: 257–272
90. Gomez GA, Sokal JE, Walsh D (1981) Prognostic features at diagnosis of chronic myelocytic leukemia. Cancer 47: 2470–2475
91. Lawler SD, Lobb DS, Wiltshaw E (1974) Philadelphiachromosome positive bone marrow cells showing loss of the Y in males with chronic myeloid leukemia. Br J Haematol 27: 247–252
92. Hossfeld DK (1980) Loss of the Y chromosome in chronic myeloid leukemia (CML). In: Tura S, Zaccaria (eds) Citogenetica Oncologica. Societa' Editrice Esulapio, Bologna, pp 177–181
93. Potter AM, Watmore AE, Cooke P, Lilleyman JS, Sokol RJ (1981) Significance of non-standard Philadelphia chromosomes in chronic granulocytic leukemia. Br J Cancer 44: 51–54
94. Sandberg AA (1980) The cytogenetics of chronic myelocytic leukemia (CML): chronic phase and blastic crisis. Cancer Genet Cytogenet 1: 217–228
95. Sadamori N, Gomez GA, Sandberg AA (1983) Chromosomes and causation of human cancer and leukemia: IL. Therapeutic and prognostic value of chromosomal findings during acute phase in Ph^1-positive chronic myeloid leukemia. Hematol Oncol 1: 77–83
96. Oláh E, Rák K (1981) Prognostic value of chromosomal findings in the blast phase of Ph^1-positive chronic myeloid leukaemia (CML). Int J Cancer 27: 287–295
97. Sakurai M, Sandberg AA (1973) Prognosis of acute myeloblastic leukemia: chromosomal correlation. Blood 41: 93–104
98. Nilsson PG, Brandt L, Mitelman F (1977) Prognostic implications of chromosome analyses in acute nonlymphocytic leukemia. Leuk Res 1: 31–34
99. Golomb HM, Vardiman JW, Rowley JD, Testa JR, Mintz U (1978) Correlation of clinical findings with quinacrine-banded chromosomes in 90 adults with acute nonlymphocytic leukemia. N Engl J Med 299: 613–619
100. Hossfeld DK, Faltermeier M-T, Wendehorst E (1979) Beziehungen zwischen Chromosomenbefund und Prognose bei akuter nicht-lymphoblastischer Leukämie. Blut 38: 377–382
101. Alimena G, Annino L, Balestrazzi P, Montuoro A, Dallapiccola B (1977) Cytogenetic studies in acute leukemias. Prognostic implications of chromosome imbalances. Acta Haematol (Basel) 58: 234–239
102. Bernard P, Reiffers J, Lacombe F, Dachary D, David B, Boisseau MR, Broustet A (1982) Prognostic value of age and bone marrow karyotype in 78 adults with acute myelogenous leukemia. Cancer Genet Cytogenet 7: 153–163
103. Fitzgerald PH, Hamer JW (1976) Karyotype and survival in human acute leukemia. J Natl Cancer Inst 56: 459–462
104. Berger R, Bernheim A, Daniel M-T, Valensi F, Sigaux F, Flandrin G (1982) Cytologic characterization and significance of normal karyotypes in t (8; 21) acute myeloblastic leukemia. Blood 59: 171–176

105. Brodeur GM, Williams DL, Kalwinsky DK, Williams KJ, Dahl GV (1983) Cytogenetic features of acute nonlymphoblastic leukemia in 73 children and adolescents. Cancer Genet Cytogenet 8: 93–105
106. Kamada N, Dohy H, Okada K, Oguma N, Kuramoto A, Tanaka K, Uchino H (1981) In vivo and in vitro activity of neutrophil alkaline phosphatase in acute myelocytic leukemia with 8; 21 translocation. Blood 58: 1213–1217
107. Fourth International Workshop on Chromosomes in Leukemia (1983) Cancer Genet Cytogenet (to be published)
108. Second International Workshop on Chromosomes in Leukemia (1980) Morphological analysis of acute promyelocytic leukemia (M3) and t (8; 21). Cancer Genet Cytogenet 2: 89–113
109. Trujillo JM, Cork A, Ahearn MJ, Youness EL, McCredie KB (1979) Hematologic and cytologic charaterization of 8/21 translocation acute granulocytic leukemia. Blood 53: 695–706
110. Tricot G, Broeckaert-van Orshoven A, Casteels-van Daele M, van den Berghe H (1981) 8/21 translocation in acute myeloid leukemia. Scand J Haematol 26: 168–176
111. Oshimura M, Ohyashiki K, Mori M, Terada H, Takaku F (1982) Cytogenetic and hematologic findings in acute myelogenous leukemia, M2 according to the FAB classification. Gan 73: 212–216
112. Fraser J, Hollings PE, Fitzgerald PH, Day WA, Clark V, Heaton DC, Hamer JW, Beard MEJ (1981) Acute promyelocytic leukemia: cytogenetics and bone-marrow culture. Int J Cancer 27: 167–173
113. Bennett JM, Catovsky D, Daniel MT, Flandrin G, Galton DAG, Gralnick HR, Sultan C (1980) A variant form of hypergranular promyelocytic leukaemia (M3). Br J Haematol 44: 169–170
114. Berger R, Bernheim A, Daniel MT, Valensi F, Flandrin G, Bernard J (1979) Translocation t (15; 17), leucémie aigue promye'locytaire et non promyélocytaire. Nouv Rev Fr Hematol 21: 117–131
115. Berger R, Bernheim A, Weh H-J, Daniel M-T, Flandrin G (1980) Cytogenetic studies on acute monocytic leukemia. Leuk Res 4: 119–127
116. Hagemeijer A, Hählen K, Sizoo W, Abels J (1982) Translocation (9; 11) (p21; q23) in three cases of acute monoblastic leukemia. Cancer Genet Cytogenet 5: 95–105
117. Dewald GW, Morrison-DeLap SJ, Schuchard KA, Spurbeck JL, Pierre RV (1983) A possible specific chromosome marker for monocytic leukemia: three more patients with t (9; 11) (p22; q21), and another with t (11; 17) (q24; q21), each with acute monoblastic leukemia. Cancer Genet Cytogenet 8: 203–212
118. Weh H-J, Kuse R, Graeven U, Hausmann K, Hossfeld DK (1983) Cytogenetic findings in patients with acute myelogenous leukemia (AML). J Cancer Res Clin Oncol 105 (abstract)
119. Secker-Walker LM, Lawler SD, Hardisty RM (1978) Prognostic implications of chromosomal findings in acute lymphoblastic leukaemia at diagnosis. Br Med J 2: 1529–1530
120. Williams DL, Tsiatis A, Brodeur GM, Look AT, Melvin SL, Bowman WP, Kalwinsky DK, Rivera G, Dahl GV (1982) Prognostic importance of chromosome number in 136 untreated children with acute lymphoblastic leukemia. Blood 60: 864–871
121. Third International Workshop on Chromosomes in Leukemia (to be published) Chromosomal abnormalities identify high risk patients with acute lymphoblastic leukemia. Cancer Res
122. Hossfeld DK, Leder L-D, Wetter O, Zschaber R, Schmidt CG (1981) Philadelphia-Chromosom-positive akute Leukämie. In: Scheurlen PG, Pees HW (Hrsg) Aktuelle Therapie bösartiger Bluterkrankungen. Springer, Berlin Heidelberg New York, S 42–45
123. Berger R, Bernheim A, Brouet JC, Daniel MT, Flandrin G (1979) t (8; 14) translocation in a Burkitt's type of lymphoblastic leukaemia (L3). Br J Haematol 43: 87–90
124. Mitelman F, Andersson-Anvret M, Brandt L, Catovsky D, Klein G, Manolov G, Manolova Y, Mark-Vendel E, Nilsson PG (1979) Reciprocal 8; 14 translocation in EBV-negative B-cell acute lymphocytic leukemia with Burkitt-type cells. Int J Cancer 24: 27–33

125. Weh J-J, Kuse R, Hausmann K, Hossfeld DK (1983) Translocation t(4; 11): prognostische Bedeutung bei akuter lymphatischer Leukämie (ALL). Verh Dtsch Ges Inn Med 89: 1005–1008
126. Neel BG, Jhanwar SC, Chaganti RSK, Hayward WS (1982) Two human c-onc genes are located on the long arm of chromosome 8. Proc Natl Acad Sci USA 79: 7842–7846
127. Taub R, Kirsch I, Morton C, Lenoir G, Swan D, Tronick S, Aaronson S, Leder P (1982) Translocation of the c-myc gene into the immunoglobulin heavy chain locus in human Burkitt lymphoma and murine plasmacytoma cells. Proc Natl Acad Sci USA 79: 7837–7841
128. Dalla-Favera R, Bregni M, Erikson J, Patterson D, Gallo RC, Groce CM (1982) Human c-myc one gene is located on the region of chromosome 8 that is translocated in Burkitt lymphoma cells. Proc Natl Acad Sci USA 79: 7824–7827

Morphology, Cytochemistry, and Ultrastructure of Leukemic Cells with Regard to the Classification of Leukemias

D. Huhn

Medizinische Klinik III, Klinikum Grosshadern, Universität München,
Institut für Hämatologie der GSF, 8000 München, FRG

Morphology and cytochemistry now play a major part in the diagnosis and subclassification of acute myeloid leukemias (AML). In acute lymphatic leukemias (ALL), however, these methods have largely been replaced by immunological membrane marker investigations.

Cytochemistry in the classification of leukemias has reached a certain standard in the last decade, and results have been published in comprehensive monographs [23, 64]. These findings will be summarized very briefly in the below, and emphasis will be placed on some recent developments.

Concerning light microscopic morphology, proposals for a uniform system of classification and nomenclature of acute leukemias (AL) were elaborated by a French-American-British (FAB) cooperative group in 1974 and published in 1976 [7]. In recent years, FAB classification has been applied in several clinical studies: its relevance for prediction of prognosis [61] and for distinction between presenting features of leukemia [14] has been variously confirmed and challenged [10, 18] by different investigators. The FAB classification is based upon morphology *and* upon some fundamental cytochemical tests. Some cytochemical methods which are important for the accurate identification of leukemic cells, therefore, will first be summarized.

Cytochemistry in the Classification of Leukemias

Myeloperoxidase (POX)

POX is most frequently demonstrated by light and/or electron microscopy, using the Graham-Knoll method simplified by Kaplow [35]. POX is localized in the azurophilic granules of both the neutrophilic and the monocytic series. In basophils and in mast cells POX can be demonstrated in the specific granules [1, 38].

In the eosinophil series, peroxidase activity is found in the eosinophil granules of all stages. Probably, in man at least, the so-called secondary granules of eosinophils with crystalline internal structures are derived directly from the homogeneous primary granules [11]. Peroxidase contained in eosinophils differs from POX of the neutrophilic series in substrate specifity and sensitivity to a variety of inhibitors. Eosinophil peroxidase, further on, is not involved in cases of POX deficiency, which may be observed rather frequently in AML [15].

POX is of great importance for diagnosis of AML: as soon as activity of this enzyme can be demonstrated even in a small percentage of blasts which unequivocally belong to the leukemic series the diagnosis of AML can be made (for further subtypes of AML, see below).

Recent Results in Cancer Research. Vol. 93

Sudan Black B Reaction

A positive Sudan black B reaction is closely related to POX reactivity [50]. In addition, the Sudan black reaction is a rather nonspecific stain for neutral fats and phospholipids.

Naphthol AS-D Chloroacetate Esterase (ASDCl)

ASDCl is positive in the granulocytic series (including basophils and immature eosinophils). The method has been published elsewhere [45]. The reaction is less sensitive than the POX reaction for the diagnosis of AML. Some of the more immature cases of AML may be totally negative for ASDCl. In particular, this enzyme may be negative in patients for whom the May-Grünwald-Giemsa stain fails to show azurophilic granules but the POX reaction is positive.

Esterases

The biochemistry of esterases is very complex, but in cytochemistry the term esterase, or nonspecific esterase, is generally restricted to enzymes capable of hydrolysing the simpler esters of N-free alcohols and organic acids. Naphthyl esters have been used predominantly in esterase cytochemistry, because the liberated naphthol will couple with an appropriate diazotized amine to give a brightly coloured azo-dye [23]. When α-naphthyl acetate or naphthyl AS (or AS-D) acetate is used as substrate [9] the enzyme reaction product is largely confined to monocytes and their precursors, whilst cells of the granulocytic and lymphocytic series exhibit weak positivity. The value of esterases for staining of cells of the monocytic series was further enhanced by the observation of Fischer and Schmalzl [17], who demonstrated that nonspecific esterase activity in monocytes is inhibited by fluoride, whereas that in granulocytes is not. The methods have been described elsewhere [51].

Acute monocytic leukemia is characterized by a strong activity of nonspecific esterase, which is inhibited by sodium fluoride. Further details are given below.

α-Naphthylacetate

When α-naphthyl-acetate is used as a substrate and a long incubation time in *acid medium* is selected, a subfraction of murine and of human resting T lymphocytes is characterized by an intense and circumscribed reaction. This subpopulation of lymphocytes marked by a "dot-like" positivity of acid α-naphthylacetate esterase (ANAE), furthermore, has been said to possess receptors for the Fc portion of IgM and to provide the required help for B cell proliferation and differentiation into plasma cells [21]. The method has been published elsewhere [28].

In some lymphatic malignancies a characteristic pattern of activity of ANAE may support the diagnosis [28]. In ALL, the percentage of patients with ANAE-positivity of leukemic blasts was significantly higher in T subtypes of ALL than in common ALL (C-ALL) [29].

Azo-Dye Techniques

With azo-dye techniques activity of *acid phosphatase* (APh) is demonstrated in most nucleated hemic cells, with stronger positivity in granulocytes and monocytes than in lymphocytes [23]. Among bone marrow cells the most intense reaction is found in reticulum cells, plasma cells, megakaryocytes, tissue mast cells, and granulocyte precursors: APh is located mainly in primary neutrophil and monocyte granules and is absent from secondary and tertiary granules [3]. The method has been described elsewhere [5].

APh activity is ordinarily greater in AML than in ALL, but seems to be variable and is not sufficiently specific to help in its diagnosis or subclassification. The APh reaction in AML is usually diffusely positive in the cytoplasm, with or without superimposed granules, while in ALL it is granular and sometimes restricted to the paranuclear region.

Concerning ALL, positivity for APh was correlated with a special subtype characterized by convoluted nuclei and by a mediastinal mass [59], and with the T subtype of ALL [2].

When 136 consecutive cases of ALL were analyzed according to immunological membrane markers and cytochemistry the following results emerged [29]: Indices (calculated from the percentage of positive blasts and the intensity of staining) and the percentage of patients showing a positive cytochemical reaction for APh were significantly higher in pre-T-ALL and T-ALL than in C-ALL and C/T-ALL (the latter defined by positivity for C and for T membrane antigen) (Fig. 1).

Periodic Acid-Schiff (PAS) Stain

PAS may give a positive reaction with several classes of naturally occurring carbohydrates, including monosaccharides, polysaccharides, glycoprotein and mucoprotein conjugates, phosphorylated sugars, cerebrosides. In normal hemic cells PAS-positive substances usually consist of glycogen. The method has been published elsewhere [6].

Early granulocyte precursors, myeloblasts and promyelocytes, show a diffuse cytoplasmic staining, usually faint, but sometimes more intense. In myelocytes and in monocyte precursors (as well as in megakaryocytes) the faint cytoplasmic coloring may be superimposed by finely scattered PAS-positive granules.

The PAS reaction is of some importance in the differential diagnosis of the various forms of AL. Myeloblasts and promyelocytes from AML tend to be substantially PAS-negative, showing at most a diffuse cytoplasmic tinge. Some monoblasts may be completely negative while others display a rather strong diffuse staining or fine to moderately coarse granules. In erythroleukemia, proerythroblasts may show intense spotted normoblasts, and intense diffuse PAS-positivity [27].

Lymphoblasts of ALL may show very marked PAS staining in the form of concentric rings of coarse granules or even heavy blocks of glycogen in a percentage of cells that is highly variable from one case to another. When the indices of PAS staining and the percentages of positive cases were determined in 136 patients with membrane marker-classified ALL [29] PAS-positivity was significantly more pronounced in C-ALL and in C/T-ALL than in pre-T- or T-ALL (Fig. 1). APh cytochemistry and PAS staining, therefore, when evaluated together, are valuable in distinguishing T-ALL (including pre-T-ALL) from C-ALL (including C/T-ALL): in the case of the constellation APh−/PAS+, T-ALL is excluded with high reliability; and APh+/PAS− is found in about 75% of patients suffering from T-ALL, but only in 28% of C-ALL cases [29].

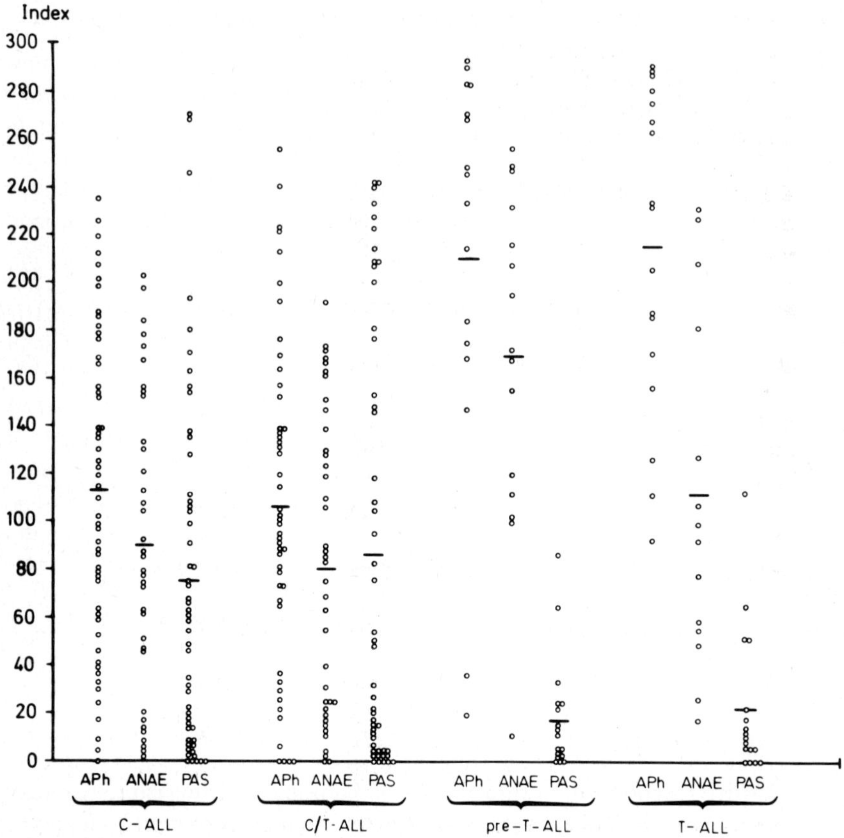

Fig. 1. Indices of enzyme positivity in leukemic blasts of 136 patients suffering from ALL and subdivided according to results of membrane markers. ———, mean values [29]

Correlation of the PAS-positivity of the leukemic blasts with a better survival has been demonstrated by several investigators [37, 43] but rejected by others [31].
The cytochemical tests discussed above have gained some significance in the diagnosis of AL and are routinely used in most hematology laboratories. Their relevance in connection with FAB classification of AL will be discussed below. Before this, some additional cytochemical investigations will be mentioned briefly.

Lysozyme

Lysozyme (muramidase) is an intracellular enzyme found in myeloid cells, monocytes, and histiocytes as well as in several nonleukemic cells. Intracytoplasmic lysozyme can be readily identified in paraffin sections of tissues fixed in formalin and in smears of peripheral blood or bone marrow by means of an immunoperoxidase technique [41]. Intracytoplasmic lysozyme is demonstrated in mature and immature neutrophilic and eosinophilic myeloid cells, in monocytic cells, and in histiocytic cells [47]. For classification in AL, detection of lysozyme is of only minor importance because of the superiority of POX and of nonspecific esterases for this purpose. Together with α_1-antichymotrypsin immunohistochemistry, however, lysozyme detection has gained importance for the delimitation of malignant histiocytic disorders from malignancies of the lymphatic system [42].

Terminal Deoxynucleotidyl Transferase (TdT)

TdT is a DNA polymerase that does not require a template to synthesize strands of DNA. Normally found in high levels in the thymus, it is found in low levels in normal bone marrow and not at all in normal peripheral blood leukocytes. When this enzyme was tested in AL, levels were raised in all 32 cases of T-ALL tested, in 108 of 115 patients who were considered to have non-T, non-B ALL on membrane marker analysis, but in only 3 of 73 patients with AML [33]. TdT can be visualized in individual cells in cytocentrifuge preparations by means of the peroxidase – antiperoxidase technique [32].

5′-Nucleotidase

5′-Nucleotidase is an enzyme of purine metabolism which is surface membrane bound and is classified as an "ectoenzyme". 5′-Nucleotidase activity has been described as decreased in T-ALL [48] but surprisingly high in the majority of 33 cases of C-ALL [22].

Morphological Classification of Acute Leukemia

Proposals for a uniform system of classification of AL were elaborated by the FAB cooperative group [7] and have since been applied in several clinical studies (Fig. 2). This classification is based entirely on the morphological appearances of the bone marrow and peripheral blood in Romanowsky-stained films, supplemented in appropriate circumstances by certain cytochemical reactions.

Lymphoblastic Leukemias

Lymphoblastic leukemias were subdivided into three subtypes (L_1, L_2, L_3) according to (a) the occurrence of individual cytological features, and (b) the degree of heterogeneity in the distribution among the leukemic cell population of some or all of these features [7]. The features considered and a summary of the characteristics of each type are given in Table 1.

L_1 represents the type of AL common in childhood. L_2 is less common in children and must be distinguished from undifferentiate myeloblastic leukemia (M_1, see below); the POX reaction may be essential for correct classification. B lymphocyte markers have been found in most cases of L_3 ALL.

In ALL classification based upon mere morphology and cytochemistry has been superseded by membrane marker investigations. When FAB classification was performed in 136 membrane marker-classified cases of ALL [29], the distribution of the L_1 and L_2 types was equal in subtypes defined by membrane markers. L_3 type was more frequent in pre-T- and T-ALL. L_1, L_2, and L_3-types according to the FAB classification will of necessity include up to 10% of heterogeneous cases of AL that are undifferentiated according to morphology, cytochemistry, and membrane marker studies (= AUL). When

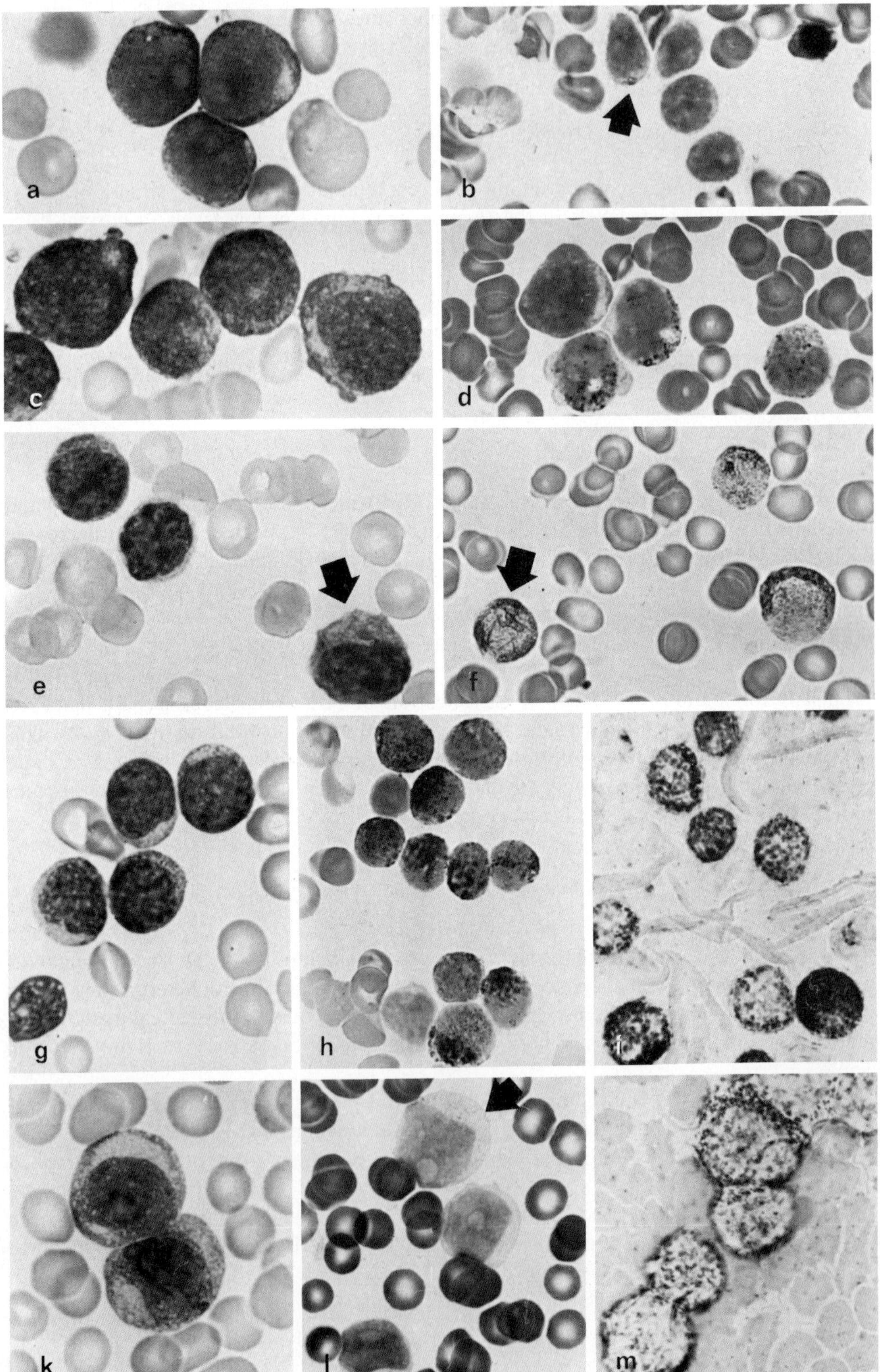
a
b
c
d
e
f
g
h
i
k
l
m

Table 1. Cytological features in subtypes of ALL [7]

Cytological features	L_1	L_2	L_3
Cell size	Small cells predominate	Large, heterogeneous in size	Large and homogeneous
Nuclear chromatin	Homogeneous in any one case	Variable heterogeneous in any one case	Finely stippled and homogeneous
Nuclear shape	Regular, occasional clefting or indentation	Irregular; clefting and indentation common	Regular; oval to round
Nucleoli	Not visible, or small and inconspicuous	One or more present, often large	Prominent; one or more, vesicular
Amount of cytoplasm	Scanty	Variable; often moderately abundant	Moderately abundant
Basophilia of cytoplasm	Slight or moderate, rarely intense	Variable; deep in some	Very deep
Cytoplasmic vacuolation	Variable	Variable	Often prominent

195 patients with AL were classified by three hematologists according to FAB criteria, all three observers recorded the same diagnosis in only 62% of the cases, and the accuracy in discriminating between lymphoid and myeloid groups was only 82% [14].

Myeloid Leukemias

In myeloid leukemia, six main types are described in the FAB classification (Table 2), according to (a) the direction of differentiation along one or more cell lines, and (b) the degree of maturation of the cells. Thus, M_1, M_2 and M_3 show predominantly granulocytic differentiation and differ from one another in the extent and nature of granulocytic maturation; M_4 shows both granulocytic and monocytic differentiation, M_5 predominantly monocytic, and M_6 erythroblastic differentiation.

Fig. 2a–m. Cytology of AL according to FAB classification. **a** M_1, May-Grünwald-Giemsa (MGG); **b** POX, one of four blasts shows deposits according to POX reactivity *(arrow);* **c** M_2, MGG; **d** M_2, POX, most of the blasts show distinct POX reactivity; **e** M_3, bundles of Auer rods *(arrow);* **f** M_3, POX, bundles of Auer rods *(arrow);* **g** M_4, transitional myelomonocytic variant, MGG; **h** M_4, transitional myelomonocytic variant, POX; **i** M_4, transitional myelomonocytic variant, NAS; all leukemic cells exhibit strong POX *and* NAS activity; **k** M_5, MGG; **l** M_5, POX, only very weak POX reactivity *(arrow);* **m** M_5, NAS, strong activity of this enzyme

Table 2. Cytological features and cytochemistry in subtypes of AML [7]

	Cytochemical features	POX	Nonspecific esterase
M_1	Myeloblastic without maturation: > 30% blasts (nongranular) in the bone marrow	≥ 3% +	(+) NaF-resistant
M_2	Myeloblastic with maturation: > 50% of bone marrow cells are myeloblasts + promyelocytes, > 30% blasts, but no heavy granulation	++	(+) or + NaF-resistant
M_3	Hypergranular promyelocytic: Great majority of leukemic cells are abnormal promyelocytes with heavy granulation or dust-like granules	+++	+ NaF-resistant
M_4	Myelomonocytic: Granulocytic and monocytic maturation present; promonocytes and monocytes > 20% and blasts > 30% in bone marrow and/or blood	> 20% +−++	> 20% ++ NaF-sensitive
M_5	Monocytic: Monoblasts or promonocytes and monocytes predominate in bone marrow and blood	< 20% +−++	> 20% ++−+++ NaF-resistant
M_6	Erythroleukemia: Erythropoietic component in the bone marrow > 50% and morphological abnormalities (when very bizarre abnormalities present: > 30%)	> 30% +−++	(+) or + NaF-resistant

In this classification the M_4 subgroup is rather heterogeneous, including two different forms of *myelomonocytic leukemia:* first, in most patients more than 20% of the leukemic cells will exhibit unequivocal differentiation into the granulocytic series (marked by a POX activity clearly outweighting the esterase activity, the latter being resistant to NaF), *and,* in addition, more than 20% of leukemic cells will show maturation into the monocytic cell line (characterized by an esterase that is inhibited by NaF and that clearly outweighs the POX). According to morphology and cytochemistry the leukemic cells in this variant of M_4 leukemia mirror the normal granulocyte and monocyte precursors.

Transitional Myelomonocytic Leukemia

In some patients, however, the *same* leukemic cell will exhibit morphological and cytochemical signs of a granulocytic and of a monocytic precursor. Most or nearly all of the leukemic cells in these patients show a morphology which renders the unequivocal diagnosis of either granulocytic or monocytic precursors rather difficult; and they are marked by an equally strong activity of both POX- and NaF-sensitive esterase. A normal counterpart of these leukemic cells is not observed in the bone marrow of healthy persons [26, 52]. To differentiate it from myelomonocytic leukemia, as defined above, this particular subtype of M_4 leukemia has been named the *"transitional myelomonocytic variant"*.

When 39 patients suffering from different subtypes of M_4 and M_5 leukemia were evaluated [30] the *transitional myelomonocytic variant* as classified above was seen in 8 patients. In clinical findings and survival these 8 patients did not differ markedly from the remaining cases of M_4 and M_5 leukemia. To avoid misunderstanding and incorrect classification, however, this special variant of M_4 morphology will have to be defined unequivocally: the transitional myelomonocytic variant will be misinterpreted as M_2 subtype if only POX staining is used, and it will be classified as M_5 if only esterase cytochemistry is performed. To guarantee the exact and reproducible subclassification of myeloid leukemias, therefore, the routine application of POX *and* of nonspecific esterase (with exposure to NaF) ought to be obligatory.

When blood and bone marrow smears from 194 patients suffering from AL were re-evaluated by the Dutch Leukaemia Working Group, application of the original FAB criteria resulted in disagreement of 14% between three investigators, while the additional introduction of a "maturation index" reduced this discrepancy to only 2% [49].

Myelodysplastic Syndromes

A standardized classification of the so-called *myelodysplastic syndromes* was also proposed by the FAB cooperative group [8]. Morphologic features relevant for diagnosis and subclassification are summarized below. Most of these morphologic abnormalities are identical with those described in previous publications dealing with the preleukemic syndrome [24, 36, 39]. Morphologic abnormalities may involve more or less any of the hemic cell lines and are summarized below.

Dyserythropiesis may include one or several of the following qualitative changes: ringed sideroblasts, multinuclearity, abnormal nuclear shape and nuclear fragments, abnormal cytoplasmic features.

In *dysgranulopoiesis,* neutrophils may appear agranular or hypogranular or show persistence of basophilia in mature cells. Nuclei may show hypo- or hypersegmentation. In the bone marrow, azurophilic granules may be of abnormal shape or stain abnormally; secondary granules may be absent or reduced. Cytochemical tests may show defects of POX or of alkaline phosphatase [55].

Dysmegakaryocytopoiesis includes micromegakaryocytes, large mononuclear megakaryocytes, and megakaryocytes with multiple small separated nuclei. In addition, megakaryocytes may contain giant or abnormally shaped granules [58]. With great regularity abnormalities of the platelets can be demonstrated [40].

Blast cells in myelodysplastic syndromes may be augmented (see below) and are subdivided into two subtypes:

Type 1 blasts vary from cells indistinguishable from myeloblasts to cells which may be unclassifiable. Cytoplasmic granules are absent. Nucleoli are prominent, the chromatin pattern appears uncondensed.

Type 2 blasts have a few azurophilic granules; the nuclear/cytoplasmic ratio tends to be lower than in type 1 and the nucleus remains in a central position.

The following five conditions are classed as myelodysplastic syndromes:

Refractory Anemia. Anemia and dyserythropoiesis are present; dysgranulopoiesis or dysmegakaryocytopoiesis are infrequent. Blasts in the bone marrow are less than 5%.

Refractory Anemia with Ringed Sideroblasts. The findings are as described for refractory anemia, but in addition ringed sideroblasts are present, accounting for more than 15% of all nucleated cells in the bone marrow.

Refractory Anemia with Excess of Blasts. Conspicuous abnormalities are common in all three cell lines. Ringed sideroblasts may be present. The percentage of blasts (type 1 and 2) in the bone marrow is 5%–20%.

Chronic Myelomonocytic Leukemia. There is an absolute monocytosis ($> 1 \times 10^9$/liter) in the blood, often associated with an increase in mature granulocytes with or without dysgranulopoiesis. The percentage of blasts in the blood is $< 5\%$. The bone marrow is similar to that in refractory anemia with excess of blasts, but may show a significant increase in monocyte precursors.

Refractory Anemia with Excess of Blasts in Transformation. Patients of any age may be involved, often with symptoms of brief duration. The morphological features are similar to those in refractory anemia with excess of blasts, but can include any of the following: 5% or more blasts in the blood; 20%–30% blasts in the bone marrow; presence of Auer rods in granulocyte precursors.

It is hoped that the classification of myelodysplastic syndromes proposed by the FAB cooperative group will clarify the rather confused nomenclature in this field of hematology. In addition, insight into the development of AML and better understanding of subtypes of AML can be expected. The chronic myelomonocytic leukemia subtype, in particular, will have to be distinguished from somewhat different cases of leukemia described by Miescher [44] and Zittoun [63] and designated with the same term.

Electron Microscopy

The fine structure of leukemic blood cells has been published in various monographs [13, 60, 64]. Some recent aspects that are of significance for the diagnosis or understanding of certain subtypes of AL are summarized below.

Acute Lymphatic Leukemia

Electron microscopic features of 29 cases of immunologically classified ALL were investigated [19]. No clear-cut differentiation between non-T, non-B neoplasms and T-ALL appears to be possible on morphological grounds.

The *"hand mirror" variant* of ALL was described by Schumacher [57]: In 15% of 134 patients with ALL this variant was observed in more than 5% of the bone marrow cells. Prognosis was not affected by hand mirror morphology of the leukemic cells. The striking features of hand mirror cells are the presence of increased numbers of mitochondria, glycogen, microspikes on the terminal uropod, and polyribosomes. The true nature of this peculiar cell awaits further elucidation, and even a relation to the "large granular lymphocyte" subgroup of lymphatic cells will have to be discussed.

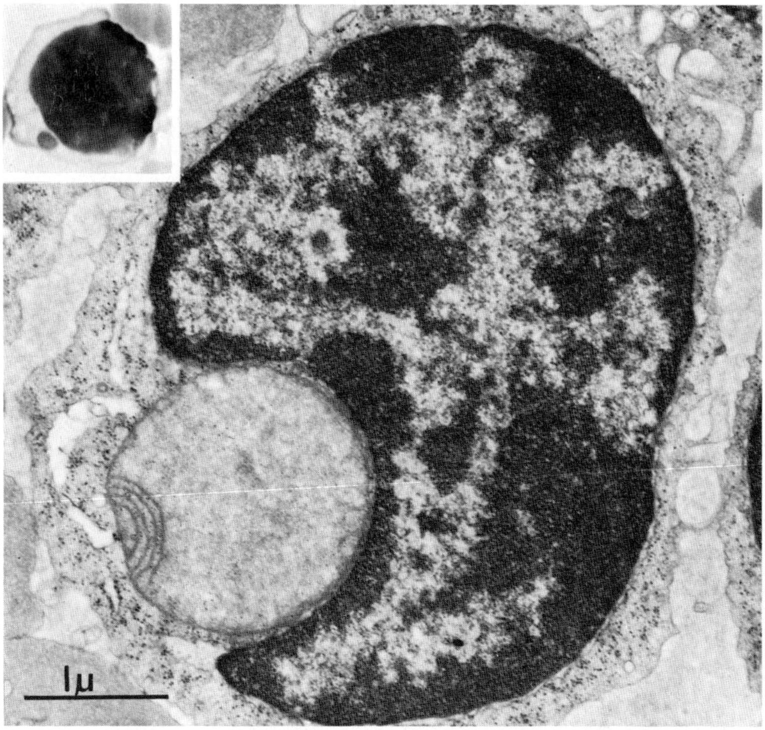

Fig. 3. Leukemic cell from centrocytic-centroblastic lymphoma: distended mitochondrium with deposits of a finely granular material and remnants of cristae. *Inset:* Corresponding cell, blood film, MGG

Leukemic mitochondria in ALL are of special interest [56]; and giant forms as well as special mitochondrial inclusions have been described. Rather frequently in ALL (as well as in other lymphatic malignancies, especially of centroblastic and/or centrocytic type), large cytoplasmic inclusions are observed (Fig. 3), which contain a finely granular material of moderate electron density and are enclosed by a double membrane (like mitochondria). Their origin from mitochondria is further confirmed by remnants of mitochondrial cristae [54]. These cytoplasmic inclusions may be observed even in light microscopic preparations and are characterized by a faint red PAS staining. Investigators not familiar with this phenomenon might mistake them for PAS-positive deposits of glycogen. The significance of these mitochondrial changes in connection with the pathogenesis of ALL is still unknown.

Acute Myeloid Leukemia

In AML the most prominent fine-structural peculiarities are defects in granule production, which may lead to reduction of granular enzymes and to a partial or complete failure of the production of a given type of granules, which may result in abnormally shaped granules and granular inclusions [4, 25, 53] (Fig. 4). Frequently, an abnormal configuration of azurophilic or of secondary granules is already observed in preleukemic states.

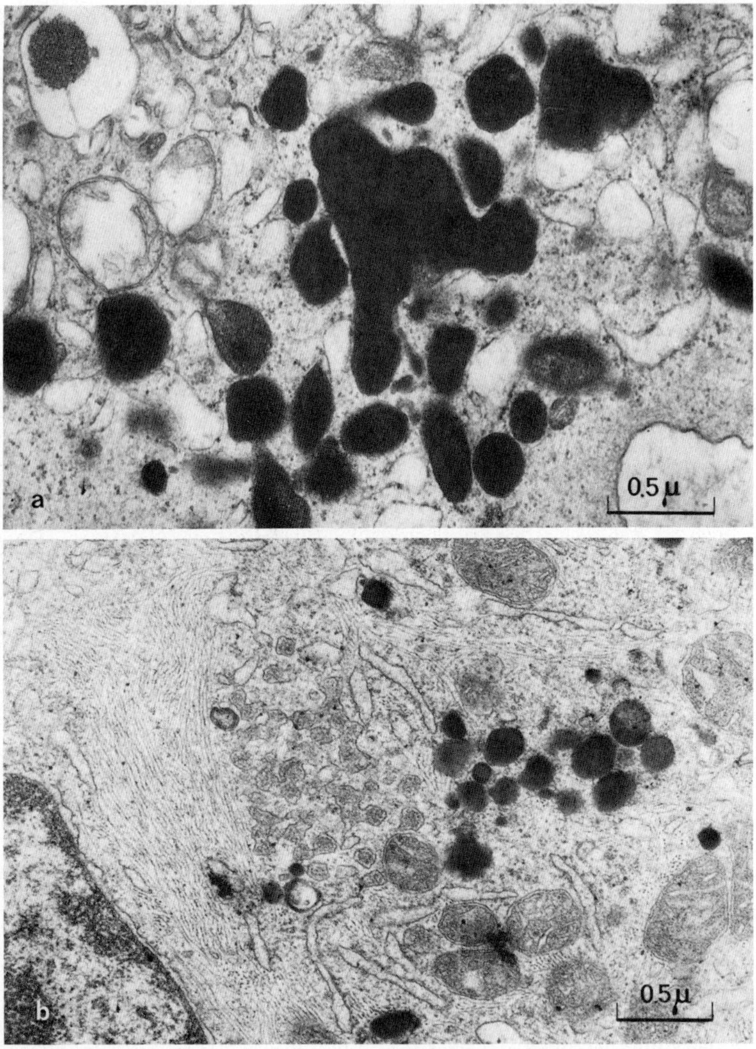

Fig. 4a, b. Abnormalities of primary granules in AML. **a** Unusually large primary granules occasionally showing bizarre structures. **b** Leukemic myelocyte; primary granules, stained for POX activity, and *(left)* small POX-negative granules which probably represent atypical secondary granules

Microgranular Acute Promyelocytic Leukemia

Special diagnostic importance attaches to the abnormally formed granules in so-called microgranular acute promyelocytic leukemia. In this variant of promyelocytic leukemia the average granule size is less than 200 nm (Fig. 5), which is significantly less than the 250-nm resolution of light microscopy. Azurophilic granules, therefore, cannot be recognized by light microscopy, and the diagnosis of promyelocytic leukemia might be missed [20]. According to its clinical course, this special variant is similar to promyelocytic leukemia, and disseminated intravascular coagulation is frequent. Interestingly, in many such cases a specific acquired chromosome abnormality, t (15 : 17), has been observed.

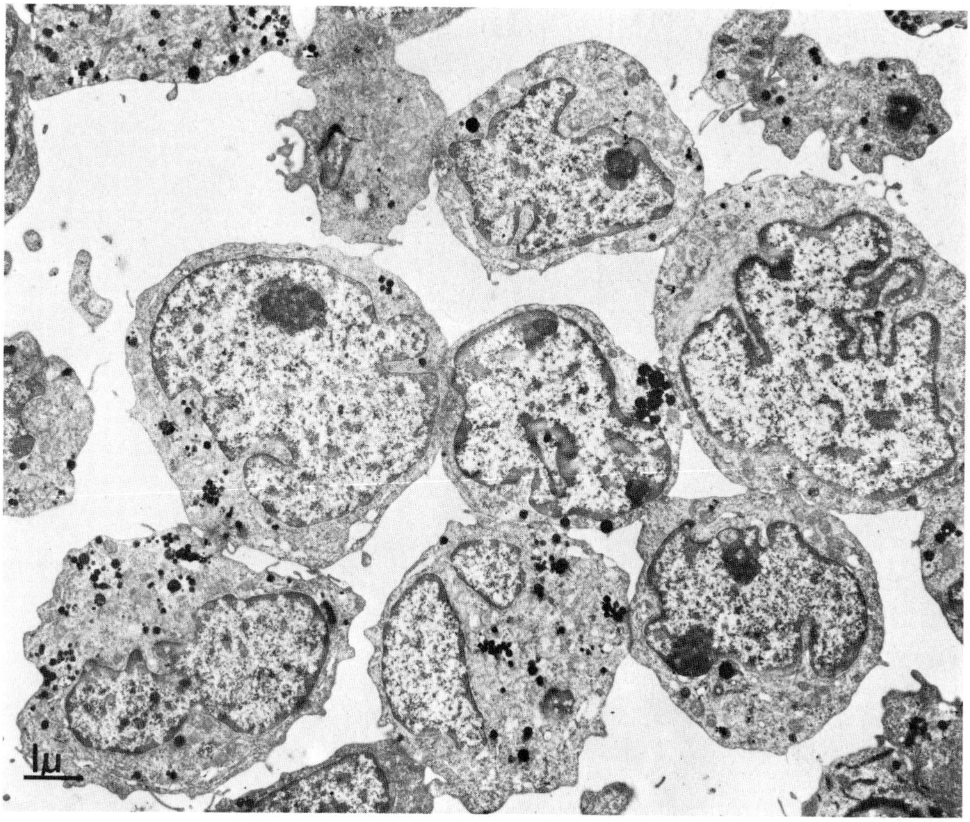

Fig. 5. Micrugranular leukemic promyelocytes stained for demonstration of POX activity. Most of the cells contain several small primary (POX-positive) granules not exceeding 200 μm in size

Early Monoblastic Leukemias

The value of ultrastructural cytochemistry of leukemic cells for the recognition of early monoblasts, was emphasized by Catovsky's group [46]. In early monoblastic leukemias, a small lysosomal granule characterized by APh activity and lack of POX activity is present in the majority of cells. These granules range from 50 to 200 nm in size and are distributed mainly at the periphery of the cells; they appear in early monoblasts before POX-positive granules (Fig. 6) can also be recognized. [This is in contrast to early myeloblasts which are characterized by larger (200–600 nm) POX-positive granules.] The study cited shows that ultrastructural cytochemistry may be helpful in the recognition and classification of AL by demonstrating the early differentiation features of monocytic (and granulocytic) percursors.

Apparently Undifferentiated Leukemias

In some rare cases of that are thought to be undifferentiated the true nature of the leukemic cells can be elucidated when the plate let peroxidase technique of Breton-Gorius [12] is

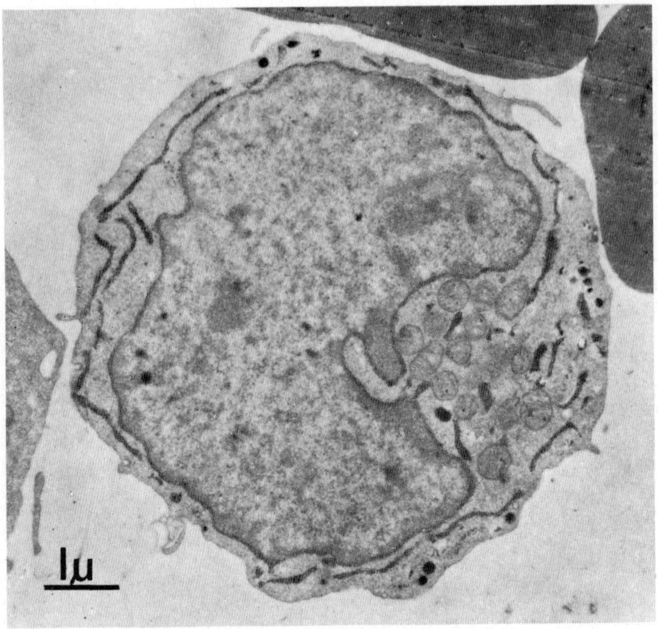

Fig. 6. Leukemic monoblast, stained for POX activity. POX activity is demonstrated in the perinuclear space, cisterns of the rough endoplasmic reticulum, and small granules

applied, using a higher concentration of 3,3′-diaminobenzidine and a different fixation method. By this method, which can only be used in electron microscopy, megakaryoblasts may be recognized on the basis of a peroxidase activity confined to the perinuclear space, rough endoplasmic reticulum, and some small granules which cannot be demonstrated when the Kaplow POX staining technique is applied (Fig. 7).

Acute Undifferentiated Leukemias

When cases of AL are classified using by means of light microscopic cytochemistry and membrane marker tests for C-and T-ALL antigen, a percentage of 10%–20% of *acute undifferentiated leukemias* will be left. This percentage can be reduced considerably when electron microscopic cytochemistry is applied, especially with demonstration of POX at the ultrastructural level. The value of electron microscopic POX cytochemistry for this purpose has been impressively demonstrated in recent publications [16, 34, 62]. As therapeutic regimens considered as optimal for the treatment of leukemias are different in ALL and AML, the application of electron microscopic cytochemistry is important in all cases of AL which remain unclassified after the application of light microscopic cytochemistry and immunological membrane marker studies.

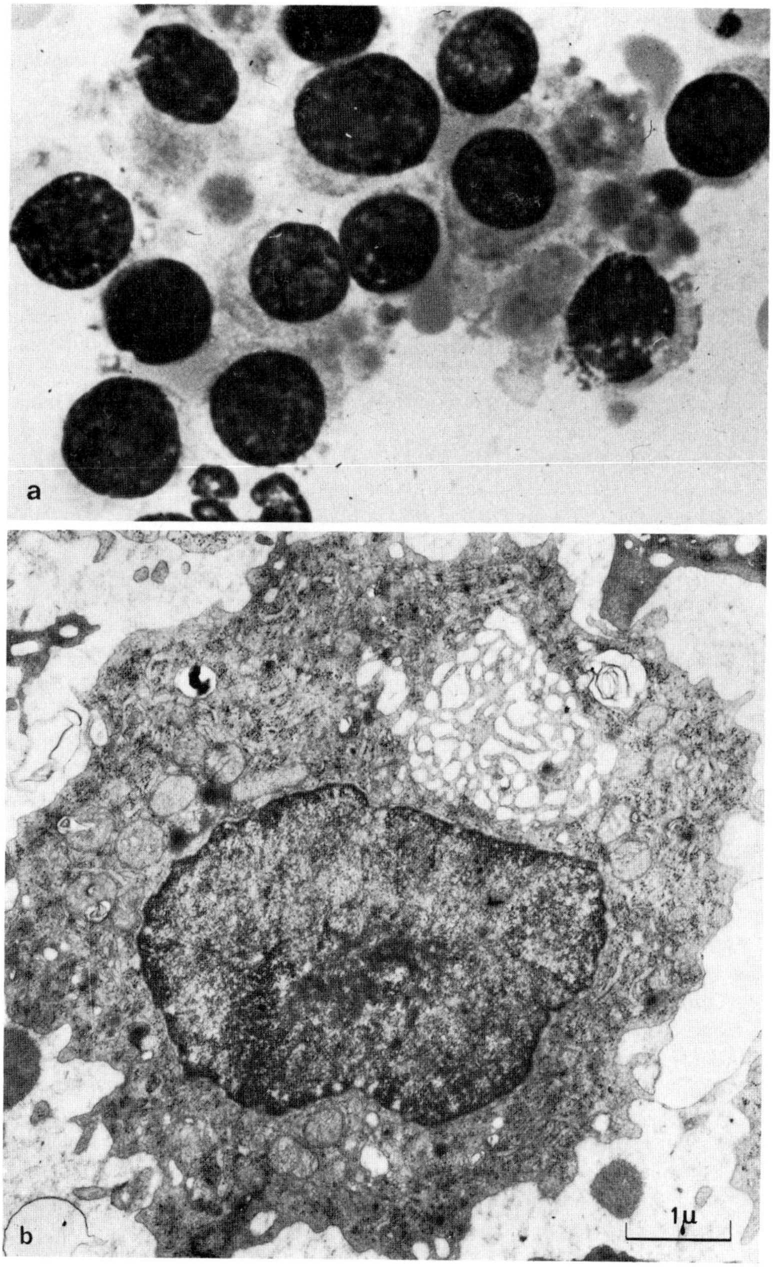

Fig. 7a, b. Atypical leukemic (micro-) megakaryocytes. **a** MGG and **b** corresponding cell showing fine structural signs of megakaryocytes, in particular some granules with a central dense core and a "prospective platelet field"

References

1. Ackermann GA, Clark MA (1971) Ultrastructural localization of peroxidase activity in normal human bone marrow cells. Z Zellforsch 117: 463–475
2. Andreewa P, Huhn D, Thiel E, Rodt H (1978) Comparison of enzyme-cytochemical findings and immunological marker investigations in acute lymphatic leukemia (ALL). Blut 36: 299–305
3. Bainton DF, Farquhar MG (1968) Differences in enzyme content of azurophil and specific granules of polymorphonuclear leukocytes. II. Cytochemistry and electron microscopy of bone marrow cells. J Cell Biol 39: 299–317
4. Bainton DF (1975) Abnormal neutrophils in acute myelogenous leukemia: Identification of subpopulations based on analysis of azurophil and specific granules. Blood Cells 1: 191–199
5. Barka T, Anderson PJ (1961) Acid phosphatase and reticuloendothelial system. Lab Invest 10: 590–595
6. Barka T, Anderson PJ (1965) Histochemistry. Theory, practice, and bibliography. Harper and Row, New York
7. Bennett JM, Catovsky D, Daniel M-T, Flandrin G, Galton DAG, Gralnick HR, Sultan C (1976) Proposals for the classification of the acute leukaemias. Br J Haematol 33: 451–458
8. Bennett JM, Catovsky D, Daniel MT, Flandrin G, Galton DAG, Gralnick HR, Sultan C (1982) The French-American-British (FAB) co-operative group. Proposals for the classification of the myelo-dysplastic syndromes. Br J Haematol 51: 189–199
9. Braunsteiner H, Schmalzl F, Asamer H, Abbrederis K, Huber H (1969) Die Diagnose der Monozytenleukämie. Wien Z Inn Med 50: 223–230
10. Brearly RL, Johnson SAN, Lister TA (1979) Acute lymphoblastic leukaemia in adults: clinicopathological correlations with the French-American-British (FAB) co-operative group classification. Eur J Cancer 15: 909–914
11. Breton-Gorius J (1970) Morphological aspects of granulopoiesis. Pathol Biol 18: 433–440
12. Breton-Gorius J, Reyes F, Duhamel G, Najman A, Gorin NC (1978) Megakaryoblastic acute leukemia: identification by the ultrastructural demonstration of platelet peroxidase. Blood 51: 45–60
13. Breton-Gorius J, Gourdin MF, Reyes F (1981) Ultrastructure of the leukemic cell. In: Catovsky D (ed) The leukemic cell. Livingstone, London
14. Burns CP, Armitage JO, Frey AL, Dick FR, Jordan JE, Woolson RF (1981) Analysis of the presenting features of adult acute leukemia: the French-American-British classification. Cancer 47: 2460–2469
15. Catovsky D, Galton DAG, Robinson J (1972) Myeloperoxidasedeficient neutrophils in acute myeloid leukemia. Scand J Haematol 9: 142–148
16. Catovsky D, de Salvo Cardullo L, O'Brien M, Morilla R, Costello C, Galton D, Ganeshaguru K, Hoffbrand V (1982) Cytochemical markers of differentiation in acute leukemia. Cancer Res 41: 4824–4832
17. Fischer R, Gropp A (1964) Cytologische und cytochemische Untersuchungen an normalen und leukämischen in vitro gezüchteten Blutzellen. Klin Wochenschr 42: 111–118
18. Foon KA, Naiem F, Yale C, Gale RP (1979) Acute myelogenous leukemia: morphologic classification and response to therapy. Leuk Res 3: 171–173
19. Glick AD, Vestal BK, Flexner JM, Collins RD (1978) Ultrastructural study of acute lymphocytic leukemia: comparison with immunologic studies. Blood 52: 311–322
20. Golomb HM, Rowley JD, Vardiman JW, Testa JR, Butler A (1980) "Microgranular" acute promyelocytic leukemia: a distinct clinical, ultrastructural, and cytogenetic entity. Blood 55: 253–259
21. Grossi CE, Webb SR, Zicca A, Lydyard PM, Moretta L, Mingari MC, Cooper MD (1978) Morphological and histochemical analysis of two human T-cell subpopulations bearing receptors for IgM or IgG. J Exp Med 147: 1405–1417
22. Gutensohn W, Thiel E (1981) High levels of 5′-nucleotidase activity in blastic chronic myelogenous leukemia with common ALL-antigen. Leuk Res 5: 505–510

23. Hayhoe FGJ, Quaglino D (1980) Haematological cytochemistry. Livingstone, London
24. Heimpel H, Drings P, Mitrou P, Queißer W (1979) Verlauf und prognostische Kriterien bei Patienten mit "Präleukämie". Klin Wochenschr 57:21–29
25. Huhn D, Schmalzl F, Krug U (1971) Unreifzellige myeloische Leukämie. Zytochemie, Elektronenmikroskopie und Zytogenetik. Blut 23:189–206
26. Huhn D, Schmalzl F, Demmler K (1971) Monozytenleukämie. Licht- und elektronenmikroskopische Morphologie und Zytochemie. Dtsch Med Wochenschr 96:1594–1605
27. Huhn D (1978) Di Guglielmo-Syndrom (akute erythrämische Myelose, akute Erythroleukämie). In: Begemann H (ed) Leukämien. Springer, Berlin Heidelberg New York (Handbuch der inneren Medizin, vol 2, pt 6)
28. Huhn D, Thiel E, Rodt H (1980) Classification of normal and malignant lymphatic cells using acid phosphatase and acid esterase. Klin Wochenschr 58:65–71
29. Huhn D, Thiel E, Rodt H, Andreewa P (1981) Cytochemistry and membrane markers in acute lymphatic leukaemia (ALL). Scand J Haematol 26:311–320
30. Huhn D, Twardzik L (1983) Acute myelomonocytic leukemia and FAB-classification. Acta Haematol (Basel) (to be published)
31. Humphrey GB, Nesbit ME, Brunning RD (1974) Prognostic value of the periodic acid-Schiff (PAS) rection in acute lymphoblastic leukemia. Am J Clin Pathol 61:393–397
32. Jäger G (1981) A simple test for the terminal deoxynucleotidyl transferase using the peroxidase-antiperoxidase technique. Blut 42:259–261
33. Janossy G, Hoffbrand AV, Greaves MF, Ganeshaguru K, Pain C, Bradstock KF, Prentice HG, Kay HEM, Lister TA (1980) Terminal transferase enzyme assay and immunological membrane markers in the diagnosis of leukaemia: a multiparameter analysis of 300 cases. Br J Haematol 44:221–234
34. Jansson S-E, Gripenberg J, Vuopio P, Teerenhovi L, Andersson LC (1980) Classification of acute leukaemia by light and electron microscope cytochemistry. Scand J Haematol 25:412–416
35. Kaplow LS (1965) Simplified myeloperoxidase stain using benzidine dihydrochloride. Blood 26:215–219
36. Koeffler HP, Golde DW (1980) Human preleukemia. Ann Intern Med 93:347–353
37. Kurz R, Haas H (1974) Value of the combined cytological and cytochemical classification in the management of acute childhood leukemia. Acta Haematol (Basel) 52:1–7
38. Lennert K, Parwaresch MR (1979) Mast cells and mast cell neoplasia: a review. Histopathology 3:349–364
39. Linman JW, Saarni MI (1974) The preleukemic syndrome. Semin Hematol 11:93–100
40. Maldonado JE (1975) The ultrastructure of platelets in refractory anemia ("preleukemia") and myelomonocytic leukemia. Ser Haematol 8:101–125
41. Mason DY, Taylor CR (1975) The distribution of maramidase in human tissues. J Clin Pathol 28:124–132
42. Meister P, Huhn D, Nathrath W (1980) Malignant histiocytosis. Immunohistochemical characterization on paraffin embedded tissue. Virchows Arch [Pathol Anat] 385:233–246
43. Melvin SL (1979) Comparison of techniques for detecting T-cell acute lymphocytic leukemia. Blood 54:210–215
44. Miescher PA, Farquet JJ (1974) Chronic myleomonocytic leukemia in adults. Semin Hematol 11:129–139
45. Moloney WC, McPherson K, Fliegelmann L (1960) Esterase activity in leukocytes demonstrated by use of naphthol AS-D chloracetate substrate. J Histochem Cytochem 8:200–206
46. O'Brien M, Catovsky D, Costello C (1980) Ultrastructural cytochemistry of leukaemic cells: Characterization of the early small granules of monoblasts. Br J Haematol 45:201–208
47. Pinkus GS, Said JW (1977) Profile of intracytoplasmic lysozyme in normal tissues, myeloproliferative disorders, hairy cell leukemia, and other pathologic processes. An immunoperoxidase study of paraffin sections and smears. Am J Pathol 89:351–362

48. Reaman GH, Levin N, Muchmore A, Holiman BJ, Poplack D (1979) Diminished lymphoblast 5′-nucleotidas activity in acute lymphoblastic leukemia with T-cell characteristics. N Engl J Med 300: 1374–1380
49. van Rhenen DJ, Verhulst JC, Huigens PC, Langenhuijsen MMAC (1980) Maturation index: a contribution to quantification in the FAB classification of acute leukaemia. Br J Haematol 46: 581–586
50. Schaefer HE, Fischer R (1970) Peroxydaseaktivität als Ursache der stabilen Sudanophilie in Granulocyten. Klin Wochenschr 48: 1424–1430
51. Schmalzl F, Braunsteiner H (1968) Cytochemische Darstellung von Esteraseaktivitäten in Blut- und Knochenmarkszellen. Klin Wochenschr 46: 642–650
52. Schmalzl F, Huhn D, Asamer H, Abbrederis K, Braunsteiger H (1972) Atypical (monomyelocytic) myelogenous leukemia. Acta Haematol (Basel) 48: 72–88
53. Schmalzl F, Huhn D, Asamer H, Rindler R, Braunsteiner H (1973) Cytochemistry and ultrastucture of pathologic granulation in myelogenous leukemia. Blut 27: 243–260
54. Schmalzl F, Huhn D, Abbrederis K, Braunsteiner H (1974) Acute lymphocytic leukemia. Cytochemistry and ultrastructure. Blut 29: 87–95
55. Schmalzl F, Konwalinka G, Michlmayr G, Abbrederis K, Braunsteiner H (1978) Detection of cytochemical and morphological anomalies in preleukemia. Acta Haematol (Basel) 59: 1–18
56. Schumacher HR, Szekely IE, Fisher DR (1975) Leukemic mitochondria. III. Acute lymphoblastic leukemia. Am J Pathol 78: 49–58
57. Schumacher HR, Champion JE, Thomas WJ, Pitts LL, Stass SA (1979) Acute lymphoblastic leukemia – hand mirror variant. An analysis of a large group of patients. Am J Hematol 7: 11–17
58. Smith WB, Ablin A, Goodman JR, Brecher G (1973) Atypical megakaryocytes in preleukemic phase of acute myeloid leukemia. Blood 42: 535–540
59. Stein H, Petersen N, Gaedicke G, Lennert K, Landbeck G (1976) Lymphoblastic lymphoma of convoluted or acid phosphatase type – a tumor of T precursor cells. Int J Cancer 17: 292–295
60. Tanaka Y, Goodman JR (1972) Electron microscopy of human blood cells. Harper and Row, London
61. Vecchi V, Rosito P, Vivarelli F, Mancini AF, Pession A, Paolucci G (1980) Prognostic significance of lymphoblast morphology in acute lymphoblastic leukaemia (ALL) in childhood. Br J Haematol 45: 178–181
62. Youness E, Trujillo JM, Ahearn MJ, Mc Credie KB, Cork A (1980) Acute unclassified leukemia. A clinicopathologic study with diagnostic implications of electron microscopy. Am J Hematol 9: 79–88
63. Zittoun R (1976) Subacute and chronic myelomonocytic leukaemia: a distinct haematological entity. Br J Haematol 32: 1–7
64. Zucker-Franklin D, Greaves MF, Grossi CE, Marmont AM (1981) Atlas of blood cells. Lea and Febiger, Philadelphia

"Atypical" Leukemias: Preleukemia, Smoldering Leukemia and Hypoplastic Leukemia

D. Hoelzer, A. Ganser, and H. Heimpel

Abteilung Hämatologie, Zentrum Innere Medizin, Universität Ulm, Steinhövelstrasse 9, 7900 Ulm, FRG

Introduction

The term "atypical leukemia" covers a wide range of heterogeneous disorders whose classification has hitherto been controversial. This controversy has arisen from the use of different criteria for the definition of the various entities. The application of morphological criteria has led to the separation of conditions without recognizable leukemic blasts, e.g., refractory anemia [11] and refractory anemia with ring sideroblasts [11], from subentities with a definite leukemic population, for which the terms refractory anemia with excess of blasts (RAEB) [38], oligoblastic leukemia [81], and hypoplastic acute leukemia [10, 78, 132] are used. Laying the emphasis on the disease stage at clinical presentation has allowed the differentiation of preleukemic states in which the diagnosis of leukemia has not yet been possible because of the lack of a definite leukemic cell population from overt acute leukemia [16, 17, 62, 114, 206]. Observation of the disease course has allowed separation of a further group of patients with a slowly progressing course, in whom the terms "subacute leukemia" [30] and "smoldering leukemia" [44, 74, 75, 83, 194] have been applied. The combination of morphological and anamnestic criteria, finally, has led to the definition of "subacute" and "chronic myelomonocytic leukemia" [11, 210].

Owing to the different criteria used for classification, there has been a considerable overlap between reports from different authors, rendering comparison a difficult, if not impossible, task. In an attempt to improve this situation the FAB cooperative group has proposed a classification of the myelodysplastic syndromes, which is based solely on morphological criteria [11] (Table 1). There is room for doubt as to whether these morphological definitions based on a single criterion will lead to any clarification unless other biological features are incorporated [61].

Such biological parameters could be the in vitro growth pattern and karyotype of the bone marrow cells. Comparison with the new FAB classification [11] will reveal the value of these parameters with respect to pathogenesis, diagnosis, and prognosis, leading to the ultimate conclusion that only the combination of several parameters will enable clinicians to evaluate the prognosis of individual patients and to find the appropriate therapeutic approach.

Definitions

Atypical leukemias can be broadly separated into the myelodysplastic syndromes, with no or only a limited percentage of blast cells in the bone marrow, and hypoplastic acute leukemia, where the blast cell percentage and clinical course are diagnostic of acute

Recent Results in Cancer Research. Vol. 93

Table 1. Definition of the myelodysplastic disorders and comparison of the terms used by different authors

FAB classification [11]	% Blasts in bone marrow	Other findings	Other terms
a) Refractory anemia (RA)	< 5%	< 1% Circulating blast cells	Preleukemia, hematopoietic dysplasia, myelodysplastic syndrome, dysmyelopoietic syndrome
b) Refractory anemia with ring sideroblasts (acquired idiopathic sideroblastic anemia)	< 5%	< 1% Circulating blast cells > 15% Ring sideroblasts in bone marrow	Preleukemia, acquired sideroachrestic anemia
c) Refractory anemia with excess of blasts (RAEB)	5%–20%	< 5% Circulating blast cells	Refractory anemia, preleukemia, myelodysplastic syndrome, hematopoietic dysplasia, dysmyelopoietic syndrome, oligoblastic leukemia, smoldering (acute) leukemia, subacute myeloid leukemia
d) Subacute and chronic myelomonocytic leukemia	< 20%	> 1×10^9/liter monocytes and promonocytes in peripheral blood	Preleukemia, oligoblastic leukemia, RAEB, smoldering leukemia, subacute myeloid leukemia, subacute myelomonocytic leukemia, myelodysplastic syndrome, dysmyelopoietic syndrome
e) RAEB in transformation	20%–30%	> 5% Circulating blast cells, Auer rods	Preleukemia, hematopoietic dysplasia, RAEB, myelodysplastic syndrome in transformation to acute leukemia, oligoblastic leukemia, subacute myeloid leukemia, smoldering leukemia, acute leukemia

leukemia. Since it is impossible to reclassify the published cases of myelodysplastic syndromes retrospectively according to a single scheme, an attempt has been made to separate the myelodysplastic syndromes with most overlapping, i.e., preleukemia, RAEB, and smoldering leukemia [105], from the well defined 5q- syndrome and from subacute and chronic myelomonocytic leukemia (SMML, CMML).

Preleukemia. The historical term "preleukemia" first introduced by Hamilton-Peterson in 1948 [62] and by Block et al. in 1953 [16] can describe any syndrome that precedes the onset of acute leukemia but in which the criteria for the diagnosis of acute leukemia are not fulfilled. Preleukemic states have been separated into two categories [96, 206]:

1. Congenital or acquired conditions with an increased risk of developing acute leukemia:
   Down's syndrome, Bloom's syndrome, Fanconi's anemia, Louis-Bar syndrome, the chronic myeloproliferative disorders, aplastic anemia, paroxysmal nocturnal hemoglobinuria, status after exposure to ionizing radiation, chemicals or cytostatic drugs, and being an identical twin of a leukemic patient [206].
2. Rather ill-defined syndromes characterized by pancytopenia and dysfunctional bone marrow changes that are highly likely to evolve to overt acute leukemia and are suspected of being an "unrecognizable phase" of this disease [72]. These disorders include the categories refractory anemia (RA) and, to a certain extent, refractory anemia with ring sideroblasts, as proposed by the FAB cooperative group [11].

Although the clinical presentation in cases of idiopathic acquired sideroblastic anemia (IASA) is similar in many ways to that in other forms of preleukemia (Tables 2 and 3), a distinction can be made between patients with true IASA and those with refractory anemia and increased ring sideroblasts according to the new FAB classification [11]. Eastman et al. [41] and Hast and Reizenstein [70] differentiated between true IASA, which appears as a consequence of disturbances of the porphyrin metabolism and only involves the red cell line, from a second form that is accompanied by involvement of two or more cell lineages. This is reflected by pure erythroid hyperplasia of the marrow in IASA [28, 41, 103], in contrast to dysfunctional marrow changes involving all lines in refractory anemia with increased ring sideroblasts [11].

Refractory Anemia with Excess of Blasts (RAEB). In contrast to the preleukemic states, RAEB is characterized by peripheral cytopenia and marrow dysplasia, including a moderate increase in blast cells to 5%–30% [11, 38]. Recently the FAB group has introduced the additional subentity of "RAEB in transformation" for patients with 20%–30% blasts in the marrow [11]. Another morphological term used, stressing the leukemic nature and reflecting the controversy with regard to this point, is "oligoleukemia" [81].

Smoldering Leukemia. The term smoldering leukemia [44, 74, 75, 83, 194] has been applied in patients with a definite leukemic blast cell population but with a prolonged and slowly progressing course of the disease extending without therapy over a period of 3–6 months [44, 74, 153]. The bone marrow changes are similar to those in RAEB. Another term that has been used in similar patients is "subacute leukemia" [30].

Subacute and Chronic Myelomonocytic Leukemia (SMML, CMML). SMML and CMML are believed to be separate entities within the myelodysplastic syndromes [11, 210],

Table 2. Clinical findings in patients with myelodysplasia

	Authors' designation	FAB classification[b]	Number of patients	Median age (range)	Male: female ratio
Saarni et al. [160]	Preleukemia	a, c, d	34	58 (16–80)	7.5 : 1
Fisher et al. [49]	Preleukemia	a, c, d	14	64 (48–79)[c]	2.5 : 1
Fischer & Mitrou [48]	Preleukemia	a, c	17	62	
Pierre[a] [145]	Preleukemia	a, b	284		
Greenberg and Mara[a] [60]	Preleukemic syndrome	a	43	61	
Heimpel et al.[a] [73]	Preleukemia	a, c, d	33		2 : 1
Hast et al. [68]	Preleukemia	a, b, c	45	71	0.55 : 1
Weber et al.[a] [99]	Preleukemic syndrome	a, b, c, d	151	73 (39–101)	0.9 : 1
Economopoulos et al. [10]	Myelodysplastic syndrome	a, b, c d, e	37		2.7 : 1
Kanatakis et al. [87]	Preleukemia	a, b, c	20	68 (55–74)	
Izrael et al. [81]	Oligoblastic leukemia	c, d, e	120		2.3 : 1
Dreyfus [38]	RAEB	c, d	29		1 : 1
Najean and Pecking[a] [130]	RAEB	c, e	90		2.8 : 1
Evenson and Stavem [44]	Smoldering leukemia	c	11	66 (48–77)	1.8 : 1
Cohen et al. [30]	Subacute myeloid leukemia	c, d	31	61 (17–86)	2.8 : 1
Streuli et al. [181]	Dysmyelopoietic syndrome	c, d	8	61.5 (45–70)	1.7 : 1
Heimpel and Hoelzer [74]	Smoldering leukemia		62	63 (22–88)	1.1 : 1
Joseph et al. [83]	Smoldering leukemia	c, d, e	45	60.5 (44–77)	0.95 : 1
Van Slyck et al. [194]	Smoldering leukemia	c, e, f	24	62.5 (45–92)	3.8 : 1
			814		1.6 : 1 (442 : 279)

[a] Prospective studies
[b] See Table 1; f, acute leukemia
[c] Mean

characterized by a distinct involvement of the monocytic lineage [11, 210]. The blast cell percentage in the marrow can range up to 30% [210, 211] and the peripheral monocyte count is $> 1 \times 10^9$/l [11, 210]. The definition proposed by the FAB cooperative group should permit comparison of reports published by different authors, since in the past patients whose condition did not fulfil these criteria were included [53, 79, 115, 210] and compared with patients in whom these criteria had been applied [53, 119, 211]. Whereas

Anemia (%)	Thrombo-cyto-penia (%)	Leuko-penia (%)	Leuko-cytosis (%)	Spleno-megaly (%)	Leukemic transfor-mation (%)	Median time to transfor-mation (months)	Median survival after diagnosis (months)
85	68	53	18	18	100	12	
93	21	86		29	64	7	23
94	65	82			24	5	15
					22		24
84	56	56		33	44	19.1	18.9
100	61	67		24	42		30
100	64	76			27		
89	40	37	10	7	27	36	
				32	52		
100	65	35	5				
73					14		14
100	29	55	0	0	24		20[c]
100	63	50	31	2	42		12
91	64	55	18	9	63		29
82				39			6
88	100	50	25	63	25		8
83	42	33					
80	76	51	13	7	38		17
92	79	71	4		8	15.5	9.3
83 (665/802)	54 (350/654)	48 (318/657)	15 (61/445)	15 (78/526)	31 (297/962)		

the FAB classification does not recognize subacute myelomonocytic leukemia [11] as a separate class, Zittoun, in 1976, proposed the term "subacute" for a separate group of patients in whom death generally occurs within 12 months from diagnosis, mainly due to infection or hemorrhage [211]. In this subgroup leukocytosis with numerous immature cells is present from the beginning, as against the chronic form in which monocytosis and blast counts are lower. In the chronic form progression is slow, with death occurring later than 12

Table 3. Clinical findings in patients with acquired idiopathic sideroblastic anemia

Authors	Number of patients	Age at diagnosis median (range)	Male: female ratio	Anemia (%)	Thrombo-cytopenia (%)
Cheng et al. [26]	28	67 (19–88)	1.9 : 1	97	10
Lewy et al. [103]	25	70[a]	1.8 : 1	100	8
	54		1.8 : 1	98	9

Authors	Leuko-penia (%)	Leuko-cytosis (%)	Spleno-megaly (%)	Leukemic transform. (%)	Median survival from diagnosis (months)
Cheng et al. [26]	28	10	48	14	57.5
Lewy et al. [103]	32	12		24	50
	30	11	48	18	

[a] Mean

months from diagnosis [211]. Other authors have distinguished CMML from SMML by blastic infiltration of the bone marrow of less than 10% [115], stressing that the prognosis in the myelodysplastic syndromes depends on the blast cell load of the marrow [73]. It is questionable whether these two subentities should be separated rather than regarded as different modes of evolution of a single disease entity.

5q − Syndrome. Cytogenetic analysis has identified a well defined disorder that is characterized by a deletion of the long arm of chromosome 5 in preparations from hematopoietic cells [192]. We will use the term "5q − syndrome" only for patients with a myelodysplastic syndrome, and not for those in whom the cytogenetic abnormality is first detected at the stage of acute leukemia.

Hypoplastic Acute Leukemia. In contrast to the syndromes discussed above, there is hardly any controversy about the leukemic nature of hypoplastic acute leukemia. It is characterized by a blast cell percentage in the marrow of > 30% combined with markedly reduced bone marrow cellularity [10, 132], an uncommon feature of typical acute leukemia [17].

Etiology and Pathogenesis

Recent studies with the G6PD isoenzyme marker [147] and cytogenetic [161] and in vitro cell culture studies [82] suggest that the preleukemic syndromes and the atypical leukemias are clonal disorders involving the hematopoietic stem cells, thereby resembling acute leukemia [46]. Therefore, they are probably not distinct entities but stages in a multiphasic myeloproliferative disorder which may eventually evolve to acute leukemia [108]. The difference between the myelodysplastic syndromes may be related to the different target cells involved. Whereas the heterogeneity of stem cell origin has been demonstrated in patients with ANLL, in some of whom only the myelomonocytic progenitor and in others a multipotent stem cell were transformed [47], similar studies have not yet been performed in patients with preleukemia or smoldering leukemia. Cytogenetic data suggest [161] that the myelodysplastic syndromes occur as a consequence of replicable somatic mutations, but up to now the exact gene defect has not been identified.

Myelodysplastic Syndromes

Preleukemia, RAEB, Smoldering Leukemia

While patients with preleukemia by definition do not exhibit a recognizable leukemic blast cell population [154, 206], smoldering or subacute leukemia is diagnosed if more than 5% blasts are present in the marrow, with an upper limit of about 30% [30, 44, 83, 194]. Preleukemia is in no way a rare disorder. The frequency has been reported to range between 6% and 12% of all cases with acute leukemia [44, 74, 83]. The incidence of a preleukemic phase preceding overt acute leukemia is difficult to assess but has been put at between 6% and 30% [17, 38, 160]. These percentages are certainly underestimates, since in patients with newly diagnosed ANLL an undetected preleukemic phase might have existed [107, 109].

The incidence of smoldering leukemia among patients with ANLL ranges from 5% to 30% [14, 44, 74, 83, 177], and certainly depends on the individual decision to withhold therapy for a certain period of time. Since the clinical presentation of patients is quite similar for preleukemia, RAEB [38], smoldering leukemia [44, 74, 83, 194], subacute myeloid leukemia [30], and oligoblastic leukemia [47, 81], they will be analyzed together.

Clinical and Hematological Findings

At first diagnosis the patients are usually middle-aged or elderly, with a median age of about 65 years, although preleukemic states in children are occasionally seen [170]. The male : female ratio is 1.6 : 1 (Table 2). Signs and symptoms at presentation are the sequelae of bone marrow failure and include weakness, easy bruising, and infection. Splenomegaly occurs in about 15% of the patients (Table 2).

Erythropoiesis. Nearly all patients are anemic with a normal to low reticulocyte count. The *anemia* most often is normochromic and normocytic or macrocytic, although rare patients may present with microcytosis, hypochromia, and reticulocytosis [190]. The anemia results mainly from ineffective erythropoiesis, with some contribution from shortened red cell survival [152]. Abnormal activities of erythrocyte enzymes, the most common being a decrease in the pyruvate kinase activity [18, 191], may be found. In about 80% of the patients the hemoglobin F level is increased to up to 6% [157], and an association with severe anemia or pancytopenia has been reported [87]. Acquired hemoglobin H has been observed [207]. The expression of the blood group antigens may be altered, with an increase of erythrocyte i antigen and a decrease in A_1 and H substance [39]. These changes are not regular findings, and individual patients with low expression of Hb F and i antigen are seen [190]. *Inefficiency of hemopoiesis* is especially prominent in the erythroid series with hyperplasia and megaloblastic changes. Nuclear and cytoplasmic maturation are dissociated and dysplastic changes are common, such as nuclear budding, bizarre multinucleated forms with occasional intranuclear bridges, karyorrhexis, and cytoplasmic vacuoles.

Sideroblastic Changes. About 20% of patients with preleukemia have sideroblastic changes [70, 108, 160]. Refractory anemia with ring sideroblasts can be diagnosed if the ringed sideroblasts account for more than 15% of all nucleated cells in the marrow [11, 151], a lower percentage than the limit of 40% that has been proposed by other authors [98]. The excessive accumulation of iron within the perinuclear mitochondria accounting for the ringed sideroblasts results from defective heme synthesis [203, 204]. Impaired hemoglobinization of some of the red blood cell precursors will often cause a dimorphic picture in the peripheral blood.

Kinetic studies with ^{3}H-TdR [67, 124, 150] or ^{14}Tdr and fluorodeoxyuridine [35] have shown an abnormally low labeling index and an increase of cells in G_1 phase. In addition, the generation times are abnormally long [152]. Ferrokinetic studies with ^{59}Fe, whose incorporation reflects the proliferative capacity of the erythroid bone marrow compartment, revealed a largely ineffective erythropoietic activity in patients with IASA, while reduced incorporation of ^{59}Fe was characteristic for RAEB and CMML, demonstrating the relative marrow failure with erythroid hypoproliferation in the last two disorders [26]. In terms of erythropoietic activity, the ^{59}Fe incorporation was intermediate in patients with RA and in a few with IASA.

Serum ferritin levels and bone marrow iron stores were found to be increased only in patients with marked ineffective erythropoiesis, not in patients with severe anemia combined with hypoplastic erythroid marrow [176].

Granulopoiesis. Leukopenia, usually neutropenia, is found in half the patients at the time of diagnosis (Table 2). The neutrophils show specific abnormalities, including pseudo-Pelger cells and so-called mature mononuclear neutrophils [72]. Immature granulocytes, including blast cells, may be found in the blood. Cytochemical abnormalities similar to those in acute myeloid leukemia have been noted in preleukemic conditions. The neutrophil myeloperoxidase is decreased in some patients [101] or may reveal a dual population with positive and negative neutrophils [25]. Leukocyte alkaline phosphatase may be normal or decreased, but is not specific for preleukemia and may even be increased [162, 163]. Chemotaxis and phagocytic capability of the neutrophils are defective in some preleukemic patients, leading to reduced resistance to infection [19, 158]. With combined cytogenetic investigations this deficiency could be related to partial or complete loss of a chromosome 7 [159], a common chromosome abnormality in preleukemia and acute leukemia.

There is usually a shift to higher percentages of immature granulopoietic cells in the marrow, including myeloblasts, the percentage of which is used for the morphological definition of the various subentities of the myelodysplastic syndromes as proposed by the FAB group [11, 12] (Table 1). Sequential trephine biopsies have demonstrated an increase in the blast cells during leukemic transformation, which was not paralleled by a change in the degree of the initial hypo- or hypercellularity [188]. In a retrospective study, Lidbeck and Manson [106] observed that progression towards acute leukemia was most apparent in changes in the promyelocytes, which exhibited both increasing nuclear irregularity and increasing nucleolar size and irregularity.

In ^{3}H-TdR studies the granulopoietic cells exhibit an abnormally low labeling index and a concomitant increase of the fraction of cells in G_1 [124, 165]. Similar findings have been obtained with ^{14}C-TdR and fluorodeoxyuridine [35]. A maturation defect has been demonstrated in vitro [55, 94]. Whether patients with blasts containing Auer rods should be included in the group with myelodysplastic disorders has been the subject of controversy, but blasts containing Auer rods have been described in patients with RAEB [117, 201] and are a recognized characteristic of RAEB in transformation according to the new FAB classification [11]. In a retrospective analysis no difference in survival between the Auer rod-positive and -negative subgroups was found [201].

Thrombopoiesis. Thrombocytopenia is seen in about 50% of patients with myelodysplastic disorders (Table 2). Giant platelets are frequently present, with defective granule formation [112]. On electron microscopy the microtubules are found to be dilated as in acute myeloid leukemia [112]. Adhesion and aggregation of the thrombocytes may be abnormal [110, 183].

The number of megakaryocytes can be normal or increased. They are usually smaller than normal with reductions in the number and size of the granules [101, 172, 205]. The mean nuclear DNA content is reduced [150]. The presence of more than 10% micromegakaryocytes within the megakaryocyte population is suggestive for a preleukemic condition, although it has no predictive value regarding the interval to development of overt leukemia [205]. Occasionally megakaryocytes with multiple small nuclei are present [38, 108]. The question as to whether the megakaryocyte count has prognostic value in patients with IASA has not yet been answered [103, 180].

Lymphopoiesis. The involvement not only of the myelopoietic but also of the lymphopoietic system has been demonstrated by low-normal or reduced natural killer cell activity [146, 186] and by low responses of lymphocytes to T cell mitogens [92, 146]. The number of T helper cells in the peripheral blood was shown to be reduced with reversal of the helper : suppressor ratio [23, 92]. It remains to be investigated whether it is true for all patients that the abnormal T cells belong to the same clone as the abnormal myeloid cells, as has been found in one patient with sideroblastic anemia by the use of the X-linked G6PD isoenzyme marker [147]. A further question is the role of the T cell disturbances with respect to the derangement of myelopoiesis, since there is evidence that T cells or T cell factors are required for in vitro CFU-C and BFU-E growth [8, 113, 213].

Course and Prognosis

The risk, in patients with myelodysplastic syndromes, of developing overt acute leukemia is difficult to assess, since they are mostly older patients and often die of infection or bleeding before progressing to acute leukemia. Patients with leukemic transformation usually develop acute nonlymphoblastic leukemia (ANLL), but occasionally their condition progresses to acute lymphoblastic leukemia [3, 9] or acute mixed lymphoblastic-myelomonoblastic leukemia [71]. In a review of 197 patients with sideroblastic anemia about 10% were reported to have developed acute leukemia, with a median time interval from diagnosis of 4 years [28], but this might be an overestimate [70]. Whereas patients with true IASA rarely develop acute leukemia [41, 70], those with RA with ring sideroblasts according to the FAB classification [11] do, especially in the presence of intermediate sideroblasts defined as erythroblasts with more than six iron grains in the cytoplasm [70]; in one study over 50% of such patients had acute leukemia at the time of death [66]. In addition, more severe anemia, lower reticulocyte counts [28], and a lesser degree of

hyperferremia [103] were found in patients whose condition had progressed to acute leukemia. Whether a high platelet count is a good prognostic sign [28, 149, 180] has been questioned [102] and will require further studies.
The prognosis in patients with RA according to the FAB classification is also difficult to ascertain, since large series with homogeneous defined groups of patients are rare. The mean overall rate of development of acute leukemia in patients with refractory anemia and a hyperplastic bone marrow with or without an increased blast cell population, according to reports on the larger series, is 31% (range 8%–100%) with a median survival after diagnosis of 6–30 months (Table 2).
The best estimates are presumably derived from the prospective studies. In 22%–44% of patients with refractory anemia without an increased percentage of blast cells in the marrow studied by Pierre [145] and Greenberg and Mara [60], this condition evolved into overt acute leukemia, with a median time to transformation of 19.1 months after diagnosis [60]. Within the observation period, 37% and 26% of the patients had died from other causes, mostly infections and bleeding [60, 145]. In prospective studies that also included patients with a definite leukemic blast cell population, transformation to aggressive acute leukemia occurred in 23%–60% [73, 131, 199], i.e., in a higher proportion than in retrospective studies, with a median survival after diagnosis ranging from 12 [131] to 30 [73] months.
In a retrospective analysis in which the new FAB classification was applied, the rate of leukemic transformation was 12.5% for 17 patients with RA and 13.3% for 16 patients with RA and ring sideroblasts, with a median of 4 years until progression to ANLL [195]. The degree of blast count elevation in the bone marrow has been cited as a bad prognostic sign in several reports [69, 73, 104, 130, 131], as has a high degree of depression of normal hematopoiesis as estimated from iron kinetic studies [36]. Independent biological parameters for evaluation of the risk of leukemic transformation in patients with a myelodysplastic syndrome are the in vitro growth pattern of the bone marrow cells and the cytogenetic findings, as will be discussed below.

Therapy

Therapy for the myelodysplastic syndromes is still inadequate, and will be considered under the therapeutic approaches during the *preleukemic, subacute,* and *acute leukemic* stages.

Preleukemia. In the preleukemic states therapy has been directed towards alleviation of peripheral cytopenia. Individual patients with sideroblastic anemia may respond to pyridoxine [76], corticosteroids [108], or androgens [108]. In one small study, corticosteroids appeared to be of value only in the treatment of those patients whose bone marrow cells showed increased CFU-C growth after exposure to cortisol [7]. In another study, despite an improvement of in vitro CFU-C growth, nonspecific immunotherapy with BCG did not relieve the cytopenia [68]. On the other hand, immunosuppressive therapy with daily azathioprine reduced the degree of anemia in a patient with sideroblastic anemia [209].

RAEB, Smoldering Leukemia. In a prospective study of 58 patients with RAEB comparing symptomatic maintenance therapy with either daily androgen therapy or low-dose cytosine arabinoside for 2 days at monthly intervals, no difference was observed between these three different approaches with respect to leukemic evolution or survival [131].

Table 4. Results of cytostatic therapy in myelodysplastic syndromes

Authors	Agents used[b]	Number of patients	CR	Median survival from diagnosis (months)
Dreyfus [38]	DNR	3	2/7	
	Ara-C, DNR	4		
Najean and Pecking [130]	Ara-C	20	–	12
	No treatment	21	–	12
Heimpel et al. [73]	VCR, 6-TG			
	Ara-C, ADR	4	–	
Cohen et al.[a] [30]	DAT	9	–	
	COAP	3	–	
	COP	2	–	5.6
	VCR, PRED	2	–	
	DNR, PRED	1	–	
	PRED	3	–	
	No treatment	15	–	11.2
Mertelsmann et al. [117]	Ara-C, 6-TG			
	AAFC, 6-TG	47	40%	
	DAT			
Streuli et al. [181]	HU, BUS	1	–	
	Ara-C, 6-TG	1	–	
	Ara-C, 6-TG, DNR	2	–	
Armitage et al. [4]	Ara-C, 6-TG	5		
	HAT	2		
	TADPO	2	3/13	1[c]
	DNR, PRED	2		
	OAP	1		
	6-MP, PRED	1		
	No treatment	12	–	14
Heimpel and Hoelzer [74]	Ara-C, 6-TG	8		
	Ara-C, DNR	3		
	ViDAP	3	1/22	3.8
	Ara-C	4		
	Other agents	4		
	No treatment	20		11
Joseph et al. [83]	Ara-C, 6-TG	5	–	

[a] 13 patients treated in all

[b] Abbreviations used for chemotherapeutic agents: *DNR,* daunorubicin; *Ara-C,* cytosine arabinoside; *VCR,* vincristine; *6-TG,* 6-thioguanine; *ADR,* adriamycin; *AAFC,* 2,2-anhydro-1-B-D-arabinofuranosyl-5-fluorocytosine; *HU,* hydroxyurea; *BUS,* busulfan; *6-MP,* 6-mercaptopurine. Definitiona of drug combinations: *DAT,* daunorubicine, cytosine arabinoside, 6-thioguanine; *COAP,* cyclophosphamide, vincristine, cytosine arabinoside, prednisone; *COP,* cyclophosphamide, vincristine, prednisone; *HAT,* adriamycine, cytosine arabinoside, 6-thioguanine; *TADPO,* 6-thioguanine, cytosine arabinoside, daunorubicin, prednisone, vincristine; *OAP,* vincristine, cytosine arabinoside, prednisone; *ViDAP,* vincristine, daunorubicin, cytosine arabinoside, prednisone

[c] Median survival after therapy

Aggressive mono- and polychemotherapy is usually delayed until the development of overt acute leukemia. Prognosis in these patients, i.e., the probability of obtaining a complete remission (CR) is significantly poorer than in de novo acute leukemia [90, 171] (Table 4). Experience with chemotherapy has been disappointing, and patients who were treated mainly with single- or multiple-drug regimens containing cytosine arabinoside, 6-thioguanine, daunorubicin, and vincristine did not survive longer than the untreated patients [4, 30, 74, 80] (Table 4). Complete remissions were rarely achieved. This of course might have been a reflection of the poor clinical condition and the advanced age of the patients, but it could also result from a too long delay before chemotherapy was instituted.

Improved CR rates were reported by Mertelsmann et al. [117], who treated 31 patients with RAEB and 16 with so-called myelodysplastic syndromes in transformation using the L-6, L-12, or L-14 protocols (Table 4). CR was achieved in 45% and 31%, respectively, with a median survival for the whole group of 9.0 and 3.8 months, respectively. Auer rod-positive patients definitely did better.

Armitage et al. [4] retrospectively analysed the effect of chemotherapy in 13 patients with RAEB, 3 of whom achieved CR lasting 14, 34+, and 36+ months, with survival times of 31, 35+, and 37+ months. These three patients belonged to a subgroup of four patients characterized by younger age, no previous cytostatic therapy, and an aggressive regimen including daunorubicin and/or cytosine arabinoside. Maintenance therapy consisted of intermittent courses of cytarabine and 6-thioguanine. The nonresponding patients with RAEB survived from less than 1 to 9 months, with a median of 1 month. In 12 untreated patients the median survival time was 14 months, with a range of 1–14+ months.

All this indicates that definition of subgroups with better response to conventional chemotherapy could improve the therapeutic results. This could be accomplished by analysing clinical data, but also by further investigations of the significance of changes in the in vitro CFU-C growth [59] and the in vitro sensitivity of leukemic cells to CSF [51].

A still more or less experimental approach to the treatment of patients with RAEB is the induction of differentiation and maturation by continuous infusion of Ara-C at a low dosage [43]. Baccarani et al. [6] improved the hematological status of a patient with RAEB by continuously administering Ara-C at a dosage of 0.7 mg kg^{-1} d^{-1} IV for 7 consecutive days. A second identical course administered to the same patient several months later had the same effect.

Moloney et al. [125] achieved CR in two patients with early de novo ANLL by administering Ara-C SC over 20–21 days at a dose of 0.8–1.0 mg kg^{-1} d^{-1}. Three patients with ANLL in the course of sideroblastic refractory dyserythropoietic anemia failed to respond to several courses of low-dose ara-C, and four additional patients with ANLL following refractory anemia (2 IASA, 2 RA) were not evaluable because of too-short follow-up periods.

Housset et al. [77] administered Ara-C SC at a dose of 10 mg/m^2 every 12 h for 17–25 days and achieved CR in a patient with ANLL developing in the course of RAEB, in one patient with AML in relapse and resistant to *m*-AMSA, and in a 74-year-old patient with previously untreated ANLL. Because of the progressive evolution of CR without aplasia and simultaneous presence of leukemic cells and islets of regenerating promyelocytes, the authors concluded that low-dose Ara-C works by differentiation induction rather than by the usual antimitotic mechanism. Using a similar regimen, Cazzola et al. [27] were unable to induce remissions in six patients with ANLL and a past history of RAEB.

An alternative to aggressive chemotherapy in the young patients with increased myeloproliferation might be total-body irradiation followed by isogeneic or allogeneic bone marrow transplantation (BMT), provided that a suitable donor is available [15, 89, 97, 200]. BMT should not only be considered when transformation to overt acute leukemia is imminent but also in the young patient with severe pancytopenia and an isogeneic or allogeneic HLA-identical donor [97, 200].

Subacute and Chronic Myelomonocytic Leukemia

Clinical and Hematological Findings

The diagnosis of subacute and chronic myelomonocytic leukemia is based on the bone marrow changes characteristic for the myelodysplastic syndromes and is defined by a blood monocytosis of $> 1 \times 10^9$/l, usually $5-10 \times 10^9$/l [11, 211], with immature and atypical circulating monocytes. Blast cells in the blood are common. The disease occurs mainly in the elderly, with a mean age of about 65 (Table 5). Males are slightly more often affected. The onset is insidious, and patients are diagnosed because of symptomatic anemia, splenomegaly, and hepatomegaly. Leukopenia occurs in one-fourth and leukocytosis in about one-half of the patients (Table V), but counts are rarely below 2×10^9/l or above 5×10^9/l [119, 169]. Thrombocytopenia is seen in nearly 60% (Table 5).

The monocytes commonly exhibit nuclear abnormalities with marked convolutions or hypersegmentations, but nucleoli are absent. The changes in the bone marrow otherwise resemble those in preleukemia. The percentage of blasts is higher than 5% and ranges up to 30% according to the older definition [211] and up to 20% according to the most recent proposals of the FAB cooperative group [11]. As a reflection of the increased turnover of monocytes and granulocytes [63], the lysozyme levels are increased in the serum [212] and in the urine [25, 212]. The uric acid in the serum is often elevated [119], as are the serum B_{12} levels [212].

Course and Therapy

A quarter of the patients with CMML will eventually enter the blastic phase (Table 5), which may be heralded by an increase in the blastic infiltration of the marrow spaces and infiltration of the skin by monocytoid cells [40]. Patients with an increased risk of evolution to overt acute leukemia are characterized by leukocytosis with many circulating immature cells from the beginning, and death from infection and bleeding usually occurs within 6–12 months after diagnosis [210, 211]. However, chronic courses with long survival have been seen [211].

The value of chemotherapy (Table 6) is difficult to assess, since there are no controlled trials. In CMML prolonged periods of marrow aplasia after chemotherapy are common, especially after daily doses of 6-MP as low as 50 mg [20, 212]. The use of VP 16-213 resulted in a complete remission in one patient with CMML [99], but the response in patients with SMML was poor [212]. A better response in a (presumably) mixed group of patients with SMML and CMML was reported by Mertelsman et al. [117], who achieved CR in 9 out of 14 patients with combinations of 6-thioguanine and Ara-C, AAFC, or Ara-C and daunorubicin. The median remission duration was 6.2 months, with a median survival for the whole group of 11.4 months.

Since up to now chemotherapy has not been successful in CMML it should be avoided, and low-dose 6-MP and HU are recommended only for patients with progressive myelopro-

Table 5. Clinical findings in patients with subacute and chronic myelomonocytic leukemia

Authors	Number of patients	Median age (range)	Male: female ratio	Anemia %	Leuko-penia %	Leuko-cytosis %	Thrombo-penia %	Spleno-megaly %	Transfor-mation to overt ANLL %	Median survival from diagnosis (months)
Zittoun et al. [212]	27	65.5	1.3 : 1	100	33	56	59	44	7.5	18
Hurdle et al. [79]	6	73 (64–80)	6 : 0	100	0	66	17	33	0	16.5
Miescher and Farquet [119]	12	78 (50–90)	2 : 1	58	8.5	42	58	33		17
Sexauer et al. [169]	10	64 (44–81)	1.5 : 1	100	40	30	60	60	0	3
Geary et al. [53]	18	68.5 (47–78)	0.6 : 1	56	17	56	67	35	66	40
Mende et al. [115]	22	74 (60–85)	0.6 : 1					27	27	
Dresch et al. [37]	24	69 (52–78)						29	61	
Zittoun [211]	31	68 (25–83)	1.6 : 1					32	35	16
	150		1.2 : 1 (69 : 57)	82% (60/73)	23% (17/73)	51% (37/73)	58% (42/73)	36% (28/78)	27% (36/123)	

Table 6. Cytostatic therapy of subacute and chronic myelomonocytic leukemia

Authors	Agents used[a]	Number of patients	CR	Median survival from diagnosis (months)
Zittoun et al. [212]	Me-GAG + Ara-C	4	1/4	
Hurdle et al. [79]	BUS	1	–	24[b]
	No treatment	5		16
Sexauer et al. [169]	6-MP	3		
	Ara-C, 6-TG	1		
	COAP	1		
Geary et al. [53]	PRED	1	–	
	6-MP	2	–	
	6-MP, PRED	4	–	
	PRED, Ara-C, 6-TG	1	–	42
	PRED, azathioprine	1	–	
	BUS	1	–	
	TRAP; COAP; 6-MP, PRED	1	1/1	
	No treatment	7	–	32
Mende et al. [115]	Ara-C, 6-TG	3	–	1.5[b]
Labedzki and Illinger [99]	VP 16-213	1	1/1	
Streuli et al. [181]	6-MP	1	–	
Mertelsmann et al. [117]	Ara-C, 6-TG (L 6)	5		
	AAFC, 6-TG (L 12)	8	9/14	11.4[b]
	DNR, Ara-C, 6-TG (L 14)	1		
Zittoun [211]	6-MP	15	?	
Armitage et al. [4]	Ara-C, 6-TG, DNR	1	–	
	Ara-C, 6-TG	1	–	
	VCR, PRED	2	–	1[b]
	DNR, PRED	1	–	
	HU, PRED	1	–	
	BUS	1	–	
	No treatment	1	–	1

[a] Abbreviations used for chemotherapeutic agents: *BUS,* busulfan; *VP 16-213,* etoposide; *Me-GAG,* methylglyoxal-bis-guanylhydrazone; *AAFC,* 2,2-anhydro-1-β-D-arabinofuranosyl-5-fluorocytosine. Definition of drug combinations: *COAP* cyclophosphamide, vincristine, cytosine arabinoside, prednisone; *TRAP,* 6-thioguanine, rubidizone, cytosine arabinoside, prednisone

[b] Median survival after therapy

Table 7. Clinical and cytogenetic findings in 76 patients with the 5q− syndrome (review from the literature)[a]

Age (years)	
Median	66
Range	25−84
Male : female ratio	0.4 : 1
Blood	
Anemia	96%
Leukopenia	41%
Leukocytosis	11%
Thrombocytopenia	32%
Thrombocytosis	21%
Bone marrow	
< 5% Blasts	70%
> 5% Blasts	30%
Cytogenetic findings	
5q− only	50%
Leukemic evolution	16%
5q− plus further changes	50%
Leukemic evolution	39%

[a] [24, 34, 54, 64, 65, 84, 88, 91, 93, 111, 129, 134, 142, 155, 173, 174, 181, 184, 185, 187, 192, 193, 196, 197]

liferation or marrow insufficiency [212]. In contrast, it has been proposed that patients with SMML should be treated in the same way as acute leukemia patients, with regimens including anthracycline drugs, Ara-C, and VP 16 [211].

5q− Syndrome

Cytogenetic and Clinical Findings

A distinct dysmyelopoietic syndrome characterized by a specific chromosome abnormality, the deletion of the long arm of chromosome 5, was originally reported in 1974 [192]. It is characterized by erythroid hypoplasia in the bone marrow with macrocytic anemia, poorly lobulated megakaryocytes with normal or elevated platelet count, normal or decreased leukocyte count, and absence of ring sideroblasts. The growth of CFU-GM from bone marrow is normal or only slightly reduced [111, 129]. The 5q− anomaly, which is almost always caused by an interstitial deletion, has also been observed in de novo ANLL and in ANLL secondary to cytostatic drugs, prior irradiation, or exposure to mutagenic agents, and is then frequently associated with further aberrations [122, 143, 155, 202]. There is a female preponderance of about 70% (Table 7), in contrast to the usual findings in the myelodysplastic syndromes (Table 2).

Course and Therapy

Despite the small number of patients so far reported with the 5q− syndrome, there is evidence that in a total of 18% the condition will eventually progress to acute nonlymphoblastic leukemia (Table 7). It can also be seen from Table 7 that in about 50% of cases the 5q− is the only abnormality at the time of cytogenetic investigation. These patients seem to have a lower risk of leukemic transformation, with 16% of them developing acute leukemia in the course of the disease as against 39% of the patients who have additional chromosome aberrations at the first investigation (Table 7). These data certainly do not support the conclusion drawn by Mahmoud et al. [111] that the 5q− syndrome does not represent a preleukemic disorder. It is only in the patients with an isolated 5q− and an additional normal stem line that the transition to acute leukemia seems to be unlikely [91], probably due to either detection in an early phase of the disease or an inherent slow evolution of the 5q− clone. Even without progression to acute leukemia the median survival of patients with an isolated 5q− and a normal cell line is longer than that of patients without any remaining normal metaphases [91] and those with additional abnormalities. Therapy in these patients is mainly symptomatic, with blood transfusion if necessary. There are no reports on the response to cytostatic therapy once leukemic transformation has occurred, but probably it is not better than in the other dysmyelopoietic syndromes. Whether isolated patients might respond to corticosteroids must await further investigations [120].

Hypoplastic Acute Leukemia

Clinical and Hematological Findings

In a subgroup of patients reported to account for about 5%−10% of all newly diagnosed patients with acute leukemia [10, 78, 132] the bone marrow is hypocellular on biopsy but contains a blast cell population diagnostic of acute leukemia. This condition has been called hypoplastic acute leukemia [10, 132] and hypocellular acute leukemia [78], but there is some overlap with the myelodysplastic disorders [10, 78] and oligoleukemia [14, 81]. The median age at diagnosis is over 60 years. Males are more often affected than females (Table 8). Almost all patients are anemic at first presentation and two-thirds are thrombocytopenic. The leukocyte count is low with few circulating blast cells or none at all. Leukocytosis has never been seen, and splenomegaly, hepatomegaly, and lymph node enlargement only sometimes.

In some patients the condition develops after antecedent hypoplastic anemia [132]. Development after prior irradiation has been reported [132]. Although nearly all patients have ANLL, the occurrence of hypoplastic ALL has been documented [132]. The marrow failure often leads to life-threatening infection or hemorrhage. Bone marrow aspirations from several sites and biopsy from one site are necessary for the diagnosis. The correct diagnosis depends on a representative biopsy specimen. The pathogenesis of the bone marrow hypocellularity is not yet clear, although leukemic cells [21, 22, 136] seem to release inhibitors of normal hematopoiesis, suppressing the proliferation of normal granulocyte-macrophage progenitor cells in vitro. In a study of in vitro granulopoiesis, there were low numbers of granulopoietic progenitor cells. CFU-GM, per aspirated bone marrow volume, and the prognosis was as dismal for these patients (5 out of 41 with acute leukemia that were examined) as for those with macrocluster growth [32].

Therapy

There are few published reports on therapeutic results of chemotherapy, and no controlled or randomized trials have been published. Furthermore, the patient characteristics of the

Table 8. Clinical findings in patients with hypoplastic acute leukemia

Authors	Number of patients	Median age (range)	Male: female ratio	Anemia %	Leuko-penia %	Leuko-cytosis %
Beard et al. [10]	9	63 (37–67)	3.5 : 1	100	100	0
Needleman et al. [132]	15	68 (40 : 82)	2 : 1	–[a]	93	0
Howe et al. [78]	29	~ 63 (15–79)	3 : 1	97	97	0
	53		2.8 : 1	97%	96%	0%

Authors	Thrombo-penia %	Spleno-megaly %	Hepato-megaly %	Enlarged lymph nodes %	Bone marrow cellu-larity	% Blasts in bone marrow
Beard et al. [10]	66	0	0	0	↓	25–85
Needleman et al. [132]	73	6.5	13	0	↓	30–68
Howe et al. [78]		7	14	17	↓	5.4–70
	71%	6%	11%	9%		

[a] Not given; median Hb, 9.0 g/dl

Table 9. Cytostatic therapy in acute hypoplastic leukemia

Authors	Agents used[a]	Number of patients	CR	Median survival from diagnosis (months)
Beard et al. [10]	Ara-C, DNR	7	5/7	24
Needleman et al. [132]	HAT	4		
	OAP	1	2/7	9.1
	TADPO	2		
	No treatment	7	–	6
Howe et al. [78]	No treatment	8	–	5
	PRED or VCR or HU or 6-MP or DNR or Ara-C	10	1/10	17.5
	Anthracycline drugs + Ara-C + additional	11	8/11	> 40

[a] Abbreviations used for chemotherapeutic agents: *Ara-C,* cytosine arabinoside; *DNR,* daunorubicin; *PRED,* prednisone and related glucocorticosteroids; *VCR,* vincristine; *HU*, hydroxyurea; *6-MP,* 6-mercaptopurine.
Definitions of drug combinations: *HAT,* adriamycin, cytosine arabinoside, 6-thioguanine; *OAP,* vincristine, cytosine arabinoside, prednisone; *TADPO,* 6-thioguanine, cytosine arabinoside, daunorubicin, prednisone, vincristine

reports summarized in Table 9 are not comparable. Some of the patients studied by Beard et al. [10] and Howe et al. [78] actually had a myelodysplastic syndrome. Antileukemic therapy has been proposed when recurrent and severe infection or hemorrhage might lead to life-threatening conditions [10]. Although the numbers considered are low it follows from the data in Table 9 that combinations of Ara-C and an anthracycline drug might be superior to single-agent therapy. CR has been reported to occur in 30%–70% of cases. Median survival times of treated patients vary from 9.1 to 40 months [78], with the longest survival in the group subjected to aggressive treatment by Howe et al. [78] (Table 9). The authors concede that this could be due to inherent patient characteristics, and it should be noted that in contrast to the reports by Beard et al. [10] and Needleman et al. [132], patients with less than 20% blast cells in the bone marrow were included by Howe et al. [78].

Alternatively, low-dose Ara-C has been used in a number of patients with hypoplastic leukemia, but despite a reduction in the peripheral blast count no complete remissions were obtained [27]. Young patients should certainly be considered for either isogeneic or allogeneic bone marrow transplantation if a suitable donor is available; this offers an actuarial survival after 1–2 years of 63% [50].

In Vitro Culture Studies

Useful information on the pathophysiology, which is also helpful in the diagnostic and prognostic evaluation of patients with myelodysplastic disorders, has been provided by in vitro studies of hematopoiesis using clonogenic assays of bone marrow cells [57].

In the assay for *granulocytic-monocytic progenitor cells (CFU-GM),* normal marrow progenitor cells will predominantly form colonies of more than 40 cells in response to colony-stimulating factors (CSF), whereas ANLL is characterized by the growth of mainly micro- or macroclusters of up to 40 cells, an increased cluster-to-colony ratio or no colony growth [126, 127]. Furthermore, the number of CFU-GM of abnormally light density is increased in ANLL [126]. The culture studies in patients with myelodysplastic syndromes have shown a characteristic growth pattern. Normal colony growth is seen in patients with IASA [59, 167], whereas a decreased incidence of normal CFU-GM is regularly found in patients with RA [58, 60, 105, 121, 166, 210], RAEB [13, 36, 45, 168], subacute myeloid leukemia [59], and oligoblastic leukemia [178]. The incidence of CFU-GM is normal or increased in patients with SMML and CMML [121, 182, 211] in whom marrow culture and cell cycle kinetics have demonstrated a growth pattern similar to that seen in chronic myeloid leukemia, although in CMML the cell cycle status is normal, as against the increased fraction of CFU-GM in S-phase found in chronic myeloid leukemia [37].

Derangement of granulopoiesis furthermore expresses itself in a higher proportion of light buoyant density CFU-GM in RA [59], subacute myeloid leukemia [59], and smoldering leukemia [127] and in increased serum and urine levels of CSF [59], in contrast to the findings in patients with IASA [59]. An increased urinary output of CSF combined with low colony-forming capacity of the bone marrow cells have been related to an impending acute transformation [59].

Use of the CFU-GM assay and of in vitro coculture experiments with normal marrow cells suggested three pathophysiologic mechanisms for cytopenia: an inherent stem cell defect, a defect of the hematopoietic environment, and the presence of suppressor cells [86]. Insight into the clonal evolution was provided by the demonstration of progressive loss of normal CFU-GM in a black female with RA who was heterozygous for the X-linked enzyme G6PD

Table 10. Bone marrow colony growth in patients with myelodysplastic syndromes

Authors	Authors designation	FAB[a] classification	Number of patients	% Leukemic growth pattern[b]	% Patients progressing to ANLL with	
					nonleukemic	leukemic
					growth pattern	
Linman et al. [108]	Preleukemic syndrome	a, b, c	10	50	0	60
Faille et al. [45]	RAEB	c, e	17	77	0	54
Beran and Hast [13]	Preleukemia	a, b, c, e, f	23	83	0	30
Greenberg et al. [59]	Preleukemic syndrome	a	43	42	40	50
Verma et al. [198]	Preleukemia	a	19	26	21	80
Spitzer et al. [178]	Oligoleukemia	c, d, e, f	65	74	29	50
Mertelsmann et al. [116]	Myelodysplastic syndrome	a, b, d	66	45	0	63
Lidbeck et al. [105]	Hemopoietic dysplasia	a, b, c	23	48	8	27
Coiffier et al. [31]	Dysmyelopoiesis	a, b, c, d, e	96	25	18	67
Coiffier et al. [32]	Dysmyelopoietic syndromes	a, b, c, d, e	79	27	3	38
			441	43 (194/441)	23 (34/147)	51 (99/193)

[a] See Table 1

[b] Term used differently by different authors: may include reduced colony growth and/or increased micro-/macro-cluster growth and/or increased cluster-colony ratio

[82]. Over a period of 17 months normal-type A progenitors were gradually lost despite minimal changes in the clinical status. The in vivo suppression of proliferation and/or maturation of normal CFU-GM were also demonstrated by the manifestation of type-B activity only in the circulating granulocytes, proving their derivation solely from the malignant clone despite the presence of normal CFU-GM in the marrow.

The *prognostic value* of the in vitro growth pattern has been demonstrated by an increased risk of developing acute leukemia when leukemic growth occurred, being about 50%, as against 23% in patients with a nonleukemic growth pattern (Table 10).

As to patients with SMML and CMML, micro- or macrocluster growth is usually a poor prognostic sign and is seen only in SMML [37]. In addition, a leukemic growth pattern as opposed to normal in vitro growth is associated with a decrease in median survival time [13, 32, 45, 60, 178, 198]. Whereas in patients with a leukemic growth pattern death occurred most frequently after leukemic transformation, in the group with low or zero growth death was generally due to pancytopenia, probably as a consequence of a reduced normal stem cell reserve [32]. Follow-up studies in patients with RA [60, 198] and oligoblastic leukemia [178] have demonstrated the alteration to a leukemic growth pattern with progression of the disease.

Recently, the presence of *blast cell progenitors* not present in normal persons has been described in the peripheral blood of five of seven patients with IASA, two of three with RAEB, and 11 of 15 with RA [168], with the aid of a conditioned medium that is produced by leukocytes after stimulation by phytohemagglutinin. The frequency of their growth was lower than in overt acute leukemia but the cell cycle activity was similar. There are as yet too few data to assess the prognostic significance in relation to the development of acute leukemia.

Since anemia and dyserythropoiesis are predominant features of the myelodysplastic syndromes, the immature and mature *erythroid progenitor cells,* BFU-E und CFU-E, have been studied in the bone marrow and in the peripheral blood using in vitro culture systems [29, 168]. No growth of BFU-E-derived colonies was seen in the bone marrow and only greatly reduced growth or none at all in the peripheral blood. Elimination of T cells did not reverse the growth failure, ruling out – at least in the four patients studied – the presence of suppressor T cells [29]. Growth of CFU-E was normal or decreased [29, 95, 121].

It is important to note the considerable overlap of the cell culture data in these disorders, partly because of the various definitions used for the different subentities (Tables 1 and 10), and partly because of methodological differences that are inherent in these nonstandardized culture systems. Despite the variations of the in vitro culture methods, a leukemic growth pattern allows not only the identification of a preleukemic condition and its separation from nonpreleukemic conditions, but also the identification of high-risk patients with regard to the progression from smoldering to overt acute leukemia (Table 10). Certainly more data are needed for determination of the influence of cell-cell interactions and microenvironmental changes; long-term marrow culture systems are required and investigations must be extended to the pluripotent progenitor cell CFU-GEMM [118]. Early results indicate that the incidence of CFU-GEMM in the peripheral blood might be reduced in preleukemia and RAEB [168], but improved culture conditions should increase the validity of these data [5].

Cytogenetic Studies

The significance of chromosome abnormalities in patients with myelodysplastic disorders has repeatedly been reviewed [133, 161, 175]. With banding techniques, cytogenetically

Table 11. Cytogenetic and clinical findings in patients with myelodysplastic syndromes

Authors	Authors designation	FAB classification[a]	Number of patients	% Abnormal findings	% Progression to ANLL	
					Normal karyotype	Abnormal karyotype
Millner et al. [121]	Refractory cytopenia, smouldering leukemia	a, c, d	14	43	38	0
Pierre [145]	Preleukemic syndromes	a, b	26	50		
Harrousseau et al. [64]	Preleukemic states	a, b, c, e	24	37.5	0	21
Geraedts et al. [54]	Preleukemic syndrome	?	34	50		
Granberg-Öhmann et al. [56]	Preleukemia	a, b, c	18	33	25	83
Streuli et al. [181]	Dysmyelopoietic syndrome	c, d	8	88	0	29
Panani et al. [138]	Preleukemia	a, c, d	24	46	100	100
Second International Workshop [164]	Preleukemia	?[b]	244	51	15	27
Kardon et al. [88]	Dysmyelopoietic syndrome	b, c, d, e	15	60	6	44
Anderson and Bagby [1]	Preleukemic syndrome	a[b]	42	36	22	66
Nowell [133]	Preleukemia	a, b	80	39	37	81
			529	47% (249/528)	26% (64/250)	43% (95/219)

[a] See Table 1
[b] Including patients with prior exposure to irradiation and/or cytostatic therapy

abnormal clones can be detected in about 50% of the patients (Table 11). The abnormal clone can replace normal hematopoiesis partially or completely. The study of cytogenetic markers made it possible to document the temporary expansion and spontaneous disappearance of an abnormal clone in a patient with RAEB [179].

The chromosome aberrations follow a nonrandom pattern and appear to be similar to the changes in acute nonlymphoblastic leukemia [123, 164]. The aberrations most frequently found are monosomy 7 or 7q−, trisomy 8 or trisomy 8 plus additional abnormalities, and monosomy 5 or 5q− [1, 56, 88, 123, 137, 144, 145, 164, 181]. It should be noted that patients with previous exposure to mutagenic/carcinogenic agents have been included in some studies [1, 164]. The Ph^1 chromosome has never been seen in CMML, but loss of the Y chromosome can be a frequent event [79].

In IASA the frequency of chromosome abnormalities seems to be lower than in the other subentities, being about 33% [64, 88]. Furthermore, in these patients the presence of a cytogenetically abnormal clone does not necessarily imply an increased rate of leukemic transformation [175].

There is good evidence from the larger series [133, 164] listed in Table 11 that the presence of chromosome abnormalities increases the risk of progression to frank acute leukemia from 26%−43% in patients with preleukemia, smoldering leukemia, and CMML. With respect to the median survival time after diagnosis, the persistence of normal metaphases seems to imply a better prognosis, similar to findings in ANLL. In two studies the median survival of patients with only abnormal metaphases was 3 [138] and 4.5 months [181], as against 18.5 and 12 months [121, 141, 155, 202] for patients with both normal and abnormal metaphases. In a recent prospective study [1] it was noted that this might be due to a larger proportion of patients with prior exposure to alkylating agents in this subgroup. Furthermore, Anderson and Bagby [1] observed that it was the complex chromosome abnormality that predisposed to leukemic transformation, whereas in patients with simple abnormalities the probability of acute transformation was not unusually high. Since complex chromosome changes have been observed especially in ANLL secondary to exposure to alkylating agents or irradiation, it may be that the two predictive factors observed by Anderson and Bagby [1] were interrelated and not independent, which would indicate some exposure to mutagenic or carcinogenic agents as etiological factors [2, 100, 122, 141, 155, 156, 202].

Apart from the significance of complex aberrations, the question remains as to whether the involvement of specific chromosomes involves a particular risk of developing acute leukemia. On the other hand, in combined studies in patients with preleukemia and SMML, the loss of part of the long arm or the whole of chromosome 7 (the most frequent abnormality in these disorders) could be related to defective neutrophil migrations and might be one reason for the high incidence of infectious episodes in myelodysplastic disorders [158−160]. The significance of abolished production of leukocyte interferon in patients with another frequent abnormality (5q−/−5) remains to be elucidated [140].

Future Prospects

Although there has been much progress in recent years in the understanding of the biological processes involved in the myelodysplastic syndromes, prospective definition of the risk groups that will eventually develop acute leukemia is still not possible. A large percentage of patients with no detectable abnormalities will nevertheless progress to overt acute leukemia. The combined analysis of the results of hitherto established diagnostic procedures, i.e., cytogenetic studies, in vitro culture growth, bone marrow morphology, and kinetic investigations, may reduce the present uncertainties [37, 52], but further progress using more refined methods is needed. Improved cytogenetic techniques, including high-resolution banding, might allow the identification of specific breakpoints and lead to further subgroups, as in the case of the 5q− syndrome [208]. Further progress can be expected from the combination of in vitro culture assay for marrow blast stem cells with immunological methods to test their neoplastic nature [33]. This might in fact lead to the detection of a leukemic clone in the preleukemic syndromes as well as to the detection of residual leukemia after therapy. Since the results of current therapy are discouraging, attempts should be made to develop predictive tests that will allow the rational use of androgens or corticosteroids in individual preleukemic patients [7, 120]. As to chemotherapy, testing the in vitro response of leukemic clonogenic cells to cytotoxic drugs [139] might allow the definition of subgroups that will respond to these agents. Furthermore, there is an urgent need for controlled therapeutic trials in these patients to clarify the effectiveness of intensive chemotherapy [78], including the usefulness of high-dose Ara-C [148]. The extent to which BMT can be used as a therapeutic approach needs further study, with especial reference to the point in the course of the disease at which it should be performed [189].

Alternative therapeutic agents that exhibit their effect through the induction of differentiation include low-dose Ara-C [6, 27, 125], retinoid acid [128], vitamin D analogs [128], and CSF inducers such as endotoxin [128], any of which might offer some prospects for the future.

References

1. Anderson RL, Bagby GC (1982) The prognostic value of chromosome studies in patients with the preleukemic syndrome (hepopoietic dysplasia). Leuk Res 6: 175−181
2. Anderson RL, Bagby GC, Richert-Boe K, Magenis RE, Koler RD (1981) Therapy-related preleukemic syndrome. Cancer 47: 1867−1871
3. Ariel I, Weiler-Ravell D, Stalnikowics R (1981) Preleukemia in acute lymphoblastic leukemia. Acta Haematol (Basel) 66: 50−52
4. Armitage JO, Dick FR, Needleman SW, Burns CP (1981) Effect of chemotherapy for the dysmyelopoietic syndrome. Cancer Treat Rep 65: 601−605
5. Ash RC, Detrick RA, Zanjani ED (1981) Studies of human pluripotent hemopoietic stem cells (CFU-GEMM) in vitro. Blood 58: 316
6. Baccarani M, Tura S (1979) Correspondence: differentiation of myeloid leukaemic cells: new possibilities for therapy. Br J Haematol 42: 485−487
7. Bagby GC, Gabourel JD, Linman JW (1980) Glucocorticoid therapy in the preleukemic syndrome (hemopoietic dysplasia). Ann Intern Med 92: 55−58
8. Barr RD, Stevens CA (1982) The role of autologous helper and suppressor T cells in the regulation of human granulopoiesis. Am J Hematol 12: 323−326
9. Barton JC, Conrad ME, Parmley RT (1980) Acute lymphoblastic leukemia in idiopathic refractory sideroblastic anemia: evidence for a common lymphoid and myeloid progenitor cell. Am J Hematol 9: 109−115
10. Beard MEJ, Bateman CJT, Crowther DC et al. (1975) Hypoplastic acute myelogenous leukaemia. Br J Haematol 31: 167−176
11. Bennett JM, Catovsky D, Daniel MT et al. (1982) Proposals for the classification of the myelodysplastic syndromes. Br J Haematol 51: 189−199
12. Bennett JM, Catovsky D, Daniel MT et al. (1976) Proposals for the classification of the acute leukemias. Br J Haematol 33: 451−458

13. Beran M, Hast R (1978) Studies on human preleukemia. II. In vitro colony forming capacity in a regenerative anemia with hypercellular bone marrow. Scand J Haematol 21: 139–149
14. Bernard J, Izrael V, Jacquillat L (1975) Les leucémies oligoblastiques (editorial). Nouve Presse Méd 4: 943–945
15. Bhaduri S, Kubanek B, Heit W et al. (1979) A case of preleukemia – reconstitution of normal marrow function after bone marrow transplantation (BMT) from identical twin. Blut 38: 145–149
16. Block M, Jacobson LO, Bethard WF (1953) Preleukemic acute human leukemia. JAMA 152: 1018–1028
17. Boggs DR, Wintrobe MM, Cartwright GE (1962) The acute leukemias. Analysis of 322 cases and review of the literature. Medicine 41: 163–225
18. Boivin P, Galand C, Hakim J, Kahn A (1975) Acquired erythroenzymophathies in blood disorders: study of 200 cases. Br J Haematol 31: 531–543
19. Breton-Gorius J, Houssay D, Dreyfus B (1975) Partial myeloperoxidase deficiency in a case of preleukemia. I. Studies of fine structure and peroxidase synthesis of promyelocytes. II. Defects of degranulation and abnormal bactericidal activity of blood neutrophils. Br J Haematol 30: 273–278, 279–288
20. Brière J, Dresch C, Brière JF, Faille A (1977) Leucémies myelomonocytaires subaigues ou chronique de l'adulte. Etude clinique et données cinétiques. A propos de 46 observations. Actual Hematol (Paris) 53–80
21. Broxmeyer HE, Jacobson N, Kurland J, Mendelsohn N, Moore MAS (1978) In vitro suppression of normal granulocytic stem cells by inhibitory activity derived from human leukemic cells. J Natl Cancer Inst 60: 497–511
22. Broxmeyer HE, Grossbard E, Jacobson N, Moore MAS (1979) Persistence of inhibitory activity against normal bone marrow cells during remission of acute leukemia. N Engl J Med 301: 346–351
23. Bynoe AG, Scott CS, Ford P, Roberts BE (1983) Decreased T helper cells in the myelodysplastic syndromes. Br J Haematol 54: 97–102
24. Cabrol C, Abele R (1978) Chromosome 5q– in the medullar cells of a patient with anemia which later developed into acute non-differentiated leukaemia. J Genet Hum 26: 195–202
25. Catovsky D, Galton DAG, Griffin C et al. (1971) Serum lysoenzyme and vitamin B_{12} binding capacity in myeloproliferative disorders. Br J Haematol 21: 661–672
26. Cazzola M, Barosi G, Berzuini C et al. (1982) Quantitative evaluation of erythropoietic activity in dysmyelopoietic syndromes. Br J Haematol 50: 55–62
27. Cazzola M, Chériè-Lignière EL, Gorini M, Montecucco CM, Riccardi A, Ascari E (1982) Treatment of acute myeloid leukemia with low dose cytosine arabinoside. 3rd international symposium on therapy of acute leukemias, December 11–14, Rome
28. Cheng DS, Kushner JP, Wintrobe MM (1979) Idiopathic refractory sideroblastic anemia. Incidence and risk factors for leukemic transformation. Cancer 44: 724–731
29. Chui DHK, Clarke BJ (1982) Abnormal erythroid progenitor cells in human preleukemia. Blood 60: 362–367
30. Cohen JR, Greger WP, Greenberg PL, Schrier SL (1979) Subacute myeloid leukemia. A clinical review. Am J Med 66: 959–966
31. Coiffier B, Sicard B, Germain D (1980) Culture in vitro des progéniteurs granuleux dans les dysmyélopoièses. Nouv Presse Méd 9: 1137–1140
32. Coiffier B, Bryon PA, Fière D et al. (1982) Agar culture of bone marrow cells in acute myeloid leukemia and dynsmyelopoietic syndromes. Reevaluation of its prognostic value. Nouv Rev Fr Hematol 24: 13–18
33. Davis FM, Dicke KA, Jagannath S, Rao PN (1983) Detection of leukemic cell colonies in agar plates by immunostaining for human malignancy-associated nucleolar antigen. J Immunol Methods 58: 349–357
34. DiBenedetto J, Padre-Mendoza T, Albala MM (1979) Pure red cell hypoplasia associated with long arm deletion of chromosome 5. Hum Genet 46: 345

35. Dörmer P, Hegemann F, Brinkmann W (1976) Proliferation and production of hemopoietic cells in two stages of disease: preleukemia and overt leukemia. Klin Wochenschr 54: 461–466
36. Dresch C, Faille A, Glogowski A, Najean Y (1977) Éléments de la prognose des dysplasies hématopoïétiques. Nouv Rev Fr Hematol 18: 401–414
37. Dresch C, Faille A, Poirier O, Balitrand N, Najean Y (1979) Bone marrow cell kinetics and culture in chronic and subacute myelomonocytic leukemia. Physiopathological interpretation and prognostic importance. Leuk Res 4: 129–142
38. Dreyfus B (1976) Preleukemic states I. Definition and classification. II. Refractory anemia with an excess of myeloblasts in the bone marrow (smouldering acute leukemia). Blood Cells 2: 33–55
39. Dreyfus B, Rochant H, Sultan C, Clauvel J, Yvart J, Chesneau A (1970) Les anémies réfractaires avec excèss de myéloblastes dans la moelle. Nouv Presse Med 78: 359–364
40. Duguid JKM, Mackie MJ, McVerry BA (1983) Skin infiltration associated with chronic myelomonocytic leukemia. Br J Haematol 53: 257–264
41. Eastman PM, Schwartz R, Schrier SL (1972) Distinctions between idiopathic ineffective erythropoiesis and di Guglielmo's disease: clinical and biochemical differences. Blood 40: 487–499
42. Economopoulos T, Stathakis N, Maragoyannis Z, Gardikas E, Dervenoulas J (1981) Myelodysplastic syndrome. Clinical and prognostic significance of monocyte count, degree of blastic infiltration, and ring sideroblasts. Acta Haematol (Basel 65: 97–102
43. Editor (1983) Leukaemogenesis and differentiation. Lancet 1: 33–35
44. Evensen SA, Stavem P (1978) Smouldering acute myelogenous leukemia. Acta Med Scand 203: 305–307
45. Faille A, Dresch C, Poirier O, Balitrand N, Najean Y (1978) Prognostic value of in vitro bone marrow culture in refractory anemia with excess of myeloblasts. Scand J Haematol 20: 280–286
46. Fialkow PJ (1982) Cell lineages in hematopoietic neoplasia studied with glucose-6-phosphate dehydrogenase cell markers. J Cell Physiol [Suppl] 1: 37–43
47. Fialkow PJ, Singer JW, Adamson JW et al. (1981) Acute nonlymphatic leukemia. Heterogeneity of stem cell origin. Blood 57: 1068–1073
48. Fischer M, Mitrou PS (1976) Panmyelopathie mit hyperplastischem Knochenmark und Präleukämie. Med Klin 71: 2127–2135
49. Fisher WB, Armentrout SA, Weisman R, Graham RC (1973) "Preleukemia". A myelodysplastic syndrome often terminating in acute leukemia. Arch Intern Med 132: 226–232
50. Foon KA, Gale RP (1982) Controversies in the therapy of acute myelogenous leukemia. Am J Med 72: 963–979
51. Francis GE, Tuma GA, Berney JJ, Hoffbrand AV (1981) Sensitivity of acute myeloid leukaemia cells to colony stimulating activity: relation to response to chemotherapy. Br J Haematol 49: 259–267
52. Francis GE, Wing MA, Miller EJ, Berney JJ, Wonke B, Hoffbrand AV (1983) Use of bone-marrow culture in prediction of acute leukemic transformation in preleukemia. Lancet 1: 1409–1412
53. Geary CG, Catovsky D, Wiltshaw E (1975) Chronic myelomonocytic leukaemia. Br J Haematol 30: 289–302
54. Geraerdts JPM, Weber RFA, Kerkhofs H, Leeksma CHW (1980) The preleukemic syndrome. II. Cytogenetic findings. Acta Med Scand 207: 447–454
55. Golde DW, Cline MJ (1973) Human preleukemia. Identification of a maturation defect in vitro. N Engl J Med 288: 1083–1086
56. Granberg-Öhman I, Hast R, Vass L (1980) Studies on human preleukemia. III. Chromosomal abnormalities in aregenerative anemia with hypercellular bone marrow. Haematologica 65: 421–436
57. Greenberg PL (1980) Annotation: clinical relevance of in vitro study of granulocytopoiesis. Scand J Hamatol 25: 369–381

58. Greenberg P, Nichols WC, Schrier SL (1971) Granulopoiesis in acute myeloid leukemia and preleukemia. N Engl J Med 284: 1225–1232
59. Greenberg P, Mara B, Bax I, Brossel R, Schrier S (1976) The myeloproliferative disorders: correlation between clinical evolution and alternations of granulopoiesis. Am J Med 61: 878–891
60. Greenberg P, Mara B (1979) The preleukemic syndrome. Correlation of in vitro parameters of granulopoiesis with clinical features. Am J Med 66: 951–958
61. Greenberg P, Bagby G (1983) Biologic rather than morphologic markers in myelodysplastic syndromes. Br J Haematol 53: 532–534
62. Hamilton-Paterson JL (1949) Preleukaemic anaemia. Acta Haematol (Basel) 2: 309–316
63. Hansen NE (1973) The relationship between the turnover rates of neutrophilic granulocytes and plasma lysoenzyme levels. Br J Haematol 25: 771–782
64. Harousseau JL, Smadja N, Krulik M, Audebert AA, Debray J (1978) Etude du caryotype au cours des états préleucémiques. Nouv Presse Med 7: 3431–3435
65. Hartley SE, McCallum CJ (1981) The 5q− chromosome in a case of erythroid hypoplasia. Cancer Genet Cytogenet 3: 33
66. Hast R (1978) Studies on human preleukemia IV. Clinical and prognostic significance of sideroblasts in aregenerative anemia with hypercellular bone marrow. Scand J Haematol 21: 396–402
67. Hast R, Reizenstein P (1977) Studies on human preleukaemia I. Erythroblast and iron kinetics in aregenerative anaemia with hypercellular bone marrow. Scand J Haematol 19: 347–354
68. Hast R, Beran M, Reizenstein P (1979) Studies on human preleukemia VI. Non-specific immunotherapy (BCG) in five patients with aregenerative anemia and hypercellular bone marrow. In: Schmalzl F, Hellriegel KP (eds) Preleukemia. Springer, Berlin Heidelberg New York, pp 170–173
69. Hast R, Beran M, Granberg I (1979) Studies in human preleukemia VII. Prognostic factors for the diagnosis of the preleukemic stage in aregenerative anemia with hypercellular bone marrow. In: Schmalz F, Hellriegel KP (eds) Preleukemia. Springer, Berlin Heidelberg New York, pp 133–137
70. Hast R, Reizenstein P (1981) Sideroblastic anemia and development of leukemia. Blut 42: 203–207
71. Hehlmann R, Zönnchen B, Thiel E, Walther B (1983) Idiopathic refractory sideroachrestic anemia (IRSA) progressing to acute mixed lymphoblastic-myelomonoblastic leukemia. Blut 46: 11–21
72. Heimpel H (1979) Conventional morphological examination of blood and bone marrow cells in the diagnosis of preleukemic syndromes. In: Schmalzl F, Hellriegel KP (eds) Preleukemia. Springer, Berlin Heidelberg New York, pp 4–11
73. Heimpel H, Drings P, Mitrou P, Queisser W (1979) Verlauf und prognostische Kriterien bei Patienten mit „Präleukämie". Klin Wochenschr 57: 21–29
74. Heimpel H, Hoelzer D (1982) Grenzfälle der Behandlung akuter Leukämien. In: Scheurlen PG, Pees HW (eds) Aktuelle Therapie bösartiger Blutkrankheiten. Springer, Berlin Heidelberg New York, pp 58–68
75. Heimpel H, Hoelzer D (1982) Präleukämie und atypische Leukämieformen im Alter. In: Bohnel J, Heinz R, Stacher A (eds) Hämatologie im Alter. Urban and Schwarzenberg, Wien, pp 95–99
76. Hoagland HC, Linman JW (1972) Pyridoxine-responsive anemia: a preleukemic manifestation? Min Med 55: 891–895
77. Housset M, Daniel MT, Degos L (1982) Small doses of ARA-C in the treatment of acute myeloid leukaemia: differentiation of myeloid leukaemia cells? Br J Haematol 51: 125–129
78. Howe RB, Bloomfield CD, McKenna RW (1982) Hypocellular acute leukemia. Am J Med 72: 391–395
79. Hurdle ADF, Garson OM, Buist DGP (1972) Clinical and cytogenetic studies in chronic myelomonocytic leukaemia. Br J Haematol 22: 773–782

80. Hussein KK, Salem Z, Bottomley SS, Livingston RB (1982) Acute leukemia in idiopathic sideroblastic anemia: response to combination chemotherapy. Blood 59: 652–656
81. Izrael V, Jacquillat C, Chastang C et al. (1975) Données nouvelles sur les leucémies oligo-blastiques. Nouv Presse Med 4: 947–952
82. Jacobson RJ, Raskind W, Sacher RA, Sahshaty G, Singer JW, Fialkow PJ (1982) Refractory anemia (RA), a myelodysplastic syndrome: clonal development with progressive loss of normal committed progenitors. Blood [Suppl] 60: 129a
83. Joseph AS, Cinkotal KI, Hunt L, Geary CG (1982) Natural history of smouldering leukaemia. Br J Cancer 46: 160–166
84. Jume'an HG, Libnoch JA (1979) 5q-myelodysoplasia terminating in acute leukemia. Ann Intern Med 91: 748–749
85. Kaffe S, Hsu LYF, Hoffmann R, Hirschhorn K (1978) Association of 5q– and refractory anemia. Am J Hematol 4: 269–272
86. Kagan WA, Fialk MA, Coleman M, Ascensao JL, Good RA, Valera E (1980) Studies on the pathogenesis of refractory anemia. Am J Med 68: 381–385
87. Kanatakis S, Chalevelakis G, Economopoulos T et al. (1983) Correlation of haematological, electron microscopic and cytogenetic findings in 20 patients with preleukaemia. Scand J Haematol 30: 89–94
88. Kardon N, Schulman P, Degnan TJ, Budman DR, Davis J, Vinciguerra V (1982) Cytogenetic findings in the dysmyelopoietic syndrome. Cancer 50: 2834–2838
89. Kay HEM (1982) Bone marrow transplantation in adult acute leukaemia: who should be transplanted, and when? In: Bloomfield CD (ed) Adult leukemias 1. Nijhoff, The Hague, pp 381–406
90. Keating MJ, Smith TL, Gehan EA, McCredie KB, Bodey GP, Freireich EJ (1982) A prognostic factor analysis for use in development of predictive models for response in adult acute leukemia. Cancer 50: 457–465
91. Kerkhofs H, Hagemeijer A, Leeksma CHW et al. (1982) The 5q– chromosome abnormality in haematological disorders: a collaborative study of 34 cases from the Netherlands. Br J Haematol 52: 365–381
92. Knox SJ, Greenberg BR, Anderson RW, Rosenblatt LS (1983) Studies of T-Lymphocytes in preleukemic disorders and acute nonlymphocytic leukemia: in vitro radiosensitivity, mitogenic responsiveness, colony formation, and enumeration of lymphocytic subpopulations. Blood 61: 449–455
93. Knuutila S, Vuopio P, Borgström GH, De La Chapelle A (1980) Higher frequency of 5q-clone in bone marrow mitoses after culture than by a direct method. Scand J Haematol 25: 358–362
94. Koeffler HP, Golde DW (1978) Cellular maturation in human preleukemia. Blood 52: 355–361
95. Koeffler HP, Cline MJ, Golde DW (1978) Erythropoiesis in preleukemia. Blood 51: 1013–1019
96. Koeffler HP, Golde DW (1980) Human preleukemia. Ann Intern Med 93: 347–353
97. Kolb HJ, and the Munich Cooperative Group for Bone Marrow Transplantation (1979) Bone marrow transplantation for treatment of preleukemic syndromes? In: Schmalzl F, Hellriegel KP (eds) Preleukemia. Springer, Berlin Heidelberg New York, pp 181–186
98. Kushner JP, Lee GR, Wintrobe MM, Cartwright GE (1971) Idiopathic refractory sideroblastic anemia. Clinical and laboratory investigation of 17 patients and review of the literature. Medicine 50: 139–159
99. Labedzki L, Illiger HJ (1979) Erfolgreiche Behandlung der chronischen myelomonozytären Leukämie mit VP 16-213. Blut 38: 421–424
100. Lawler SD, Summersgill BM, McElwain TJ (1982) Cytogenetic studies in patients previously treated for Hodgkin's disease. Cancer Genet Cytogenet 5: 25–35
101. Lehrer RI, Goldberg LS, Apple MA, Rosenthal NP (1972) Refractory megaloblastic anemia with myeloperoxidase-deficient neutrophils. Ann Intern Med 76: 447–453

102. Lewy RI, Kansu E (1978) Correspondence: prognostic value of platelet counts in idiopathic sideroblastic anemia. Blood 51: 766–767
103. Lewy RI, Kansu E, Gabuzda T (1979) Leukemia in patients with acquired idiopathic sideroblastic anaemia: an evaluation of prognostic indicators. Am J Hematol 6: 323–331
104. Lidbeck J (1980a) Studies on hemopoietic dysplasia (the preleukemic syndrome). Acta Med Scand 208: 459–462
105. Lidbeck J (1980b) In vitro colony and cluster growth in haemopoietic dysplasia (the preleukaemic syndrome) I. Clinical correlations. Scand J Haematol 24: 412–420
106. Lidbeck J, Manson JC (1981) Progression of bone marrow abnormalities in malignant hemopoietic dysplasia. Evaluation of cytological changes with serial bone marrow samples. Acta Med Scand 210: 293–298
107. Linman JW, Saarni MI (1974) The preleukemic syndrome. Semin Hematol 11: 93–100
108. Linman JW, Bagby GC (1976) The preleukemic syndrome: clinical and laboratory features, natural course, and management. Blood Cells 2: 11–31
109. Linman JW, Bagby GC (1978) The preleukemic syndrome (hemopoietic dysplasia) Cancer 42: 854–864
110. Lintula R, Rasi V, Ikkala E, Borgström GH, Vuopio P (1981) Platelet function in preleukaemia. Scand J Haematol 26: 65–71
111. Mahmood T, Robinson WA, Hamstra RD, Wallner SF (1979) Macrocytic anemia, thrombocytosis and nonlobulated megakaryocytes. The 5q-syndrome, a distinct entity. Am J Med 66: 946–950
112. Maldonado JE, Pierre RV (1975) The platelets in preleukemia and myelomonocytic leukemia: ultrastructural cytochemistry and cytogenetics. Mayo Clin Proc 50: 573–587
113. Mangan KF, Chikkappa G, Bieler LZ, Scharfman WB, Parkinson DR (1982) Regulation of human blood erythroid burst-forming unit (BFU-E) proliferation by T-lymphocyte subpopulations defined by Fc receptors and monoclonal antibodies. Blood 59: 990–996
114. Mayer RJ, Canellos GP (1983) Preleukemic syndromes and other myeloproliferative disorders. In: Gunz FW, Henderson ES (eds) Leukemia. Grune and Stratton, New York, p 741–757
115. Mende S, Fülle HH, Knuth A, Weissenfels I (1977) Myelomonozytäre Leukämie: klinische, zytologische und zytogenetische Studien bei akuten, subakuten und chronischen Verlaufsformen. Blut 35: 21–34
116. Mertelsmann R, Morre MAS, Clarkson BD (1979) Sequential marrow culture studies and terminal deoxynucleotidyl transferase activities in myelodysplastic syndromes. In: Schmalzl F, Hellriegel KP (eds) Preleukemia. Springer, Berlin Heidelberg New York, pp 106–117
117. Mertelsmann R, Thaler HT, To L et al. (1980) Morphological classification, response to therapy and survival in 263 adult patients with acute nonlymphoblastic leukemia. Blood 56: 773–781
118. Messner HA, Fauser AA (1980) Culture studies on human pluripotent hemopoietic progenitors. Blut 41: 327–333
119. Miescher PA, Farquet JJ (1974) Chronic myelomonocytic leukemia in adults. Semin Hematol 11: 129–139
120. Miller AM, Chen H, Combs B (1981) 5q-refractory anemia: response to corticosteroid therapy. The 6th meeting of the international society of hematology, European and African division, August 30–September 4, Athens
121. Milner GR, Testa NG, Geary CG et al. (1977) Bone marrow culture studies in refractory cytopenia and "smouldering leukaemia". Br J Haematol 35: 251–261
122. Mitelman F, Brandt L, Nilsson PG (1978) Relation among occupational exposure to potential mutagenic/carcinogenic agents, clinical findings, and bone marrow chromosomes in acute nonlymphocytic leukemia. Blood 52: 1229–1237
123. Mitelman F, Levan G (1981) Clustering of aberrations to specific chromosomes in human neoplasms IV. A survey of 1,871 cases. Hereditas 95: 79–139
124. Mitrou PS, Fischer M (1979) Cell proliferation in refractory anemia with hyperplastic bone marrow (preleukemia) In: Schmalzl F, Hellriegel KP (eds) Preleukemia. Springer, Berlin Heidelberg New York, pp 76–90

125. Moloney WC, Rosenthal DS (1981) Treatment of early acute non lymphatic leukemia with low dose cytosine-arabinoside. In: Neth R, Gallo RC, Graf T, Mannweiler K, Winkler K (eds) Modern trends in human leukemia. Springer, Berlin Heidelberg New York, pp 59–62
126. Moore MAS, Williams N, Metcalf D (1973) In vitro colony formation by normal and leukemic human hematopoietic cells: characterization of the colony-forming cells. J Natl Cancer Inst, 50: 603–623
127. Moore MAS, Spitzer G, Williams N, Metcalf D, Buckley J (1974) Agar culture studies in 127 cases of untreated acute leukemia: the prognostic value of reclassification of leukemia according to in vitro growth characteristics. Blood 44: 1–18
128. Moore MAS, Gabrilove J, Sheridan AP (1983) Myeloid leukemic cell differentiation induced by human postendotoxin serum and vitamin analogues. In: Neth R, Gallo RC, Greaves MF, Moore MAS, Winkler K (eds) Modern trends in human leukemia V. Springer, Berlin Heidelberg New York, pp 327–337
129. Mueller RA, Auf der Maur P, Beck EA, Deubelbeiss K, Bucher U (1982) Das 5q-Minus-Syndrom – eine Chromosomenaberration mit charakteristischem hämatologischem Bild: Präleukämie? Literaturübersicht und Beschreibung einer eigenen Beobachtung. Schweiz Med Wochenschr 112: 242–252
130. Najean Y, Pecking A (1977) Refractory anemia with excess of myeloblasts in the bone marrow: a clinical trial of androgens in 90 patients. Br J Haematol 37: 25–33
131. Najean Y, Pecking A (1979) Refractory anemia with excess of blast cells: prognostic factors and effect of treatment with androgens or cytosine arabinoside. Results of a prospective trial in 58 patients. Cancer 44: 1976–1982
132. Needleman SW, Burns CP, Dick FR, Armitago JO (1981) Hypoplastic acute leukemia. Cancer 48: 1410–1414
133. Nowell PC (1982) Cytogenetics of preleukemia. Cancer Genet Cytogenet 5: 265–278
134. Nowell P, Finan J (1978) Chromosome studies in preleukemic states. IV. Myeloproliferative versus cytopenic disorders. Cancer 42: 2254–2261
136. Olofsson T, Olsson I (1980) Biochemical characterization of a leukemia-associated inhibitor (LAI) suppressing normal granulopoiesis in vitro. Blood 55: 983–991
137. Panani A, Papayannis AG, Kyrkou K, Gardikas C (1977) Cytogenetic studies in preleukaemia using the G-banding staining technique. Scand J Haematol 18: 301–308
138. Panani A, Papayannis AG, Sioula E (1980) Chromosome aberrations and prognosis in preleukemia. Scand J Haematol 24: 97–100
139. Park CH, Wiernik PH, Morrison FS, Amare M, Van Sloten K, Maloney TR (1983) Clinical correlations of leukemic clonogenic cell chemosensitivity assessed by in vitro continuous exposure to drugs. Cancer Res 43: 2346–2349
140. Pedersen Bjergaard J, Haahr S, Philip P et al. (1980) Abolished production of interferon by leukocytes of patients with the acquired cytogenetic abnormalities 5q– or –5 in secondary and de novo acute non-lymphocytic leukaemia. Br J Haematol 46: 211–223
141. Pedersen Bjergaard J, Philip P, Mortensen T (1981) Acute nonlymphocytic leukemia, preleukemia, and acute myeloproliferative syndrome secondary to treatment of other malignant diseases. Clinical and cytogenetic characteristics and results of in vitro culture of bone marrow and HLA-typing. Blood 57: 712–723
142. Petit P, Van den Berghe H (1979) The 5q– and additional chromosome anomalies in two patients with acute myeloid leukemia. Ann Genet 22: 103
143. Pierre RV (1974) Preleukemic states. Semin Hematol 11: 73–92
144. Pierre RV (1975) Cytogenetic studies in preleukemia: studies before and after transition to acute leukemia in 17 subjects. Blood Cells 1: 163–170
145. Pierre RV (1978) Preleukemic syndromes. Virchows Arch [Cell Pathol] 29: 29–37
146. Porzsolt F, Heimpel H (1982) Impaired T-cell and NK-cell function in patients with preleukemia. Blut 45: 243–248
147. Prchal JT, Throckmorton DW, Carroll AJ 3rd, Fuson EW, Gams RA, Prchal JF (1978) A common progenitor for human myeloid and lymphoid cells. Nature 274: 590–591

148. Preisler HD, Early AP, Raza A et al. (1983) Therapy of secondary acute nonlymphocytic leukemia with cytarabine. N Engl J Med 308: 21–23
149. Presant CA (1977) Prognostic value of platelet count in idiopathic sideroblastic anemia: reply. Blood 50: 767–768
150. Queisser U, Olischläger A, Queisser W, Heimpel H (1972) Cell proliferation in the 'preleukaemic' phase of acute leukaemia. Acta Haematol (Basel) 47: 21–32
151. Reizenstein P, Lagerlöf B (1972) Aregenerative anemia with hypercellular sideroblastic marrow. Acta Haematol (Basel) 47: 1–12
152. Reizenstein P, Lagerlöf B, Skåberg KO, Carlmark B, Kock Y, Jores S (1975) Alterations in erythropoiesis preceding leukemia. Acta Haematol 54: 152–158
153. Rheingold JJ, Kaufman R, Adelson E, Lear A (1963) Smoldering acute leukemia. N Engl J Med 268: 812–815
154. Rothstein G, Wintrobe MM (1975) Preleukemia. Adv Intern Med 20: 363–378
155. Rowley JD (1976) 5q-acute myelogenous leukemia: reply. Blood 48: 625–626
156. Rowley JD, Golomb HM, Vardiman JW (1981) Nonrandom chromosome abnormalities in acute leukemia and dysmyelopoietic syndroms in patients with previously treated malignant disease. Blood 58: 759–767
157. Rochant H, Dreyfus B, Bouguerra M, Tont-Hat H (1972) Refractory anemias, preleukemic conditions and foetal erythropoiesis. Blood 39: 721–726
158. Ruutu P, Ruutu T, Vuopio P, Kosunen TU, De La Chapelle A (1977) Function of neutrophils in preleukaemia. Scand J Haematol 18: 317–325
159. Ruutu P, Ruutu T, Repo H, Vuopio P, Timonen T, Kosunen TU, de la Chapelle A (1981) Defective neutrophil migration in monosomy –7. Blood 58: 739–745
160. Saarni MI, Linman JW (1973) Preleukemia: the hematologic syndrome preceding acute leukemia. Am J Med 55: 38–48
161. Sandberg AA (1980) The chromosomes in human cancer and leukemia. Elsevier, Amsterdam
162. Schmalzl F, Konwalinka G, Michlmayr G, Abbrederis K, Braunsteiner H (1978) Detection of cytochemical and morphological anomalies in 'preleukemia'. Acta Haematol (Basel) 59: 1–18
163. Schmalzl F, Hellriegel K (eds) (1979) Preleukemia. Springer, Berlin Heidelberg New York
164. Second International Workshop on Chromosomes in Leukemia (1980) Chromosomes in preleukemia. Cancer Genet Cytogenet 2: 108–113
165. Seigneurin D, Hollard D (1981) Use of the tritiated thymidinelabelling index of the myeloblast-promyelocyte pool for the identification of the leukemic population n oligoblastic leukemia. Acta Haematol (Basel) 66: 181–186
166. Senn JS, Pinkerton PH (1972) Defective in vitro colony formation by human bone marrow preceding overt leukaemia. Br J Haematol 23: 277–281
167. Senn JS, Curtis JE, Pinkerton PH, Till JE, McCulloch EA (1980) The distribution of marrow granulopoietic progenitors among patients with preleukemia. Leuk Res 4: 409–413
168. Senn JS, Messner HA, Pinkerton PH, Chang L, Nitsch B, McCulloch EA (1982) Peripheral blood blast cell progenitors in human preleukemia. Blood 59: 106–109
169. Sexauer J, Kass L, Schnitzer B (1974) Subacute myelomonocytic leukemia. Clinical, morphological and ultrastructural studies of 10 cases. Am J Med 57: 853–861
170. Sills RH, Stockman JA 1981) Preleukemic states in children with acute lymphoblastic leukemia. Cancer 48: 110–112
171. Smith TL, Gehan EA, Keating MJ, Freireich EJ (1982) Prediction of remission in adult acute leukemia. Cancer 50: 466–472
172. Smith WB, Albin A, Goodman JR, Brecher G (1973) Atypical megakaryocytes in preleukemic phase of acute myeloid leukemia. Blood 42: 535–540
173. Sokal G, Michaux JL, Van Den Berghe H (1975) Anémie réfractaire et chromosome 5q–: un nouveau syndrome. Bull Acad R Med Belgique 130: 368

174. Sokal G, Michaus JL, Van den Berghe H et al. (1975) A new hematologic syndrome with a distinct karyotype: the 5q-chromosome. Blood 46: 519–533
175. Sokal G, Michaux JL, Van den Berghe H (1980) The karyotype in refractory anaemia and pre-leukaemia. Clin Hematol 9: 129–139
176. Solomon CR, Hillman RS, Finch CA (1981) Serum ferritin in refractory anemias. Acta Haematol (Basel) 66: 1–5
177. Speer JR, Freireich FJ, Hart JS (1974) Identification of smoldering leukemia by delaying chemotherapy. Clin Oncol 15: 73
178. Spitzer G, Verma DS, Dicke KA, Smith T, McCredie KB (1979) Subgroups of oligoleukemia as identified by in vitro agar culture. Leuk Res 3: 29–39
179. Stein RN, Rowley JD, LeBeau MM, Hoagland HC, Berry TM (1982) Spontaneous resolution of myelodysplastic syndrome associated with non-random chromosomal abnormality. Blood [Suppl] 60: 140a
180. Streeter RR, Presant CA, Reinhard E (1977) Prognostic significance of thrombocytosis in idiopathic sideroblastic anemia. Blood 50: 427–432
181. Streuli RA, Testa JR, Vardiman JW, Mintz U, Golomb HM, Rowley JD (1980) Dysmyelopoietic syndrome: sequential clinical and cytogenetic studies. Blood 55: 636–644
182. Sultan C, Marquet M, Joffroy (1973) Etude des dysmyélopoièses acquises idiopathiques au culture de moelle in vitro. Nouv Rev Fr Hematol 13: 431–436
183. Sultan Y, Caen YP (1972) Platelet dysfunction in preleukemic states and various types of leukemia. Ann NY Acad Sci 201: 300–306
184. Swansbury GJ, Lawler SD (1980) Chromosomes and prognosis in preleukaemia: four cases of 5q− with other karyotypic abnormality. Leuk Res 4: 611–618
185. Swolin B, Weinfeld A, Ridell B, Waldenström J, Westin J (1981) On the 5q-deletion: clinical and cytogenetic observations in ten patients and review of literature. Blood 58: 986–993
186. Takaku S, Takaku F (1981) Natural killer cell activity and preleukaemia (letter). Lancet 2: 1178
187. Teerenhovi L, Borgström GH, Lintula R et al. (1981) The 5q-chromosome in preleukaemia and acute leukaemia. Scand J Haematol 27: 119–129
188. Thiele J, Vykoupil KF, Georgii A (1980) Myeloid dysplasia (MD); a hematological disorder preceding acute and chronic myeloid leukemia. A morphological study on sequential core biopsies of the bone marrow in 27 patients. Virchows Arch [Pathol Anat] 389: 343–367
189. Thomas ED (1983) Bone marrow transplantation in leukemia. In: Neth R, Gallo RC, Greaves MF, Moore MAS, Winkler K (eds) Modern trends in human leukemia V. Springer, Berlin Heidelberg New York, pp 11–15 (Hämatologie und Bluttransfusion, vol 28)
190. Tulliez M, Testa U, Rochant H et al. (1982) Reticulocytosis, hypochromia, and microcytosis: an unusual presentation of the preleukemic syndrome. Blood 59: 293–299
191. Valentine WN, Konrad PN, Paglia DE (1973) Dyserythropoiesis, refractory anemia, and "preleukaemia": metabolic features of the erythrocytes. Blood 41: 857–875
192. Van den Berghe H, Cassimann JJ, David G, Fryns JP, Michaux JL, Sokal G (1974) Distinct hematological disorder with deletion of long arm of no. 5 chromosome. Nature 251: 437–438
193. Van den Berghe H, David G, Michaux HL, Sokal G, Verwilghen R (1976) 5q-acute myelogeneous leukemia. Blood 48: 624–625
194. Van Slyck EJ, Rebuck JW, Waddell CC, Janakiraman N (1983) Smoldering acute granulocytic leukemia. Observations on its natural history and morphologic characteristics. Arch Intern Med 143: 37–40
195. Varela BL, Chuang C, Bennett JM (1982) Clinical signficance of the new proposals for the classification of the myelodysplastic syndromes. Blood [Suppl] 60: 140a
196. Verhest A, Van Schonbroeck F, Wittek M, Naets JP, Denolin-Reubens R (1976) Specificity of the 5q-chromosome in a distinct type of refractory anemia. J Natl Cancer Inst 56: 1053–1054
197. Verhest A, Lustmann F, Wittek M, Van Schonbroeck F, Naets, JP (1977) Cytogenetic evidence of clonal evolution in 5q-anemia. Biomedicine 27: 211–212

198. Verma DS, Spitzer G, Dicke KA, McCredie KB (1979) In vitro agar culture patterns in preleukemia and their clinical significance. Leuk Res 3: 41–49
199. Weber RFA, Geraedts JPM, Kerkhofs H, Leeksma CHW (1980) The preleukemic syndrome. 1. Clinical and hematological findings. Acta Med Scand 207: 391–395
200. Weber W, Speck B, Cornu P, Nissen C, Hofer H (1979) Bone marrow transplantation a possible approach for preleukemia? In: Schmalzl F, Hellriegel KP (eds) Preleukemia. Springer, Berlin Heidelberg New York, pp 176–180
201. Weisdorf DJ, Oken MM, Johnson GJ, Rydell RE (1981) Auer rod positive dysmelopoietic syndrome. Am J Hematol 11: 397–402
202. Whang-Peng J, Knutsen T, O'Donnell JF, Brereton HD (1979) Acute non-lymphocytic leukemia and acute myeloproliferative syndrome following radiation therapy for non-Hodgkin's lymphoma and chronic lymphocytic leukemia. Cytogenetic studies. Cancer 44: 1592–1600
203. White JM, Brain MC, Ali MAM (1971) Globin synthesis in sideroblastic anaemia I. α and β peptide chain synthesis. Br J Haematol 20: 263–275
204. White JM, Ali MAM (1973) Globin snythesis in sideroblastic anaemia II. The effect of pyridoxine, δ-aminolaevulinic acid and haem in vitro. Br J Haematol 24: 481–489
205. Wiesneth M, Pflieger H, Kubanek B, Heimpel H (1980) Micromegakaryocytes in human bone marrow. Acta Haematol (Basel) 64: 65–71
206. Wintrobe B (1981) Clinical hematology, VIII. ed. Lea and Febiger, Philadelphia
207. Yoo D, Schechter GP, Amigable AN, Nienhuis AW (1980) Myeloproliferative syndrome with sideroblastic anemia and acquired hemoglobin H disease. Cancer 45: 78–83
208. Yunis JJ, Bloomfield CD, Ensrud K (1981) All patients with acute nonlymphocytic leukemia may have a chromosomal defect. N Engl J Med 305: 135–138
209. Zervas J, Geary CG, Oleesky S (1974) Sideroblastic anemia treated with immunosuppressive therapy. Blood 44: 117–123
210. Zittoun R (1976) Annotation: subacute and chronic myelomonocytic leukaemia: a distinct haematological entity. Br J Haematol 32: 1–7
211. Zittoun R (1981) Subacute and chronic myelomonocytic leukemia. Haematol Blood Transfus 27: 157–165
212. Zittoun R, Bernadou A, Bilski-Pasquier G, Bousser J (1972) Les leućemies myélo-monocytaires subaigues. Etude de 27 cas et revue de la litérature. Sem Hop Paris 48: 1943–1956
213. Zuckermann KS (1980) Stimuation of human BFU_E by products of human monocytes and lymphocytes. Exp Hematol 8: 924–932

Biological and Clinical Significance of Immunological Cell Markers in Leukemia

E. Thiel

Gesellschaft für Strahlen- und Umweltforschung mbH, Institut für Hämatologie, Abteilung Immunologie, und Medizinische Klinik Innenstadt, Ludwig-Maximilians-Universität, Landwehrstrasse 61, 8000 München 2, FRG

Introduction

In 1845, Rudolf Virchow [1] described a disease which he first called leukemia *("Weisses Blut")*. In contrast to John Hughes Bennet [2], who the same year explained another case of leukocythemia as suppuration of the blood, Virchow suggested a disturbed regulation of maturation as the underlying pathophysiologic mechanism of the disease. After a century of increasing knowledge of morphologic criteria owing to the use of the microscope and of specialized staining techniques in a never-ending guest for more precise cellular identification, this maturation arrest of leukemic cells as described by Virchow was re-emphasized. Further such emphasis occurred when the advent of immunologic techniques offered the potential for specific identification of cells by their antigenic constitution. In recent years it has become evident that various levels of leukocyte differentiation can be precisely defined by a number of immunologic parameters. Experience with lymphocytes of rodents, birds, and man has taught us that cell populations which are functionally heterogeneous yet morphologically homogeneous can be differentiated with considerable precision by virtue of the cell surface properties of the constituent subpopulations. The T/B dichotomy of the immune system has become the best model for surface marker technology, and the definition of various levels of lymphocyte differentiation by immunological means has been particularly productive and useful. Studies in several laboratories have indicated that highly specific antisera, unique surface markers, and intracellular enzymes can be used for fine differentiation of cellular identities in the hematopoietic system. Phenotypic analyses of normal and malignant lymphoid cells have provided important insights into lymphocyte differentiation and also into the origin of leukemias. It is also now well established that lymphatic leukemias and lymphomas can be further subdivided into clinically relevant subgroups by use of immunologic markers. This has been exemplified in many publications, and an early review of the subject was given at the WHO-sponsored symposium held in Munich in 1977 [3].

The definition of new subsets of leukemia has since been further substantiated, and even more important, has become generally accessible due to the introduction of monoclonal antibody-producing hybridoma technology [4]. The production and unlimited supply of highly reactive and specific monoclonal antibodies has revolutionized the identification of lymphocyte subsets. Early experiences in leukemia phenotyping with this new technology were summarized at a leukemia marker symposium held in Vienna [5]. Indeed, much of current hematophysiology and -pathology, with particular reference to the lymphocytic leukemias, is derived from investigative work based on these very methods.

In the present chapter an attempt will be made to review this investigative work, for it is essential to current understanding of leukemia. The chapter falls into four parts, the first

Recent Results in Cancer Research. Vol. 93

dealing with the classic but still useful surface markers and methods, the second with the use of monoclonal antibodies for the identification of malignant cell phenotypes and their normal counterparts in the differentiation pathway, and the third with the biological and clinical relevance of surface markers; the last part is designed to give an insight into the pathogenesis of leukemia as provided by immunological methods.

"Conventional" Cell Surface Markers

The delineation of lymphocytic subsets followed the observation that lymphoid subsets could be identified and separated on the basis of their differing membrane structures. These membrane characteristics have been called "markers". Generally, membrane surface markers can be divided into two categories: receptors and antigens. Receptors, namely surface structures responsible for the binding of defined particles such as erythrocytes, e.g., E, EA, and EAC receptors, are usually detected by rosette assays. Surface antigens, such as surface immunoglobulins, T cell antigens, or other differentiation antigens, are detected as xenoantigens with specific heterologous antibodies directed to them. A variety of markers for T cells, B cells, and their subpopulations have been described, and the most widely used and best defined will be explained below. This discussion will emphasize the populations of normal lymphocytes which express classic markers, the functional correlate of the markers, and its occurrence in the leukemias. In a later section, we will describe the expansion of the options available with surface markers with the introduction of the monoclonal antibody-producing hybridoma technology.

Immunoglobulins

Surface Immunoglobulin: Recording Methods

B Lymphocytes carry Ig (immunoglobulin) molecules on their membrane. This means that Ig molecules constitute a unique marker defining the B cell system. These structures serve as the antigen recognition unit of the lymphocyte and are an integral membrane component synthesized by the cell, as opposed to immunoglobulins that are adsorbed to the cell via Fc receptors. This structure has therefore been called surface immunoglobulin (SIg). The SIg of most B cells is IgM alone or IgM and IgD together. A much smaller proportion of B lymphocytes express either IgG or IgA. However, most cells with IgG on the membrane have acquired this passively by adsorption onto membrane receptors for the Fc part of IgG. The IgG can be removed by incubation at 37° C and is not resynthesized by the cell [6].

The most common method used to detect SIg is incubation of cells in suspension with fluorescein-conjugated anti-immunoglobulin reagents. This procedure is relatively simple and quick, and remarkably sensitive when reagents with high F/P ratios (4 or greater) and microscopes with epi-illumination are used. Certain precautions should be maintained to ensure the detection of SIg and not Ig adsorbed to lymphocytes or monocytes via Fc or C receptors. Preincubation at 37° C for at least 1 hour and the use of antiglobulin reagents without an Fc portion (Fab dimers) have proved useful. Of course, reliability is dependent on the sensitivity and specificity of the antisera used. Affinity-purified IgG F $(ab')_2$ fragments of goat anit-human Ig are very useful reagents.

Immunoperoxidase methods can also be employed but are more time-consuming, and are only preferred if detailed morphology or permanent slides are needed or if electron microscope studies are considered [7, 8]. A quantitative immunoperoxidase method has been described [9]. This procedure, like quantitative immunoautoradiography with radioiodinated antibodies [10], allows quantitation of SIg density. The density of SIg on chronic lymphocytic leukemia cells is reported to be lower than that of normal B lymphocytes, and to vary less widely from cell to cell. On the other hand, SIg is more dense on lymphocytes of prolymphocytic leukemia. Whereas quantitative immunoperoxidase and immunoradioautography techniques are not widely used, due to their greater complexity and sophistication, analysis and physical sorting in flow systems (e.g., cytofluorograph or fluorescence-activated cell sorter, FACS) are being used increasingly for both clinical and investigational phenotyping of leukemia samples [11]. With such systems, the fluorescence intensity of a large number of cells can be registered within minutes in relation to cell size as measured by the scatter. The percentage of positive-staining cells and average staining intensity are quantified, the latter by determining the fluorescence "window" on the FACS at which 50% of the cells are positive. Simultaneous staining for different cell surface antigens is also possible when antibodies coupled to different fluorochromes are used, e.g., rhodamine and fluorescein. Such double labelings are extremely useful, especially in the case of mixed cell populations.

Cytoplasmic Immunoglobulins

In animals and in man, during ontogeny of the lymphoreticular system a pre-B cell develops in the fetal liver before the appearance of SIg-bearing lymphocytes [12, 13]. The pre-B cell has IgM in its cytoplasm but lacks detectable surface immunoglobulin. Pre-B cells are found normally in adult bone marrow, and it is for this reason that the adult bone marrow is thought to be analogous to the avian bursa of Fabricius [14]. Since the cytoplasmic IgM is of weak intensity, affinity-purified IgG F $(ab')_2$ fragments of anti-human IgM are needed for demonstration. Unlike the CIg found in pre-B lymphocytes, the CIg in plasma cells and in lymphoplasmocytoid cells includes both heavy and light chains. Plasma cells, which are the most highly differentiated B lymphocytes, contain large quantities of CIg.

The detection of cytoplasmic immunoglobulin within a cell has been taken as an indicator for the B lymphocytic origin of that cell, since it is generally accepted that Ig is highly specific and still the best marker for the B cell system. However, the demonstration of Ig within a cell must be subject to qualification, for Ig may be present as a result of mechanisms other than synthesis: cells of the histiocyte/monocyte series may contain Ig by virtue of phagocytosis of immune complexes; these same cells bear Fc receptors and are capable of adsorbing and internalizing Ig by this mechanism. The detection of more than one light chain or more than one heavy chain within a single cell suggests that the cell contains Ig as a result of some mechanism(s) other than synthesis, since individual B cells synthesize only one light chain and one cytoplasmic heavy chain (though it is known that changes in the heavy chain do occur in the so-called heavy chain switch, the light chain type remains constant). Passive absorption of serum immunoglobulin through membranes that have lost their integrity is a major pitfall for analyses of cytoplasmic Ig positive cells.

Immunoglobulins and Monoclonality

It is generally accepted that monoclonality reflects the proliferative expansion of a clone of cells. The initial event may involve a single cell or several, but the end result is a dominant clone with characteristics identical with those of the parent cell. Lymphomas and leukemias of B cells are the best examples of monoclonal cell proliferation. They are commonly referred to as monoclonal, because the cells which possess detectable surface or cytoplasmic Ig express only one or two heavy chains and one light chain (e.g., IgMk), whereas a reactive or nonneoplastic lymphocyte population contains cells bearing the spectrum of heavy and light chains (polyclonal). Monoclonality can be affirmed in an absolute sense by the use of anti-idiotypic sera. For example, the identification of circulating B lymphocytes bearing idiotypes common to those produced by plasma cells in multiple myeloma supports the idea that multiple myeloma is a neoplasm of B cells with cells in different stages of differentiation [15]. Further, the target cell of malignant transformation can be assumed to be less mature than the malignant cell type of the dominant clone. Observations that individual cells within a clonal proliferation may bear two heavy chains (e.g., CLL with IgM and IgD both expressed at cell surface) are compatible with studies that have demonstrated a sequential switch in the production of heavy chains, controlled at the gene level (*C*-region genes); the antigen-combining site or idiotype (hypervariable sequence of the *V* region of the Ig molecule) is constant. It is this constancy of the idiotype expressed by the neoplastic cells [16] that holds great promise for the identification of neoplastic B cells that because of a lack of morphological identity otherwise remain undetected within a mixed polyclonal population. Thus a tumor-associated marker is detected by the use of anti-idiotype antisera. In practice, however, such antisera are rarely available, and a monoclonal pattern of surface Ig (one light chain) is relied upon as an indicator of the neoplastic nature of the proliferative process. Thus, the monotypic pattern provided by the monoclonal light chain restriction is of great diagnostic value. For example, multiple myeloma can be distinguished from reactive plasmacytosis by its monoclonal staining pattern in sections or smears of bone marrow aspirates, even at a stage when the morphologic criterial for multiple myeloma [17] are not fulfilled. Recognition of a monotypic pattern is also of value in distinguishing a reactive lymphocytosis in the blood from an incipient chronic lymphocytic leukemia. Thus, a bone marrow investigation can be circumvented by immunological blood cell typing in conditions where differential diagnosis might otherwise be difficult.

Rosetting Techniques

E Rosettes

After the first observation of spontaneous rosetting of sheep erythrocytes (E) by human lymphocytes, [18] many reports appeared dealing with this first important, commonly used marker for human T lymphocytes [19–26]. The rosetting phenomenon was not inhibited by anti-immunoglobulin sera [19], and the rosetting lymphocytes were shown to be different from those with surface immunoglobulins or complement receptors [22–24]. Rosetting cells were demonstrated in the thymus and in the thymus-dependent areas of the lymphatic tissues [21, 24]. Anti-T-cell sera inhibited the rosetting phenomenon at various dilutions [25, 26]. T cell antigens and the E receptor were shown to be located on the same cell, but to be redistributed in different areas of the membrane [26]. In contrast to most T antigens, the E receptor is trypsin sensitive [26].

Many technical variations in the rosetting procedure and different treatments of the sheep erythrocytes prior to their use (e.g., with neuraminidase or the sulfhydrylreagent AET) have been described and recently reviewed [27]. The sensitivity of the rosette procedure was increased: whereas the first reports indicated that as few as 5%–15% of blood lymphocytes formed E rosettes, by 1975 laboratories were reporting scores of 50%–80%, which is now regarded as the normal range. Many factors, however, still influence this relatively simple and therefore useful test, so that a general standardization is difficult. For instance, temperature of incubation, vigor of resuspension, media used, counting criteria, and age of sheep erythrocytes and of lymphocytes are all factors that influence the results. While the formation of E rosettes remains the standard against which the newer techniques are measured, it must be remembered that the E rosette test is not specific for T cells, since other cell types, including fibroblasts and parenchymal cells from liver and lung, also form E rosettes [28]. In addition, with reference to cell suspensions derived from leukemic blood or bone marrow, it is important to remember that the population of rosetting cells is likely to be heterogeneous, consisting of residual T lymphocytes, activated T lymphocytes, and any neoplastic E rosette-forming cells. In such instances the usual E rosette percentage score is misleading. Cytocentrifuge preparations for examination of rosette-forming cells may be useful. As reviewed in a later section, there are now monoclonal antibodies reacting with the E receptor-associated surface structure. It should be borne in mind that there may be some T cells without E receptor as recognized by specific anti-T cell sera [29]. The occurrence of leukemias consisting in the presence of T cells with "incomplete" T cell phenotype must be considered, since such leukemias were formerly misdiagnosed when the E receptor was used as the sole T marker [30].

Rosettes with Mouse Erythrocytes

Erythrocytes from several other species have been reported to form spontaneous rosettes with human lymphocytes. Whereas rhesus monkey red blood cells, goat erythrocytes, and rabbit red cells rosette primarily with portions of T lymphocytes, the first rosetting with mouse erythrocytes was observed to be caused by chronic lymphocytic leukemia cells, indicating a B cell attribute [31]. This was confirmed by double-labeling experiments showing that lymphocytes which rosetted with mouse red blood cells had IgM, IgD, or both on their surfaces [32–34]. The same authors also reported that only a subclass of B lymphocytes (around 5% of normal peripheral blood lymphocytes) rosetted with mouse red blood cells. Since mouse rosette-forming cells are present during ontogeny at least as early as surface IgM [35], the M-rosette receptor may characterize a somewhat immature stage of B lymphocytes. Accordingly, the high percentages of M-rosetting cells in chronic lymphocytic leukemia may correlate with a less highly differentiated B cell phenotype than the majority of blood cells. For this disease, the marker is useful for diagnosis and in some circumstances also has some prognostic value [36]. Interestingly, acute lymphoblastic leukemia cells of the pre-B type can be induced to express M receptors by culture in diffusion chambers implanted into irradiated mice [37].

Fc and Complement Receptors

Receptors for the Fc end of the IgG molecule are present on most hematopoietic cells, including granulocytes, monocytes, macrophages, and lymphocytes [38–41]. This marker, therefore, is not cell lineage specific and is thus of limited value for cell-type immunodiagnosis. Its more pronounced expression on B lymphocytes has been emphasized in earlier reports to discriminate them from T cells [42, 43]. Later reports, however, provided evidence for Fc receptors for IgG on activated T lymphocytes and for weak Fc receptors for IgM on the majority of T cells. This latter receptor type was detectable only by special culture techniques, again highlighting the crucial importance of the sensitivity of the method used. A variety of methods differing in sensitivity have been described for detection of Fc receptors. Those most commonly used include the EA rosette assay and binding of heat-aggregated immunoglobulin [42, 43]. Ripley (anti-CD) antibody-coated human erythrocytes do not bind to all Fc receptor-bearing lymphocytes, but rather to a subpopulation of lymphocytes which is responsible for antibody-dependent cell-mediated cytotoxicity (ADCC) [43]. Thus a third population of lymphocytes can be detected by a relatively insensitive Fc receptor technique. The function of Fc receptors on this third population of lymphocytes is to allow the cell to participate in ADCC, whereas SIg-positive Fc receptor-bearing B lymphocytes do not exhibit ADCC activity. Thus the functional relationship of this surface marker is noteworthy. For instance, the presence of Fc receptors for IgG or IgM on T lymphocytes has been correlated with their functional activity: cells with IgM receptors were shown to provide help for B cell differentiation to plasma cells, whereas cells with IgG recepors were reported to function as suppressors [44]. Besides the functional aspects of Fc receptors, information as to the maturational level of various cell types in a cell lineage can be gained by recording of FcR expression [45]. Thus, granulopoietic precursor cells become strongly FcR positive during maturation, or FcR-negative lymphocytes can differentiate to FcR-positive lymphocytes accompanied by functional maturation [45].

In 1970, a receptor of antigen-antibody complement complexes was demonstrated on some lymphocytes of various species [46]. This population was distinct from the theta-bearing population in mouse [47], and had the same tissue distribution as B lymphocytes in humans [24]. Different receptors have been defined for the split products of activated C3 (C3b, C3d) and C4 [48, 49]. Such complement receptors (CR) are typically not expressed on T lymphocytes, but have been demonstrated in double-labeling assays on a small subpopulation of T cells [50]. CR are strongly expressed on monocytes, macrophages, and granulocytes [51]. A correlation of CR expression to leukocyte differentiation has been demonstrated [51]. Also in ontogenetic studies, maturation of CR-negative Ig-positive lymphocytes to CR-positive and Ig-positive B cells has been demonstrated [52]. Thus, like Fc receptors, the CR marks certain differentiation steps within a cell lineage, without being specific.

Lymphocyte Differentiation Antigens as Defined by Classic Heteroantisera

In 1963, a system of alloantigens was described in the mouse, the expression of which is controlled by two allelic genes in thymus cells, in some leukemias, and in neural tissue [53]. This theta alloantigen is a specific and highly useful marker for the T cell system of the mouse [54]. A comparable alloantigen system has not yet been defined in humans. Many xenoantisera with reported specificity for T or B lymphocytes have been developed in the past decade, however, by injecting human thymocytes, lymphoid cell lines, brain tissue, or cell fragments to nonhuman primates or xenogeneic species. The antisera raised required extensive absorption to assure specificity. Most of these antisera are directed at stable cell surface antigens that have the nature of glycoproteins. Apparently these surface antigenic structures are related to differentiation, and they are therefore called differentiation antigens. The differentiation antigens are different from common antigens such as species-specific antigenic determinants and individual-specific histocompatibility antigens. The most widely studied differentiation antigens as defined by classic heteroantisera are discussed in the next section.

T Cell Antigens

In 1973, the first anti-human T cell antisera wer reported [25, 55, 56], which were produced in rabbits by injection of thymocytes or human (agammaglobulinemic) T lymphocytes. Extensive absorption was necessary to achieve specificity, and the remaining reactivity of the antisera was only weak. Approximately 80% of peripheral blood lymphocytes are identified by such antisera, along with over 90% of thymic cells, 50% of tonsil cells, and 20% of marrow lymphocytes. A comparatively strong and specific antiserum was prepared by hyperimmunization with thymocytes and by the application of a standardized scheme of various absorption steps [29]. The resulting antiserum was shown to be T cell specific and to be unreactive with other blood and marrow cells [29]. Immunoprecipitation studies for molecular identification of the T cell-specific antigens revealed that the antiserum reacted with six different glycoproteins of thymocytes and peripheral T cells [57]. This illustrates the known fact that classic antisera often react against various antigenic determinants covering broad reaction patterns, in contrast to the focused reaction pattern of monoclonal antibodies. Similar approaches were used to prepare antisera reacting with T cell subpopulations [58, 59]. One of the best characterized (anti-TH_2) reacted with 90% of thymocytes but only some blood T cells [58]. The reactive T cell subset was shown to have cytotoxic activity, whereas the TH_2-negative cells proliferated in MLC and functioned as amplifiers of the cytotoxic TH_2 subset [58]. Antisera reacting with antigens of the early T cell differentiation phase (thymocytes of the cortex) were prepared by immunization with ALL cells of pre-T cell type, whereas antigens on mature T cells (blood and thymus medulla) were detected by using antisera raised against CLL cells of T type [59].

B Cell Antigens and Ia-Like (HLA-DR) Antigens

Heteroantisera that identify B cell antigens that are not Ia related and are distinct from SIg and receptors for C3 and Fc have recently been described [60–63]. These antisera cross-react to varying degrees with monocytes and null cells, and some are specific only in cytotoxicity, a technique that is not suitable for diagnostic enumeration of lymphocytes in blood. Thus, similar problems to those that occur with heterologous anti-T cell sera have to be considered, and it is not possible to make such antisera on a large scale or in a reproducible manner.

Human B lymphocytes have also been reported to have immune-related antigens (Ia) on their surface. In mice, the immune response appears to be controlled by part of the central segment of the histocompatibility complex designated the *Ir* region [64–66]. The Ia antigens, which are gene products of the *Ir* region, are strongly expressed on B cells [66]. They were first defined in congenic mouse strains and are detected usually by alloantisera [67], but also by using heterologous antisera [68]. By analogy, Ia-like antigens detectable as alloantigens [69] or as heteroantigens [70, 71] have been described in man. The demonstration of a linkage to LD or to the *D* locus of the HLA system provided evidence of an analogous Ia system in man [72]. In view of the close relationship between the Ia antigens and gene products of the *HLA-D* locus, the term *HLA-D* related or *HLA-DR* is sometimes used to indicate Ia antigens on human cells. The Ia antigens are glycoproteins composed of a heavy chain of 35,000 daltons and a light chain of 27,000 daltons [73]. Preliminary data suggested that the Ia antigens were unique to B lymphocytes, but it is now evident that they are also present on monocytes [70], immature myeloid and possibly erythroid progenitor cells [74–77], activated T lymphocytes [78], a subpopulation of peripheral blood T lymphocytes [79], and some nonhematopoietic tissues such as sperm or epidermal cells. Thus, without being specific, the Ia marker provides useful information in combination with other markers, e.g., immature cell phenotypes can be identified in the myeloid cell series and cell activation can be assumed for an Ia-stained T cell.

Common ALL Antigen

Immunization of rabbits with acute lymphoblastic leukemia (ALL) cells devoid of T or B cell markers provided, after appropriate absorption procedures, an antiserum of high specificity for most of the non-T ALLs [80]. As confirmed by various groups [81–83], these antisera did not react with blood cells or any other leukemic cell type excepts cells from the "lymphoid" form of blast crisis in chronic myelogenous leukemia (CML). Thus a candidate for human leukemia antigen was assumed in earlier reports [84]. A weak expression on some fetal bone marrow cells and on cells in regenerating bone marrow was later demonstrated, indicating that it might be a normal differentiation antigen of lymphoid bone marrow progenitors [85]. Since the common ALL antigen (CALLA) is generally not detectable in blood or in great numbers in bone marrow, it is nevertheless operationally leukemia-associated and thus has a high diagnostic value. The CALLA is a glycoprotein with a molecular weight of about 100,000 [86, 87]. The gp 100 antigen has also been demonstrated on normal immature lymphoid cells by means of monoclonal antibodies [88]. An approximately 20-fold lower expression of CALLA has recently been demonstrated on granulocytes and skin fibroblasts [89].

Biochemical and Miscellaneous Markers

A large number of other lymphocyte markers and receptors have been described, which can only be briefly mentioned in this review. The reader is referred to a recent review article for additional information [27]. Hormone receptors have recently begun to be studied in lymphatic cells, whereas the suppressive effect exerted by glucocorticoids on lymphoid cells has been known for a long time. Thus, *glucocorticoid receptors* have been extensively studied. These are cytoplasmic binding proteins that are specific for glucocorticoids and appear to be required for hormone action in sensitive tissues. The binding to the receptor is followed by a series of steps, which includes nuclear transfer and inhibition of a number of biosynthetic and transport functions. Several groups have found that response to glucocorticoids in lymphoproliferative disorders correlates with glucocorticoid receptor level [90–93]. Moreover, glucocorticoid receptors have prognostic significance within certain immunologic classes of childhood ALL [90]. The non-T, non-B ALL subtype is reported to have higher receptor levels than null ALL or T-ALL [93]. Other authors, however, have questioned the possibility of a correlation with clinical response and the quantity of steroid receptors [94].

The hydrocortisone-sensitive subset of the thymus was shown to bind *peanut agglutinin* (PNA) [95]. A differential response of PNA-positive and -negative thymocytes to phytohemagglutinin led the same authors to suggest that the PNA-positive subset was less mature. Accordingly, PNA receptors were found in some cases of ALL but not in CLL. PNA receptors also occur on the surface of AML cells, indicating that PNA may define many lineages of hematopoietic cells which are in relatively early stages of differentiation.

Histamine receptors were detected on about 33% of blood cells and on 10% of peripheral T lymphocytes by using a rosette assay [96]. In later reports [97–100], the histamine H2-type receptor was shown to be phenotypic for suppressor T cells (using biochemical methods). Accordingly, histamine reactivity has been correlated with cellular maturation and modulation of cellular immune responses in vivo and in vitro [98, 99]. *Insulin receptors* are present on both T and B lymphocytes which have been stimulated with antigens or mitogens [101]. Thus the insulin receptor represents a marker for cell activation in lymphocytes. A difference in the expression of insulin receptors between T-ALL and Null ALL has been reported [102].

Receptors for catecholamines [103], *adenosine* [104], *prostaglandins* [105], and *T-cell growth factor* [106] have been described. These receptors may have important immunoregulatory functions, but have not yet been related to subclassifications of lymphocyte subsets or leukemia cell types.

Receptors for the Epstein-Barr virus (EBV) are present on B cells [107]. A close association between EBV receptors and the C3d receptor has been reported [108]. T lymphocytes have been shown to possess a *receptor for measles virus* [109]. Blood lymphocytes have also been subdivided into several categories on the basis of their ability to bind certain strains of *bacteria*. These lymphocytes were shown to differ in function [110]. Several membrane biochemical markers of leukemic cells have also been described. The glycolipid *asialo* GM_1 is found on cells from patients with acute lymphoblastic leukemia (ALL) (non-B non-T, and T-ALL), but not on cells from patients with other forms of leukemia [111]. Alterations in membrane carbohydrates, such as decreased complex gangliosides [112], carbohydrate-containing antigens [113], and receptors for cholera toxin [114], have been reported on leukemic cells.

Enzyme Markers

The determination of the presence of certain enzymes, such as myeloperoxidase or unspecific esterase, by cytochemical methods has been extremely useful for the differentiation of acute nonlymphoblastic leukemia (ANLL) from ALL. Also, the biochemical or immunological assessement of certain enzymes will continue to be of value for differentiation of ALL and AML. It should be noted, however, that enzyme marker analysis has not yet proved as useful as immunological marker analysis for the subclassification of leukemias. Specific antisera have so far been the mainstay of diagnostic management. Cytochemical studies of hematopoietic cell classes have demonstrated differing, although not unique, cellular distributions of a member of enzymes. Studies using biochemical techniques suggest that the total specific activity of enzymes also differs among immunologic cell classes. The enzymes most studied to date are terminal deoxynucleotidyl transferase, 5′-nucleotidase, adenosine deaminase, and hexosaminidase isoenzymes, which will be discussed below. They have been reviewed recently [115].

Terminal Deoxinucleotidyl Transferase (TdT)

The most widely studied intracellular enzyme is TdT, which has been reviewed recently [116]. TdT is a polymerizing enzyme that, unlike other DNA polymerases, catalyzes the addition of deoxyribonucleotide triphosphates to the 3′OH end of poly- or deoxyribonucleotide primers without requiring a template. TdT activity can be measured in populations of cells with a quantitative enzyme assay and in individual cells with specific antibodies, e.g., by immunofluorescence. TdT is found in thymocytes and in a small percentage of bone marrow cells, but not in mature lymphocytes. Increased TdT activity has been reported in most blast cells of ALL, in lymphomas of immature cell type, and in blast crisis (BC) of CML. Since common ALL, T-ALL, some pre-B ALL, and BC-CML are linked by the presence of TdT, a common pathway of differentiation has been suggested [116]. In BC-CML, TdT has been shown to be predictive of response to chemotherapy [117]. However, repeated measurements of TdT activity or antigen alone in cells from the peripheral blood or bone marrow have not yet proven of value in the management of childhood ALL [118]. TdT has proved valuable for distinguishing acute lymphoid and myeloid leukemias [116]. However, the demonstration of TdT-positive cells in 10%–20% of patients with acute nonlymphoid leukemia without the Philadelphia chromosome [119] limits the interpretation of TdT positivity concerning cell lineage affiliation when additional morphological, cytochemical, or immunological markers are lacking. The presence of graded amounts of enzyme within the T cell lineage, so that the less highly differentiated thymocytes or T lymphoblasts have the most activity and the more differentiated peripheral lymphocytes and Sézary cells have much lower activity [116], is thus of diagnostic value for assessing the stage of differentiation of T cells. B lymphocytes usually do not have the enzyme and TdT is absent or present only in low levels in Burkitt's lymphoma, chronic lymphocytic leukemia, hairy cell leukemia, and multiple myeloma [116].

5′-Nucleotidase (5′N), Adenosine Deaminase (ADA), and Purine Nucleoside Phosporylase (PNP)

Another biochemical marker of current interest is the enzyme *5′-nucleotidase (5′-N)*. This enzyme of purine metabolism is surface membrane bound, with its active center facing the extracellular space, and is therefore classified as an ectoenzyme. This ectoenzyme catalyses the dephosphorylation of 5′-nucleotides to produce the corresponding nucleosides, and has been reviewed recently with reference to its role as a biochemical marker enzyme [120]. It is expressed in many human tissues but only in some lymphocytes [121]. The activity of this ezyme was recently found to be greater in peripheral B cells than in peripheral T cells [122]. In addition, lymphocytes of patients with some forms of hypogammaglobulinemia have been reported to have reduced amounts of 5′-N [122]. A decrease of 5′-N activity in lymphocytes has been noted in studies on chronic lymphocytic leukemia [120, 121, 123] and on ALL with T cell characteristics [120, 124]. In contrast, surprisingly high 5′-N activities were recorded on ALL blasts with common ALL antigen and in lymphoid blast crisis of chronic myelogenous leukemia, whereas acute myeloid leukemia and CALLA-negative blast crisis of CML are correlated with decrease of enzyme activity on the blast cells [120, 125].

Thus, determination of 5′-N activity represents an additional highly reproducible enzyme marker for the distinction of myeloid and lymphoid blasts in CML, which can easily be tested even in material containing dead cells [125]. The finding of high 5′-N in 15 patients with lymphoid blast crisis among 44 patients with blast crisis of CML [125] has been confirmed by others in four cases of lymphoid blast crisis among nine patients with blastic CML [126]. Elevated serum-5′-N activity was frequently observed in common ALL with elevated cellular 5′-N activity [120]. There was, however, no correlation between cellular enzyme activity and serum-5′-N activity [120]. 5′-N-specific antisera strongly inhibited the 5′-N activity of leukemia cells, whereas the 5′-N activity was not affected by incubation with anti-CALL sera [125]. Thus, 5′-N and CALLA are different immunoreactive proteins which are expressed on different sites of the cell membrane of CALLA-positive blast cells [125]. A partial or complete absence of the two other purine-pathway enzymes, *adenosine deaminase (ADA)* and *purine nucleoside phosphorylase (PNP)* has been linked with characteristic immunodeficiencies [127–129]. Hypo- and agammaglobulinemia have also been reported to be linked with a deficiency of the third purine-pathway enzyme, the above-mentioned 5′-N [122, 130, 131]. *ADA,* which irreversible converts adenosine to inosine and deoxyadenosine to deoxyinosine, is essential for differentiation of lymphoid cells, particularly T cells. ADA activity reflects both the T cell or B cell origin of a cell population and its degree of maturation. ADA levels are higher in thymocytes than in unstimulated mature T cells, which have greater activity than peripheral B cells [132]. Normal or low levels of ADA have been observed in B cell ALL [133], chronic lymphocytic leukemia [132] multiple myeloma, and hairy cell leukemia [134], whereas relatively high enzyme activities were measured in non-T, non-B ALL [133]. Though distinctive patterns of ADA activity become evident in various lymphoproliferative diseases, this enzyme appears not to be so sensitive as 5′-N or TdT. However, the development of specific inhibitors of ADA suggests an avenue for selective chemotherapy. Preliminary work in phase I and II studies with one such inhibitor, 2′-deoxycoformycin, has already demonstrated that this drug is active against ALL [135].

Purine nucleoside phosphorylase (PNP) acts sequentially with ADA in purine metabolism, reversibly converting purine nucleosides, including inosine, guanosine, and their deoxy analogs to their corresponding purine bases. Complete and partial deficiencies of this enzyme have been associated with inherited defects in T cell function [128, 129]. PNP activity has also been reported to be lower in normal and immature cells of the T cell axis than in normal blood T cells. However, these decreases are not as profound as those noted for 5′-N. Although neither normal B lymphocytes nor chronic lymphocytic leukemia cells stain histochemically for PNP [136], enzymatic measurement has demonstrated that lymphoblastoid lines of B cell origin and non-T, non-B lymphoblasts have a range of PNP activity comparable to that of normal peripheral T cells [115].

Lysosomal Enzymes, Acid Phosphatase, and Lysozyme

Lysosomal enzymes have been useful in identifying hematopoietic cells, particularly normal phagocytes. *Hexosaminidase* is one of the lysosomal acid hydrolases and occurs as three isozymes (A, I, or B) that have characteristic profiles in normal granulocytes, lymphocytes, and thymocytes. The isoenzyme pattern, determined either by ion-exchange chromatography or by isoelectric focusing, has been reported by two groups to be useful in distinguishing immunologic types of ALL [137, 138]. Elevated levels have been found in common ALL and in some cases of null ALL, but not in T-ALL or B-ALL.

Absolute levels and isozyme patterns of other lysosomal enzymes have also been useful in defining subtypes of leukemia and lymphoma. The *acid phosphatase* reaction may be

Table 1. Human hematopoietic cell markers for leukemic cell analysis[a]

	Specific/selective for[b]	Problems/cross-reaction with[b]
1. Immunologic markers		
Immunoglobulin (SIg, cIg)	B, Pre-B, P	Passively adsorbed/internalized Ig
B cell antigens	B	M, varying specificity
Mouse E rosettes	B subset	–
Ia-like antigens	B, early hem. prec.	T subset, activated T
Sheep E rosettes	T	Sensitive for artefacts
T cell antigens	T	Weak antisera, varying specificity
Myelomonocytic antigens	G, M	Varying reactions with G, M
Glycophorin A	E	–
Common ALL antigen	Early L	–
2. Biochemical enzyme markers		
Terminal deoxynucleotidyl transferase (TdT)	Early L	Some early myeloid prec.
5′-Nucleotidase (5′-N)	Early L, B	Only selective by activity
Hexosaminidase isoenzyme I	Early L	G
Adenosine deaminase (ADA)	T	Only selective by activity
Muramidase (Lysozyme)	G, M	Ubiquitous except L
3. Cytochemical markers		
Myeloperoxidase	G	–
Platelet peroxidase	Pl	–
Naphtol-AS-acetate esterase, inhibition by NaF	M	–
Acid phosphatase	T blasts	G, P

[a] For details and references see text section: „Conventional“ Cell Surface Markers

[b] *B*, B lymphocytes; *T*, T lymphocytes; *P*, plasma cells; *M*, monocytes, macrophages; *L*, lymphocytes; *G*, granulocytes; *E*, erythrocytes; *Pl*, platelets; *hem. prec.*, hematopoietic precursor cells

positive in cells of T cell lineage, including T lymphoblasts, phytohemagglutinin-transformed normal lymphocytes, Sézary cells, and the atypical lymphocytes of patients with infectious mononucleosis, as well as T cell-dependent areas of spleen and lymph nodes [139, 140]. Acid phosphatase is absent in most cases of chronic lymphocytic leukemia, although a form resistant to tartrate has been found in the malignant cells of several patients with chronic B cell lymphocytic leukemia and leukemic reticuloendotheliosis [139]. A strong focal positivity in a paranuclear distribution has been shown to be characteristic for T cell ALL [140]. Similarly, *acid α-naphthyl esterase (ANAE)* is present in mature T cells and in T lymphoblasts in acute lymphocytic leukemia [141], although the specificity of this enzyme as a marker for the T axis has been questioned. It also occurs in some cases of common ALL [141].

Lysozyme, alternatively termed muramidase, is an enzyme present in certain human secretions such as tears, saliva, and breast-milk, and in certain cells, most notably granulocytes and cells of the monocyte/histiocyte series. Among mononuclear cells, therefore, detection of cytoplasmic lysozyme is indicative of the histiocytic or monocytic nature of the cell, for lymphocytes are not known to contain this enzyme. High levels of serum and urinary lysozyme have been found in patients with monocytic or myelomonocytic leukemia [142].

Information on the markers discussed is summarized in Table 1.

Monoclonal Antibodies Against Lymphocyte Differentiation Antigens

As a consequence of the various immunological cell markers of different specificity or relative selectivity discussed in the last section, it is of the utmost importance to rely on a suitable set of markers to accomplish an exact immunodiagnosis of a certain cell type with reference to cell lineage and maturation. For this purpose, specific antisera have so far been the mainstay of diagnostic management.

Thus the key to the immunodiagnosis of certain cell types depends upon the availability of heteroantisera directed against stable cell surface antigens. Traditionally prepared antisera have to be rendered specific by extensive absorption procedures. Given the diversity of the immune response and the complexity of the absorption procedure, it is difficult to reproduce such antibodies with identical specificity. Since the serum supply from one animal is naturally limited, antisera of this type are not normally used by more than a few laboratories.

Advantages and Problems of Monoclonal Antibodies

It appears that essentially all the problems associated with classic heteroantisera were solved with the introduction of the antibody-producing hybridoma technology of Köhler and Milstein [4]. With this technique immune mouse B lymphocytes are fused with myeloma cells. The resultant cell hybrids retain both the antibody-producing capacity of the B lymphocyte and the capacity for indefinite growth of the myeloma line, so that after cloning there may be an immortal cell line producing high concentrations of antibody of a single molecular species. Besides the advantage of uniformity, precision, and unlimited supply, a second merit of the technique becomes evident: antibodies against minor determinants that are hidden in conventional polyclonal antisera can be prepared in pure form by the appropriate selection procedure even though nonpurified antigens have been used for immunization. Thus renewed interest has arisen in achieving further characterization of differentiation antigens of human lymphopoiesis and in lymphatic malignancies.

The use of monoclonal antibodies (mAbs) in studies of human lymphocytes, leukemia, and lymphoma is rapidly expanding, and it is beyond the scope of this chapter to provide a comprehensive review of this field. The published proceedings of a recent conference on this subject will give access to more information [5]. Since the great majority of papers published to date deal with mAbs against antigens on lymphoid cells a somewhat arbitrary selection was necessary, which focuses on the results with well established and widely used mAbs, most of which are already commercially available.

Before a discussion of some of the mAbs which recognize differentiation antigens of human lymphocytes, a few general remarks concerning the interpretation of reactions with mAbs should be made. Since mAbs are directed against restricted determinant(s) or epitope(s) of an antigenic macromolecule, their reaction can be influenced in several ways.

Cross-reactions by epitopic identity may occur more frequently than expected and lead to erroneous interpretations. One example that stands for many others is the cross-reaction of mAbs against T cells with Purkinje neurons of various species [143]. *Genetic polymorphism* can explain some negative reactions, as evidence in some rare cases of polymorphism of OKT4 antigen on human inducer T cells [144]. *Cryptic epitope expression* or *loss of epitope* must also be taken into account for negative reactions, especially in malignancy. This is exemplified in Table 2, where the mAb BS-1 directed against kappa light chain antigen did not react with the leukemia cells of one patient among ten with kappa light chains, despite its good staining of the other nine leukemia cell samples. Also, some *technical problems* have to be considered: mAbs will not usually precipitate their target antigen because they can only cross-link antigens into dimers rather than form a lattice – hence the failure of Ouchterlony assays. Classic antisera fix complement more readily than do mAbs because complement requires at least two bound antibody molecules on neighbouring determinants [145]. One way of solving these problems is to use suitable blends of mAbs. For both precipitation and cytotoxicity it has been shown that a mixture of two mAbs is sufficient [145]. Some mAbs, however, do not fix complement at all, such as OKT5, which is IgGl, whereas OKT3, OKT4, and OKT8 fall in the IgG2 subclass and do fix complement [146, 147].

Differentiation Pathways and Tissue Distribution of Human T Cells

The most widely used anti-T mAbs are grouped according to reaction pattern in Table 3. It is obvious that most of the currently used anti-T mAbs (and a large number of others) can easily be allocated to one of these groups. It is already becoming clear that the various mAbs raised in different laboratories identify the same molecular structure, though possibly via different epitopes. Similar experiences have recently been reported at workshop held in Paris, where the anti-T mAbs were grouped in clusters.

Thymus immunophysiology has been studied extensively in animal models and to a lesser extent in humans, but it is beyond the scope of this paper to review all aspects of human thymocyte differentiation. Only a summary of recent information derived from the use of selected anti-T mAbs will be given (see Table 3). Studies in both rodents and humans have demonstrated that thymocytes originate from bone marrow precursor cells which migrate to the thymus [148]. Ninety percent of thymocytes are found in the cortex, while the remaining 10% are in the thymic medulla. Cortical thymocytes consist of a major

Table 2. Reaction pattern of monoclonal antibodies against Bence-Jones proteins with chronic lymphocytic leukemia (CLL) cells of B type

	No. of cases tested	No. of cases positive with		
		BS-1[b]	BS-3[b]	BS-4[b]
CLL K + λ − [a]	10	9	10	0
CLL K − λ + [a]	7	0	0	7

[a] As defined by FITC-labeled F $(ab')_2$ fragments of polyclonal goat antibodies (Kallestadt; Dacko)

[b] MAbs against Bence-Jones proteins of kappa type (BS-1, BS-3) or of lambda type (BS-4) (Biotest)

population of small E-rosette-positive thymocytes and a minor subcapsular population of large, rapidly dividing E-rosette-negative cells. The latter cells are regarded as thymic precursor cells and have been designated prothymocytes [149, 150]. There may be a correlation between them and the stage I thymocytes described by Reinherz et al. [151], and they may express OKT10 and OKT9 (see Table 3). Since subcapsular prothymocytes are the most rapidly dividing cells in the thymus, reactivity of these cells with OKT9 can probably be explained on this basis. Surprisingly, the common ALL antigen (CALLA) has recently been demonstrated on some clusters of subcapsular thymocytes [152], but the simultaneous expression of T differentiation antigens on these cells has not yet been determined. Stage II (common) thymocytes, found primarily in the thymic cortex, express the E receptor and, likewise, react with OKT11 and Lyt 3. More importantly, most of the cortical thymocytes strongly express the human thymocyte antigen (HTAl) as recognized by NA1/34 and OKT6. The expression of this antigen on thymocytes appears to be reciprocal to HLA, as recognized by the mAb W6/32 [153]. Some common thymocytes simultaneously display OKT4, 5, and 8 antigens. Also, the other antigens of groups II, III, IV, and V of Table 3 appear in this stage. In addition, rosette formation with rabbit red blood cells characterizes the transitional stage from common to mature thymocytes, as shown by double marker analysis with mAbs [154]. Stage III (mature) thymocytes are represented by cells in the thymic medulla. They acquire HLA-ABC antigens [155] and OKT3, lose HTA-1, and reciprocally express OKT4 and OKT5/OKT8. In the extrathymic periphery, OKT 4+, OKT5/8− cells predominate in peripheral blood, tonsil, and lymph node paracortex, and intestinal lamina propria [156]. In contrast, OKT5/8+, OKT4− cells predominate in normal human bone marrow and gut ephithelium [156]. It was previously reported that human bone marrow T cells mediate primarily suppressor activity for in vitro B cell differentiation [157]. The T cell phenotype of bone marrow T cells as recently described [156] is consistent with this finding. Furthermore, a close association has been noted between OKT4+, OKT5/8− T cells and Ia+ tissue macrophages and interdigitating cells [156]. The multiple data regarding distinct in vitro functional capabilities of T cell subsets are important and suggest the existence of discrete functional T cell substrains. The data regarding tissue distribution of subsets of T cells are particularly compelling and imply that various subsets of T cells may have different immunological functions in vivo as well.

Comparative Phenotypic Characterization of Human Malignant T Cells

Using essentially the same selected anti-T cell mAbs as outlined in Table 3, many investigators have determined the phenotype of the dominant clone in T cell malignancies of acute and chronic diseases. All authors agree that an unexpected heterogeneity among certain particular leukemic subclasses becomes evident when a battery of monoclonal anti-T cell antibodies is used.

If the composite phenotypes of leukemic cells from individual patients are assembled in a presumptive sequence of T lymphocyte differentiation (see Table 4), the first cell in line would be of prothymocyte phenotype, without the E receptor but already displaying T cell differentiation antigens. This incomplete T cell phenotype has been observed in some *acute lymphoblastic leukemias (ALL)* with the aid of conventional anti-T cell sera. This subgroup, tentatively designated "pre-T-ALL", has been shown to differ from the other non-T- and T-ALL groups clinically and prognostically [158]. The distinction of a pre-T cell ALL subgroup can, in our experience, also be made with mAbs OKT10, Leu-1, and Lyt-2 [158]. This pre-T-ALL phenotype has recently been confirmed by another group by demonstration of positivity for Leu-1 and negativity for E receptor and B cell mAbs [159].

Several studies have demonstrated that most of the T-ALL phenotypes correspond to an early common thymocyte type (mostly stage II type) [146, 160, 162]. The most immature T cell ALL type may correspond to a common thymocyte already displaying the E receptor and OKT11, Lyt-3, or Leu-5 reactivity in addition to OKT10. A good correlation with the predominating common thymocyte type is indicated by HTA-1 (OKT6, NA1/34) on the majority of T-ALL samples, which sometimes also display OKT4 and OKT8 simultaneously. More mature T cell ALL types correspond to a thymic cell expressing OKT3 without HTA-1 (OKT6, NA1/34). Interestingly, *lymphoblastic lymphoma* (LL) cells of T type were exclusively of later thymic phenotype (Nos. 3 and 4 in Table 4) in three studies [159, 160, 162].

It should be emphasized, however, that any phenotypic categorization such as is provided in Table 3 is likely to be an oversimplification, since the true extent of heterogeneity may be greater than can be accomodated by any such scheme. Also, the phenotypic features of cells from some patients studied do not coincide clearly with the common or expected characteristics.

Amongst the most interesting of these are cases of thymic ALL that were TdT negative, some mature T cell leukemias with expression of OKT10, and T-ALL with strong expression of HLA-ABC [162, 163]. In marked contrast to T-ALL, in all the *chronic T leukemias,* i.e. Sézary lymphoma/leukemia, chronic lymphocytic leukemia of T type (T-CLL), and lymphoblastic lymphomas of T type in elderly patients the cells have mature T cell phenotypes [162, 164]. Practically all examples of cutaneous T cell lymphoma (mycosis fungoides, Sézary's syndrome) studied were exclusively of helper T4+/T8,5−) phenotype, as were other cases of lymphoblastic lymphoma/leukemia with marked skin involvement [162, 164, 165]. This phenotype correlated well with earlier studies which showed that Sézary cells function as helper cells [166]. In contrast, chronic lymphocytic leukemia cells of T type (T-CLL) were mostly of suppressor (T4−/T8+) phenotype and less often of helper type [159, 164]. Interestingly, in some rare cases antibody-dependent cellular cytotoxicity (ADCC) was demonstrated, which corresponded to the Tγ phenotype (E-receptor-positive, IgG-FcR-positive) of the leukemia cells [167, 168]. Those cases illustrate that a T lineage status can be assumed for a lymphocyte subset of Tγ type with suppressor and K cell activity. The cell lineage of a leukemia with natural killer cell (NK) activity appears to be equivocal, since a reaction with OKM1 (specific for myelomonocytic

Table 3. Monoclonal antibodies reactive with human T lymphocytes and thymocytes

Group	Designation (clone)	Source[a]	Reactivity pattern	Molecular weight of antigen (daltons)	References
I	OKT3, UCHT1 (T28)	O, –	Pan peripheral T	19,000, 19,000	[190, 191]
II	OKT11, Lyt 3 (9.6) Leu 5	O, NEN, BD	Pan T, E-rosette receptor associated	55,000, 55,000	[192–194]
III	OKT1, Leu 1 (L17F12) Lyt 2 (10.2)	O, BD, NEN	Pan T and B-CLL	66,000, 67,000, 67,000	[182, 190, 195]
IV	OKT4, Leu 3a	O, BD	Inducer/helper T	62,000, 55,000	[145, 196]
V	OKT5, OKT8, Leu 2a	O, O, BD	Cytotoxic/suppressor T	33,000, 33,000, 32,000	[146, 150, 196]
VI	MAS 036 (NA1/34) OKT6	S, O	Cortical thymocytes	49,000 49,000	[150, 152]
VII	OKT10	O	Pan thymocyte[b]	37,000	[150]

[a] Commercially available from: *BD*, Becton Dickinson; *NEN*, New England Nuclear; *O*, Ortho Pharm. Co.; *S*, Serolab
[b] Not restricted to thymocytes, reactive with activated T lymphocytes and hematopoietic precursor cells

Table 4. T cell leukemia phenotypes in relation to the framework of normal T cell differentiation

Cell type	Tissue	Markers[a]							Clinical diagnosis
		OKT10	OKT6 NA1/34	OKT3 UCHT1	OKT5 OKT8 Leu 2a	OKT4 Leu 3a	HUTLA Leu 1 Lyt 2	E-R OKT11 Lyt 3	
T precursors									
1. Early/prethymic	Subcapsular thymus	+	–	–	–	–	+	–	Pre-T-ALL
2. Common thymic, immature	Thymus cortex	+	–	–	–	–	+	–	T-ALL
3. Common thymic	Thymus cortex	+	+	–	+	+	+	+	T-ALL, T-NHL
4. Mature thymic	Thymus medulla	+	–	+	+	+	+	+	T-NHL
Mature T									
5. Mature T, inducer/helper	Peripheral compartment	–	–	+	–	+	+	+	Sézary S, T-CLL
6. Mature T, suppressor	Peripheral compartment	–	–	+	+	–	+	+	T-CLL

[a] See Table 2. HUTLA is defined by a polyclonal T cell-specific absorbed antithymocyte serum [29, 157]

cells) [214] has been demonstrated besides the Tγ phenotype [168]. Strong reactions with OKT3 and OKT8, however, were indicators of some T maturation in this case. The hybrid phenotype (T lymphocytic/myelomonocytic) of leukemias with NK activity was best demonstrated by raising mAbs against such a leukemia [169]. Two different kinds of mAbs resulted: one reacting with T8 cells, one staining granulocytes. Thus a combined monocyte and T cell lineage of those NK leukemia cells was confirmed, and the leukemia phenotype helped to identify normal counterpart cells with the same phenotype and NK cell function [169]. T cell antigens were lacking on a cell line with NK cell activity established from a child with ALL: the leukemia cells were of Tγ type, positive for OKM1 and asialo GM1, but negative with all mAbs against T cells [170]. Apart from one other example of an ALL case where the leukemic cells after preculturing with normal T cells became potent inhibitors of immunoglobulin production of PWM-stimulated normal B cells [171], all examples of leukemic cells with reported functional activity have been observed in chronic diseases. A phenotype of advanced T maturation (reactive with groups IV and V of Table 2) mostly correlated with the retained function of the leukemic clone.

It is noteworthy that the recent findings of human T cell leukemia/lymphoma virus (HTLV) were always associated with chronic and mostly cutaneous T cell lymphoma cases recognized in the endemic areas of Japan, the Caribbean, and the southeastern United States [172, 173]. It is also interesting to note that mature fetal T lymphocytes are the cells most readily transfected with virus when cocultivation techniques are performed [172]. This indicates that the major phenotypes documented in different leukemias represent the level of maturation arrest imposed on the dominant subclone, and that this is determined by the target cell and associated clonogenic cell population in the leukemia/lymphoma (see section: *Target Cell for Malignant Transformation and Leukemia Phenotype*).

B Cell Leukemia/Lymphoma Phenotypes in Relation to the Framework of Normal B Cell Differentiation

A number of mAbs reacting with human B cells have been described, and some widely used ones are given in Table 5. Our list includes antibodies that are not B cell specific but nevertheless show selective reactivity within the B cell lineage. Ia antigens are present on B lymphocytes but not on plasma cells (see section: B Cell Antigens and Ia-like (HLA-DR) antigens). Many mAbs that react with Ia antigens have been produced. Most of them react with nonpolymorphic determinants, but some react with *HLA-DR*-associated polymorphic antigens. The latter may be useful for tissue typing and the former are used for phenotyping; two examples are given in Table 4. MAbs reacting with B cells in blood or secondary lymphoid tissue are of some diagnostic value. MAbs B1 and B2 show an interesting difference in their reactivity with blood B cells and B cells in lymph nodes [174, 175]. FMC1 can be used in enumerating B cells and generally parallels SIg as a B cell marker [176], whereas FMC7 reacts with a B cell subpopulation and is useful in distinguishing prolymphocytic leukemia (PLL) from CLL [177, 178]. Tü-1 shows an even more restricted distribution, being found almost exclusively on germinal-center B cells and some B cell malignancies [179]. BA-1 reacts with all B cells including ALL cells of pre-B type, but also reacts with mature granulocytes [180].

In Table 6 a simplified B cell maturation scheme is used as a framework against which to compare the mAbs with surface and cytoplasmic Ig expression. Cells with differentiation from the progenitor stem cell are considered to be committed to the B lineage when rearrangements of immunoglobulin *(Ig)* genes have been initiated, since these are

Table 5. Monoclonal antibodies reactive with human B lymphocytes, with common ALL antigen (CALLA), or with Ia (HLA-DR) antigens

Designation (clone)	Source[a]	Reaction with	References
BA-1	H	All B cells	[179]
B1, FMC1	C,–	All blood B cells	[173, 175]
B2	C	Tissue B cells	[174]
FMC7	–	B cell subpopulation	[176]
Tü 1	B	Germinal center B cells	[178]
J5, VIL-A1, BA-3	C, NEN, H	gp 100/CALLA	[197–199]
OKIa 1, L243	O, BD	Ia(p28, 33), monomorphic HLA-DR	[190, 200]

[a] Commercially available from: *BD*, Becton Dickinson; *B*, Biotest; *C*, Coulter; *H*, Hybritech Inc.; *NEN*, New England Nuclear; *O*, Ortho Pharm. Co.

characteristic of the B lineage [181]. Rearranged *Ig* heavy chain genes are detected in the majority of *common ALL* (cALL) cases but not in T-ALL. Thus, the CALLA+ cell type prior to the expression of cytoplasmic μ is taken as a pre-pre-B cell, which is mostly BA-1 or B1 positive, but can be induced to become B1 positive [182]. The next cell type in line, also inducible by in vitro treatment of cALL cells with phorbol diester, is the "true" pre-B cell type with cytoplasmic μ. The virgin or early B cell phenotype as characterized by CALLA, weak cytoplasmic and surface IgM heavy chains without light chains, is a transitional stage of development between pre-B and B cells. A cell line of this early B cell type has recently been established [161]. All these pre-B cell types reside in the bone marrow. Some cross-reactions with anti-T cell mAbs (Group III, Table 2) even occur at this early stage [161]. A cross-reacting T 65,000-dalton antigen has been shown to be weakly expressed on *chronic lymphocytic leukemia* (CLL) cells of B type [183, 184]. The same cell phenotype, with weak expression of Slg, excess light chains, and weak T 65, has recently been identified in some infrequent B lymphocytes in the normal human tonsil and lymph nodes [185]. These putative early memory cells also rosette mouse erythrocytes, in contrast to *prolymphocytic leukemia* (PLL) cells. This cell type is also derived from the medullary cord, has a higher density of Slg than CLL cells, has Ia, BA-1, and B1 antigens, and reacts strongly with the FCM 7 mAb, while cells from CLL patients bind this antibody only exceptionally [178]. *Hairy cell leukemia* (HCL) cells also stain with FCM 7, but they have a low percentage of mouse erythrocyte rosettes and only 20% react with BA-1.

Nodular or follicular lymphomas most probably represent a neoplastic proliferation of lymph node follicular-center B lymphocytes. This cell type, which is often small and cleaved, has high-density monoclonal Slg and, unlike CLL cells, a low percentage of mouse rosette formation. BA-1, B1, and mostly B2 antigens are expressed, and especially Tü-1, which is expressed almost exclusively on germinal-center B cells. Furthermore, maturation from primary to secondary follicles is accompanied by changes in the relative expression of B1 and B2. Finally B cells can be stimulated to differentiate into plasma cells, the functional end cells of the B lineage. Malignant B cells found in Waldenström's macroglobulinemia, heavy chain disease, and multiple myeloma may represent a further stage in the maturation of medullary cord B cells. Cells from patients with *Waldenström's macroglobulinemia,* like CLL cells, express monoclonal Slg, Ia, and B1 antigens. Unlike CLL cells, however, these cells do not express the B2 antigen or rosette with mouse erythrocytes, but sometimes already have cytoplasmic Ig of complete type with light chains,

Table 6. B cell leukemia-lymphoma in relation to the framework of normal B cell differentiation

Cell type	Tissue	Markers[b]									Clinical diagnosis
		CALLA	Cytopl. Ig	Surface Ig	BA-1	B1	B2	FMC1	FMC7	Tü1	
1. Pre-Pre B	Bone marrow	+	–[a]	–	+	+	–	–	–	–	C-ALL
2. Pre-B	Bone marrow	+	+μ	–	+	+	+	–	–	–	Pre-B ALL
3. Virgin/early B	Bone marrow	(+)	–	+μ	+	+	ND	ND	ND	–	Pre-B-ALL
4. B blast	Periphery	–	–	+μ, k, λ	+	+	ND	+	ND	–	B-ALL, Burkitt-like NHL
5. B 1 cell	Lymph node	–	–	+μδ kλ	+	+	+	+	–	+	B-CLL
6. B 2 cell	Lymph node	–	–	+μδ kλ	+	+	+	+	–	+	B-NHL follicular
7. Prolymphocyte	Lymph node	–	–	+μδ kλ	+	+	ND	–	+	–	B-PLL, B-HCL
8. Lymphoplasmo-cytoid	Lymph node	–	+μk	+μδ kλ	+	+	–	ND	ND	ND	Waldenström's macroglobulinemia
9. Plasma cell	Bone marrow/periphery	–	+γkλ	–	–	–	–	ND	ND	ND	Multiple myeloma

[a] Gene rearrangement for μ chains detectable [34]
[b] See Table 4

like myeloma cells. *Myeloma cells* have cytoplasmic Ig but usually lack SIg, the B1, B2, BA-1, and Ia antigens. They do not form rosettes with mouse erythrocytes. Interestingly, myeloma cells stain intensively with OKT10. It should be noted that several mAbs detect antigens present on most cells of the B lineage, but none encompasses the entire maturation sequence. None of the mAbs described so far is restricted to stem cells or the B-committed progenitor. This probably reflects the screening panels that have been used to detect the reactive mAbs. Screening on a panel of tumors including new tumors, or functional screening may provide new answers.

Current Status of Clinical Utility of Monoclonal Antibodies Against Lymphocytes

Experiments with mAbs provide some insight into the basic biology of hematopoietic malignancy differentiation. The panel of mAbs listed in Tables 3 and 5 allows determination of the composite phenotypes of various T and B cell malignancies, and there is a clear association between clinical/hematological subgroup and the maturity of B or T cell phenotype. Obviously, the composite phenotype of leukemia cells can be interpreted as an indicator of the leukemia-"specific" maturation arrest or as an indicator of the target cell for malignant transformation. "Target cell" and "associated clonogenic cell population" may not necessarily be synonymous, as best evidenced in the situation of CALLA-positive lymphoid blast crisis in CML, where the leukemia is derived from a pluripotential stem cell. In contrast, CALLA-positive common ALL probably reflects the malignant transformation of B lineage-committed precursor cells, since cALL very rarely transforms intraclonally to AML and never to T-ALL (see section: Target Cell and Maturation Arrest of the Clonogenic Cell Population) [186]. Besides the information relating to target cell and maturation arrest of leukemias, mAbs appear to be useful for studies of maturation induction in vitro (see section: Modulation of Leukemic cell Phenotype. In Vitro [187]). Hereby, changes of cell phenotype during maturation can best be monitored by means of mAbs.

Some more direct or practical applications of mAbs to patient management can also be considered. These include differential diagnosis, serial monitoring, and immunotherapy. Cell type-specific mAbs directed against unique structures, e.g., gp 100 CALL antigen, have replaced conventional sera. The main categories of lymphatic leukemias that were defined with conventional markers can easily be diagnosed by anyone with essential mAbs. This has been illustrated in ALL, where T/pre-T-ALL, common ALL including pre-B-All, B-ALL, and null ALL (see section: Diagnostic Value of Immunologic Markers for Classification of Nonmyeloid Leukemias) can also be classified by using mAbs [159, 186, 188]. In addition, new subsets in between the T or cALL subgroups become evident [151, 162, 189]. The clinical usefulness of such subclassification with mAbs was recently demonstrated in children with non-T ALL [189]. Clinical features such as splenomegaly and high white blood cell counts (WBC) were significantly related to BA-1- and CALLA-negative children, and high WBC was less significant than phenotype in predicting outcome.

Since cell differentiation is associated with topographical compartmentalization of cells (see Tables 4 and 6), mAbs detecting differentiation-linked features may have an operational leukemia specificity when applied to certain tissues. Good examples are the detection of cells expressing the gp 100/CALLA or the common thymocyte antigen HTA-1 in blood, cerebrospinal fluid, or testicular biopsies. It remains to be shown whether serial tests of this kind, which now include mAbs, have a therapeutic impact.

Finally, mAbs have a potential in therapy, e.g., for serotherapy, for targeting of drugs, toxins, and radioisotopes in vivo, or cell selection in vitro prior to allogeneic or autologous marrow transplantation. This perhaps most interesting and innovative clinical aspect has already been pursued by many investigators, as recently reviewed [190]. Many obstacles limiting the use of mAbs in vivo must be considered, and such specific factors as circulating antigen, antigenic modulation, and reactivity of mAbs with normal cells have been identified that result in the development of resistance to antibody-mediated lysis in vivo. Current research is now being directed towards developing methods of circumventing these obstacles. Many of the obstacles limiting the use of mAbs in vivo may be circumvented through carefully controlled use of these reagents in vitro. In a manipulated environment, blocking factors can be removed, modulation can be inhibited, human complement can be replaced by more active rabbit complement, and the total number of cells eliminated can be controlled.

This potential has already been studied in relapsed CALLA-positive ALL by using ex vivo marrow treatment with J5 following ablative chemotherapy prior to autologous retransplantation, and in ex vivo marrow conditioning for allogeneic bone marrow transplantation by eliminating T lymphocytes with mAbs.

Although it is too early to draw any conclusions, preliminary results are encouraging. In the near future mAbs may prove to be an additional important therapeutic modality for patients with hematopoietic malignancy.

Monoclonal Antibodies Against Granulocytes, Monocytes, Erythrocytes, and Platelets

Nonlymphatic cell elements of the hematopoietic tissue are still primarily classified according to their morphological appearance and histochemical reactivity. Accordingly, the most widely used FAB classification of acute leukemias is based essentially on morphological criteria with cytochemical staining [202]. This classification distinguishes subgroups of myeloid leukemia cells that appear to correlate with specific states of differentiation and maturation of their normal cellular counterparts. Although later stages of myeloid maturation are readily identifiable by changes in morphology and histochemistry, the detailed study of early myeloid differentiation and the diagnosis of poorly differentiated myeloid leukemias has been difficult because of their lack of distinctive morphological or biochemical features. The immunological identification of specific surface antigens of myeloid cells may be helpful in this situation. In addition, a standardization of diagnosis may also be achieved in leukemias, where morphological signs of maturation are recognizable according to subjective criteria.

Differentiation Antigens of Myelopoiesis and of Myeloid Leukemias

Several investigators have described heteroantisera, mostly from rabbits, that react with granulocytes, monocytes, and acute myelogenous leukemia cells [203–206]. While the myelomonocytic antigens described are not leukemia specific, they may be useful in distinguishing myeloid and lymphoid leukemias. The less pronounced expression on immature myeloid cells [203, 204], however, limits their usefulness.

A number of monoclonal antibodies that react with myeloid cells have been described as reviewed recently [20]. Some of these antibodies are restricted to granulocytes [208, 210] or to monocytes [211, 212], while others react with both [213–215]. The one that reacts with

both, i.e., OKM1 [215], also reacts with platelets and a subset of T cells. Although most of these reagents clearly distinguish myeloid from lymphoid leukemias, some may distinguish the granulocyte subtypes of AML (M1, M2, and M3) from the monocytic subtypes (M4 and M5) as defined by FAB criteria; the monocytic antibodies Mol and 63D3, for example, react predominantly with M4 and M5 [211, 212], whereas the granulocyte-reactive antibodies My-1 and VIMD5 stain the M1, M2, and M3 subgroups [208, 209].
It must be emphasized, however, that in some relatively immature myeloid leukemias of M1 type no staining by monoclonal antibodies is available. This situation resembles that described in earlier reports when conventional heterologous antigranulocyte antisera were used for AML diagnosis. A monoclonal antibody which is specific for or reacts predominantly with the earliest myeloid differentiation stage up to CFUc does not yet exist. The My7 antibody, which is reported to react with 79% of all AML patients tested [213], appears to at least partly fulfill the desire to have a myeloblast-directed monoclonal antibody. Up to now, the determination of ultrastructural peroxidase appears to be more sensitive [216], but its application is hampered by its technical complexity.

Erythroid Membrane Antigens and Erythroid Lineage Leukemias

The introduction of antisera against a major sialoglycoprotein of erythrocytes, namely glycophorin A, has provided a specific marker of the erythroid cell lineage [217]. It has been suggested that immature erythroleukemias diagnosed incorrectly as AML (M1) or even ALL can be identified with glycophorin A [217]. With the aid of monoclonal antibodies to glycophorin and band 3 [218], the expression of these antigenic determinants during normal erythroid [219, 220] differentiation and in acute leukemia has been investigated. Surprisingly, neither the band 3 nor glycophorin determinants were detected on erythroid precursor cells provided in BFU-E and CFU-E culture techniques [219]. Thus, the glycophorin expression can be suggested to happen at a post-CFU-E stage of erythroid ontogeny. Accordingly, acute leukemias of a very early maturation arrest, i.e., at the BFU-E/CFU-E equivalent level, would probably not be readily detectable by glycophorin antisera. Indeed, only a very small number of acute leukemias (7 of 157 ALL/AUL plus 105 AML) which were not diagnosed as erythroleukemias were also glycophorin positive [220]. Interestingly, the Ph^1-positive myelogenous cell line K562, which has been established from a patient in blast crisis of CML [221], has been shown to be reactive with anti-glycophorin [222]. In keeping with this, erythroid developmental potential has been demonstrated in this cell line [222].

Platelet Antigens and Megakaryoblastic Leukemias

Megakaryoblastic leukemia as a malignant transformation of platelet precursors is probably relatively rare, although cases have been recorded. Thus, no special category has been provided for this leukemia type in such classifications as that produced by the FAB group. In a considerable proportion of Ph^1-positive CML in blast crisis, a dominant subclone in maturation arrest at the small megakaryoblast level of differentiation has been demonstrated by platelet peroxidase staining and electron microscopy [223]. Recently, a monoclonal antibody (AN51) restricted in its pattern of reactivity to platelets has been described [224]. In initial studies, a minor AN51-positive population of blast cells has been detected in 4 of 16 patients tested with blast cell crisis of CML [220]. In only 1 of 60 cases of lymphoblastic/undifferentiated leukemia tested was a major AN51-positive population present [220]. So far, the more sensitive demonstration of platelet peroxidase by electron microscopy should be reserved for the apparently nonmyeloid leukemias with negative lymphoid immunologic markers.

Clinical Relevance of Leukemic Cell Phenotypes

The introduction of immunologic cell markers for diagnosis of the underlying malignant cell phenotype has allowed greater objectivity in the classification of acute and chronic forms of the clinical entity of leukemia. It was tempting to speculate that characteristic clinical signs would emerge for immunologically defined subgroups of leukemia that were formerly assigned to a group of leukemias collected according to morphological criteria alone and not admitting of any finer classification. In the meantime, clinical peculariaties concerning presentation signs and – even more important – response to therapy have been linked with some leukemia or lymphoma subtypes as defined by immunologic criteria. Examples of this in chronic lymphocytic leukemia, acute lymphocytic leukemia, and blast cell crisis of chronic myelogenous leukemia are given below.

Clinical Significance of T-Cell Chronic Lymphatic Leukemia Subtypes

The recognition of a T cell variant of chronic lymphocytic leukemia (CLL) defines a rare subgroup of CLL occurring in fewer than 2% of patients with CLL in Western countries [225, 226]. T-CLL is marked by clinical peculiarities such as skin lesions, massive splenomegaly, moderate marrow infiltration, sometimes major neutropenia, and a rather poor prognosis [225, 226]. Refined morphological, ultrastructural, and immunological studies, however, have indicated that there is still a marked heterogeneity in the T-CLL subgroup [226]. This has also been observed in Japanese patients, in whom helper surface phenotype was suggested by reaction with monoclonal antibodies (OKT3+, T4+, T8−) in some patients without demonstrable helper activity in vitro [227]. The clustering of the birthplaces of the Japanese patients with adult T cell leukemia was most striking, as were other characteristics such as frequent skin involvement and rapidly progressive terminal course [228]. This new type of T cell malignancy reported from Japan has an adult onset and is apparently closely related to the classic CLL of T cell origin and the typical Sézary syndrome [228]. A subsequent report described six patients from the West Indies who had a similar type of T cell malignancy with hypercalcemia as a prominent clinical feature [229]. In the United States also, some patients with T cell lymphoma in whom hypercalcemia developed with or without lytic bone lesions have been described [230]. Patients with these T cell lymphoma-leukemias were later shown to have antibodies to human T cell lymphoma virus (human type C retrovirus), and viral isolates from the United States, Japan, and the Caribbean had nucleic acid homologies [231]. Recently, the aggressive clinical course with rapid onset of disseminated skin lesions or symptoms related to hypercalcemia with metabolic bone abnormalities has been summarized in 11 patients with adult T cell lymphoma with T cell lymphoma virus [232]. Thus the recognition of a lymphoma with malignant T cells of mature phenotype by immunological means helped, in connection with clinical and epidemiologic studies, to identify a possible etiologic agent for this homogeneous lymphoma-leukemia subtype. Since the phenotype of malignant cells appears to be influenced by the transforming agent [233], precise records of patients with identical phenotype of the malignant cell may in turn help to identify etiologic agents. Hereby mean the mechanisms of leukemogenesis can be studied further [234].

Diagnostic Value of Immunologic Markers for Classification of Nonmyeloid Leukemias (Acute Lymphatic or Undifferentiated)

One of the most fruitful applications for surface markers has been and still is the phenotyping of acute leukemia cells. Numerous reports have discussed the diagnostic value of a large number of surface markers in acute leukemia, and this has been reviewed recently [27, 159, 235, 236]. Summaries have been provided in the reports from leukemia marker conferences [3, 5].

Three major tasks are reserved for immunodiagnosis in leukemia: (a) To provide an accurate aid for the diagnosis of leukemia; (b) to unmask otherwise undetectable differentiation signs of leukemia cells, particularly for the decision of myeloid versus lymphoid differentiation; and (c) to provide new subclasses of leukemias, hopefully related to clinical signs and prognosis. The first aim relates to the still unresolved question on the existence of leukemia-specific antigens. This point has been discussed in detail elsewhere [85], starting from the detection of the common ALL antigen (CALLA), which was initially believed to be leukemia specific. The hypothesis that there is no leukemia-specific phenotype which cannot be explained as normal gene product has been elegantly demonstrated by the identification of infrequent CALLA-positive normal precursor cells. Accordingly, all so-called leukemia-specific markers can be explained as normal gene products occurring in some rare and therefore overlooked normal cell counterparts. The "operational" leukemia-specific or, better, leukemia-associated attribute should be emphasized, however, in view of its nonetheless high diagnostic value. The occurrence of some rare cells with CALLA in normal bone marrow allows no doubt of the obvious diagnosis of common ALL when a large proportion of positive cells is demonstrated in a marrow sample. Since cell differentiation is associated with topographical compartmentalization of cells, operational leukemia specificity can be afforded by marker demonstration in certain tissues. Good examples of this are single CALLA- or TdT-positive cells in cerebrospinal fluid or testicular biopsies, and the detection of cells of thymic phenotype (e.g., HTA-1, positive with OKT6 or NA 1/34) in the bone marrow in T-ALL patients. In these situations the diagnosis and the type of leukemia can be determined without clinical or morphological information.

The second point relates to the crucial question whether the rate of so-called acute undifferentiated leukemias (AUL, a term based on conventional hematologic criteria including negative morphologic and cytochemical differentiation, particularly peroxidase and PAS) can be diminished by using immunologic markers. The proportion of acute leukemias that are camouflaged by morphologic anonymity is usually around 5%–15% [186, 237]. According to the experience of some groups which have analysed with immunologic methods a number of AULs, lymphatic differentiation is demonstrable in about two-thirds of AULs [158, 186, 216]. This is of particular importance in adults, in whom the proportion of AUL in the nonmyeloid leukemias is relatively high [158, 238, 239]. When ultrastructural peroxidase is determined in addition to immunologic methods, the remaining third of AUL cases are revealed as poorly differentiated acute myelogenous leukemia (AML) [216]. After the inclusion of antisera already available (see section: Monoclonal Antibodies Against Granulocytes, Monocytes, Erythrocytes, and Platelets) in the typing set against myeloid, erythroid, and megakaryoblastic precursor cells, a proper cell lineage affiliation of nearly every case of AUL can be expected. The exact allocation of this ill defined group of acute leukemias (up to 50% of acute nonmyeloid leukemias in adults) appears to be of great importance both for current therapy and for planning of therapy trials. In some trials, the AUL group was lumped together with AML in the so-called acute nonlymphatic leukemia (ANLL) group, though at least two-thirds can have immunologic ALL differentiation. Thus, application of immunologic methods in diagnosis appears to be mandatory for acute leukemia therapy trials.

The third task, namely the recognition of new subclasses of leukemia, has been most convincingly fulfilled in ALL during the last decade. The practice of classification into three major groups by using two markers, i.e., the E receptor and surface immunoglobulin, had been adopted worldwide by the mid-1970s. This classification, namely into a T-cell ALL subgroup, a minor group of B cell origin, and a major group without T-B marker, referred to as non-T, non-B ALL, not only revealed that ALL is a heterogeneous disease, but proved to be of prognostic significance [239–243]. A positive identification of most cases of the non-T, non-B ALL group was accomplished by the introduction of specific antisera against the common ALL antigen [80]. Thus, the non-T, non B ALL group was divided into a large common ALL group and a residual small group called null ALL, since the blast cells were lacking any marker [80–83]. The application of specific anti-T cell sera revealed, however, that some cases of the latter null ALL group reacted with anti-T without having the E receptor [30]. This All type with blast cells of incomplete T cell phenotype was referred to as pre-T ALL [30, 187]. Both the common ALL type and the pre-T ALL subclass were later confirmed by using monoclonal antibodies [159, 186, 189, 198]. A pre-B cell phenotype analogous to normal cell counterparts in human bone marrow and fetal liver was identified in a quarter of patients with common ALL [244] and this was confirmed by others [245].

Thus, a classification into at least six well defined subgroups of ALL was evident by the late 1970s: (a) common ALL, (b) pre-B ALL, (c) B-ALL (d) null ALL, (e) pre-T ALL and (f) T-ALL [158, 235]. This classification, with its six ALL subclasses, has been used as the framework for further classifications up to now. The introduction of monoclonal antibodies confirmed these major subgroups, but also revealed some heterogeneity within single subclasses. The variance of T antigenic sites suggested different subsets of T-ALL when polyclonal anti-T sera were used [158]. This was further substantiated with the aid of a battery of monoclonal anti-T reagents, when a series of T-cell ALL subsets was defined that correlated with discrete stages of intrathymic differentiation [151]. This and other studies clearly indicated that the blast cells in most cases of T-ALL correspond to relatively immature thymus cell types [150, 159, 162, 164], whereas T lymphoblastic lymphoma cells tend to correlate with more mature thymocytes [160]. The subdivision of the larger non-T-ALL group by means of monoclonal antibodies has already been shown to be of prognostic significance [189], whereas the subclassifications of T-ALL still await vindication with reference to clinical usefulness.

Relation of ALL Subgroups to Morphology and Cytochemistry

Morphology

In recent years several groups have classified ALL on the basis of cytomorphology, mainly using the FAB classification [201], with the object of identifying subgroups having different prognoses. The majority of children with ALL, i.e., 84%, were reported to have the L1 morphologic form, whereas only 15% had the L2 type and 1% the L3 type [246]. In contrast, only 29%–41% of adults with ALL had the L1 type, but 49%–64% had the L2 type, and 7%–8% had the L3 type [247–251]. In most studies, patients with L3 leukemia have a particularly dismal outlook with reference to survival. L1 cytology was superior to L2 in survival analyses [246–248].

The L3 type, with its outstanding and most characteristic morphology, was shown to be almost exclusively of B-cell type, through some few exceptions were reported [158, 251]. Among children with common ALL, 71% had L1, 28% L2, and 0% L3 [235]. In contrast, among 21 adults with common ALL, 33% had L1 and 67% L2 [249]. T-ALL appears to have a distribution of L1 and L2 similar to that of common ALL in both children and adults. In pre-T ALL, the L2 type prevailed with 62%, the L1 type accounting for 38% [158]. At least one case of adult T-ALL with L3 morphology has been reported [251].

Without discussing all aspects and problems with morphology in great detail, some generalities can be drawn from the studies on morphology and surface markers in ALL: (a) Except in B-ALL, which commonly has L3 morphology, there is no clear relation between immunologic subtype and morphology; (b) the occurrence of certain morphologic blast cell forms is different in children and adults, even within the same immunologic subtypes; and (c) in some studies a prognostic significance has been shown for blast cell morphology in children [247, 251], though objective lymphoblast cell size measurements revealed no correlation with subtype or outcome [252].

Cytochemistry

Among the various cytochemical stains, periodic acid-Schiff (PAS) has been most extensively studied in ALL. The degree of PAS positivity has been suggested to correlate with survival, and patients with higher counts of lymphoblasts with PAS-positive coarse granules in blocks had longer remissions [250]. The PAS stain is positive in various immunologic ALL subtypes and relations have been studied by several groups [158, 235, 253–255]. A block PAS positivity is seen in 56%–77% of patients with common ALL (Table 7). It is somewhat less frequent in null ALL, lying around 50%. Lower frequencies were recorded for pre-B ALL (25% of patients), pre T ALL (10%–20%), and T-ALL (9%–25%). B-ALL lymphoblasts appear to be generally PAS negative.

Acid phosphatase (APh) is the cytochemical stain most frequently suggested to discriminate immunologic classes of ALL. APh in strong focal positivity in a paranuclear distribution has been reported to be a marker for T-ALL [140]. This has been confirmed in many studies [158, 235, 253–255]. APh is mostly positive in pre-T-ALL, also [158, 253]. However, APh has also been demonstrated in up to 40% of patients with common ALL (Table 7) and in 28% of children with pre-B-ALL [158, 254]. The few cases of B-ALL that have been studied have generally been reported to be negative for APh [235, 254, 255].

Acid α-naphthyl esterase (ANAE) was initially reported to be useful in distinguishing T-ALL from non-T-ALL [256]. When larger groups of patients were studied, however, it turned out that ANAE occurs in around 80% of T-ALL, 70% of pre-T-ALL, but also in 25% of common ALL [141, 253].

The following general conclusions can be drawn from the studies on cytochemistry and surface markers in ALL: (a) APh is the most useful enzyme for staining T-ALL and

Table 7. Cytochemistry in subtypes of ALL[a]

Immunologic class	No. of patients	PAS	APh	ANAE	APh+ PAS−	APh− PAS+
		Percent of patients with positive blasts[b]				
1. Common ALL	133	58	38	41	25	44
2. pre-T-ALL	17	19	88	93	73	0
3. T-ALL	32	18	94	87	82	0
P values (Student's *t*-test) for						
Common ALL vs pre-T ALL		< 0.01	< 0.001	< 0.001		
Common ALL vs T-ALL		< 0.01	< 0.001	< 0.4		

[a] Taken from references 158 and 253

[b] Distinct positivity, granular and paranuclear pattern of staining

pre-T-ALL; (b) PAS stains cells in about two-thirds of common ALL; (c) ANAE is less suited than APh for T/pre-T-ALL staining; and (d) positivities in the alternate classes prevent a substitution of immunologic markers by enzymes despite significant differences (Table 7): Thus cytochemical reactions play an important supplementary role to immunologic marker investigations and can be helpful when immunological data are not available or doubtful, e.g., interpretation of T markers in probes with T lymphocyte contamination. Some combinations provide exclusive results; for example, APh-PAS+ excludes a T/pre-T ALL (Table 7). The clinical and prognostic relevance of cytochemical subtypes within immunologic classes, e.g., common ALL PAS+ versus common ALL PAS−, is still unsettled.

Relation of ALL Subgroups to Cytogenetics, Aneuploidy, and Proliferative Activity

Cytogenetics

Clonal chromosome abnormalities are common in ALL. In the largest series reported to date abnormalities were found in 66% of 330 newly diagnosed patients [248]. A number of specific chromosomal subgroups of ALL have been recognized, including Ph1+ (22q−) ALL, t (4; 11) ALL, 8q−ALL, 14q+ALL, and 6q−ALL. Other chromosome abnormalities have been grouped by the predominant number of chromosomes in cells. Some of these karyotypic subgroups appear to have distinct clinical features and response to treatment. In a recent large study of 136 patients, chromosome number was shown in multivariate analysis to be the strongest single predictor of outcome and to be the only variable that added significant prognostic information to leukocyte count [257]. Children in the hyperdiploid (more than 50 chromosomes) category had the best response to treatment, and those in the pseudodiploid category had the poorest.

Several studies have recently correlated karyotype with immunologic phenotype [248, 257–259]. All cases of B-ALL so far reported had abnormalities (8q− or 14q+), compared with 68% of non-T-, non-B-ALL and only 45% of T-ALL. The most common chromosomal abnormality in non-T-, non-B-ALL is a Philadelphia chromosome (Ph^1), most commonly t (9; 22) (q 34; q 11). The next most commonly occurring abnormality is the translocation t (4; 11) (q 21; q 23). ALL with a modal number > 50 is usually restricted to non-T-, non-B ALL accounting for as many as 20% of cases of this condition, and appears to carry an usually good prognosis [257]. Recurring specific chromosome abnormalities have rarely been reported in T-ALL. Most cases of T-ALL have a modal number of 46. Rare cases with the Ph^1 or the t (4; 11) have been reported [248, 260].

Aneuploidy

Clonal abnormalities of the DNA content of leukemia cells can be assessed by flow cytometry (FCM) after staining with specific fluorochromes. Aneuploidy detected by FCM is a specific marker of malignant cells in many types of human cancer [261]. The degree of DNA content abnormality detected by FCM is correlated with the number of whole chromosome gains (hyperdiploidy) or losses (hypodiploidy) [262]. It should be noted, however, that the prognostically important pseudodiploid karyotypes caused by translocations are not detected by FCM. The method provides results in every patient analysed however, and is less time-consuming than cytogenetic methods, which are sometimes not feasible when metaphases are in low proportion to other cells. In a recent large study of 225 children with acute leukemia there was an aneuploidy rate of 24% [262]. Aneuploidy was significantly correlated with the cell phenotype: 46 of 127 cases with common ALL were aneuploid, as against 2 of 21 cases with T-ALL [262].

Proliferative Activity

With the aid of FCM, the percentage of cells in the S-phase of the cell cycle can also be assessed. The pretreatment ^{3}H-thymidine labeling index is another measure for proliferative activity of cells. The median percentage of cells in S-phase or the labeling indices were significantly higher for B cell and T cell ALL compared with non-T-, non-B ALL in several studies of children [240, 262, 263].
A correlation of cytokinetic data with prognosis was questioned in earlier studies [264, 265]. In a large recent study, however, the pretreatment proliferative activity of blood and marrow blasts added significant prognostic information to leukocyte count, as shown by Cox's regression analysis [262].

Relation of ALL Subgroups to Clinical Characteristics

The next two sections relate mainly to data drawn from our own studies on patients with ALL phenotyped at diagnosis. Essential parts of these studies have been published elsewhere [158, 238, 266]. The results of those studies are discussed with the data from some selected reports from the literature.

Age and Sex Distribution

In all reports except one [267] there is a male preponderance and a characteristic age distribution for T-ALL [158, 235, 239–243, 254, 268]. Since E-rosette-positive T-ALL makes up only 11%–14% of all cases of ALL (Table 8), a sufficiently large number of

Table 8. Immunologic ALL subgroups in children and adults in two large series [158, 235, 238, 266][a]

	Children		Adults		Phenotypic pattern				
	Greaves et al.	Thiel et al.	Greaves et al.	Thiel et al.	CALLA	Ia	T	E-R	SIg
Total (*n*)	701	694	103	191					
Common ALL	75.6%	71.5%	50.5%	49.2%	+	+	–[b]	–	–
T-ALL	11.7%	14.4%	9.7%	15.1%	–[c]	–	+	+	–
pre-T-ALL	n.d.[d]	7.8%	n.d.[d]	8.1%	–	–[e]	+	–	–
B-ALL	0.5%	1.1%	2%	2.1%	–	+	–	–	+
Unclassified or null ALL	12.1%	5.2%	37.8%	25.5%	–	+	–	–	–

[a] Some unpublished data are included
[b] Blast cells in some patients express T antigens simultaneously (C/T type); another common ALL subset is characterized by the presence of cytoplasmic IgM (pre-B type, in one-third of cases of common ALL)
[c] A minor T subset (10%–20%) also has CALLA+ Ia– blast cells
[d] Not determined; probably included in the null ALL category
[e] Sometimes weakly positive

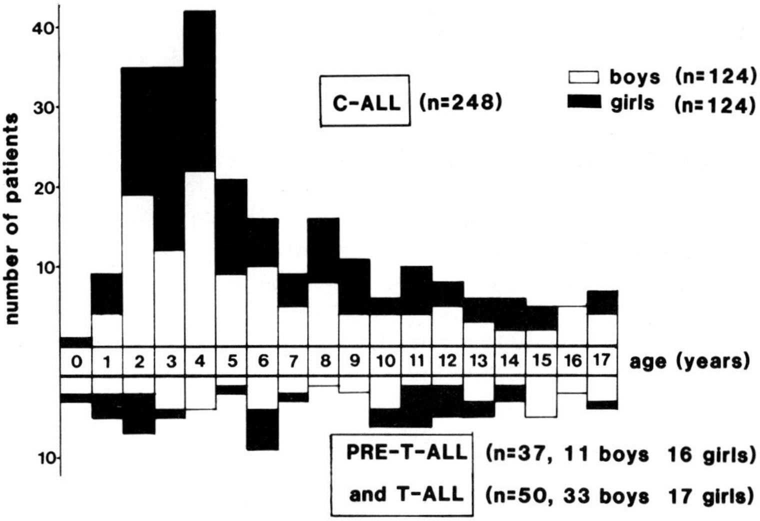

Fig. 1. Age and sex distribution in 335 children with newly diagnosed ALL of common or pre-T-/T-cell phenotype

patients has to be phenotyped for relevant results. As shown in Fig. 1, the very pronounced peak at age 2–10 years in CALL is not evident in T-ALL [158, 235]. The great majority of patients with T-ALL were aged 10–20 years, while no patient with T-ALL was recorded who was older than 35 [158]. Common ALL occurred up to the age of 80, but ALL is rare in patients over 20 years of age. Differences in sex and age distribution were statistically significant between CALLA-positive and CALLA-negative ALL.

Table 9. Clinical correlates of ALL subclasses in children at presentation

Feature	Total	C-ALL	T-ALL	Pre-T-ALL	Null-ALL	Significant differences[a]
No. of patients	329	237	50	27	18	C vs pre-T, T; T vs null
M:F ratio	1.15	1.0	1.9	0.7	1.1	T vs C, pre-T, null
Mediastinal mass (%)	12.2	1.6	55.8	33.3	5.5	C vs pre-T, T; T vs null
Lymphadenopathy (%)	54.8	52	69	69.6	33.3	C vs pre-T, T
Splenomegaly (%)	58.3	55	68.3	76	71.4	C vs pre-T
CNS leukemia (%)	6.1	2.9	12.8	16.7	7.7	C vs pre-T, T
WBC $> 50 \times 10^9$/l	25.6	17.4	52.2	46.2	41.2	C vs pre-T, T, null
Hemoglobin < 8 g/dl (%)	53.3	61	29.5	56	37.5	C vs T; pre-T vs T
Platelets $< 50 \times 10^9$/l (%)	56.1	57.1	56	51.2	64.7	n.s.

[a] Computed according to Kruskal-Wallis test

Unclassified or null-ALL occurred more often in adult patients, in whom common ALL made up a markedly smaller group than in childhood. The frequencies of CALL in children and adults were quite similar in two large studies (Table 8). In part the differences for null ALL frequency between the studies may be explained by the fact that the pre-T ALL type was assessed only in one study.

Clinical Features at Presentation

An analysis of the clinical data recorded in 347 children whose blast cells were typed between 1975 and 1980 will now be given (Table 9). Organomegaly was less frequent in common ALL. A mediastinal thymic mass was recorded in more than half the patients with T-ALL, in a third of those with pre-T-ALL, in 1 of 18 with null-ALL, and in 4 of 248 with documented CALLA-positive blast cells. This symptom was therefore significantly associated with T-ALL with E-R. Splenomegaly and lymphadenopathy were less pronounced in common ALL. The lower WBC in common ALL than in T- and pre-T-ALL may be explained in the light of a lower tumor cell burden in this subgroup. CNS leukemia, which was a relatively rare complication, was more frequent in T-ALL and pre-T-ALL than in common ALL. On the other hand, anemia and thrombocytopenia were more pronounced in common ALL than in T-ALL. The lack or relatively low grade of hematopoietic insufficiency observed in T-ALL (Table 9) has been explained as consequence of tumor origin outside the marrow [239]. The more lymphomatous form of T-ALL, with organomegalies of spleen, liver, and lymph nodes, fits in with this interpretation. Thus the marrow may be invaded secondarily in T-ALL. In contrast, pre-T-ALL, like the other non-T ALL forms, may originate in the marrow, since anemia and thrombocytopenia are mostly present at diagnosis [158].

In the rare cases of B-ALL in this study ($n = 4$, not shown in Table 9) and in the few cases reported in the literature [158, 251, 269, 270], quite a characteristic clinical pattern also becomes evident. Splenomegaly and hepatomegaly are particularly common, and half the patients present with CNS leukemia. The patients frequently have low leukocyte counts and a low percentage of circulating blasts. Abdominal lymphomatous masses are often encountered, sometimes with infiltration of the gut. Thus the clinical spectrum of B-ALL may represent peripheralizing lymphoma, and the term "ALL" may be a misnomer for a

Table 10. Results of treatment in 328 children, evaluated by immunological subclasses

	Total	Common ALL	T-ALL	Pre-T-ALL	Null ALL	B-ALL
Number evaluable	329	237	46	26	16	4
Complete remission rate (%)[a]	84.8	87.8	76.1	80.8	81.3	50
Relapse rate up to 1 year (%)	9.4	5.9	17.4	23.1	18.7	0
Relapse rate up to 2 years (%)	19.5	16.8	23.9	34.6	25	0
Relapse rate after 2 years (%)	6.4	7.2	4.3	0	12.5	0
In lasting CR (%)	59	63.7	47.8	46.1	43.7	50
Death rate observed (%)	31.9	27	50	46.1	25	50

[a] Early death included

rapidly disseminating lymphoma. In conclusion, characteristic clinical patterns are becoming evident for the immunologic subclasses. Thus a relation between differentiation status of tumor cells as measured by its immunologic phenotype and in vivo behavior as recorded by growth rate, homing properties, and infiltration pattern, is also emerging in human ALL. Such relations have been convincingly demonstrated in animal models, e.g., IgM-producing tumors in the BALB/c mouse [271].

Relation of ALL Subgroups to Response to Treatment

ALL is the most successfully treated leukemia, and has served as a model for designing strategies for other leukemias. The stepwise introduction of combined-modality treatment protocols with CNS prophylaxis during the late 1960s and early 1970 led to spectacular successes: complete remissions (CRs) in well over 90% of children and in up to 80%, of adults, and survival for 5 years or more in over 50% of children [272, 273]. In view of this therapeutic breakthrough, which is valid for a substantial proportion of patients though not for all, the immediate recognition of responders and nonresponders at diagnosis became mandatory. Some clinical risk factors such as male sex, age less than 2 or more than 10 years, high white cell count, and mediastinal mass, are known to indicate poor prognosis [272, 274]. Immunologic typing of leukemic blasts has indicated that both children and adults with T-ALL have a considerably worse prognosis than those with non-T, non-B, or common ALL [158, 235, 239–243, 248, 268, 275]. In some studies, the phenotype appears to be an independent variable [268, 276], whereas in others there was only a marginal independent significance for the immunologic phenotype [277]. Except for the few cases of B-ALL, where a poor prognosis was generally observed despite a low WBC, it appears to depend on the particular form of therapy and on methodological differences whether an important prognostic factor or only a strong association with clinical risk factors has been ascertained for the immunologic phenotype.

In our study of 329 children followed up for response to treatment there were only smal differences in remission rate for the immunologic subgroups (Table 10). CR rates were significantly different for common ALL and T-ALL, but not for other subgroups. The majority of patients, namely 274 (see Fig. 2), were treated according to two protocols in two variations each (BFM 76/79, BFM 79/81; 7701, 7702) [278–280]. Allocation to the protocols depended on the hospital of admission. The distribution of the various

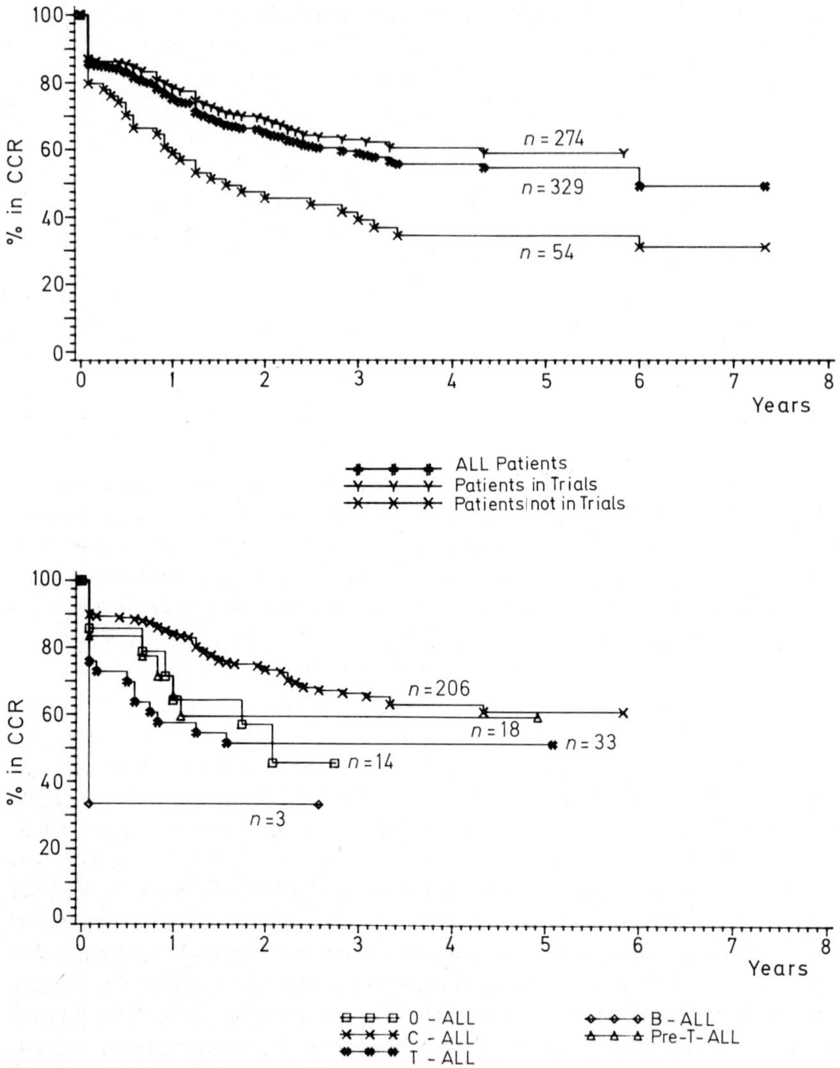

Fig. 2. Remission duration for 329 children with ALL. The *curves* are plotted according to a life-table analysis program. *Upper part:* 54 children were treated according to various protocols, whereas 274 children were treated according to trial protocols (see text). In the *lower part* of the figure, the remission curves of trial children are given according to immunologic subgroup

immunologic subclasses within the treatment groups was similar. Each protocol contained prednisone, vincristine, asparaginase, daunorubicin, or doxorubicin for induction therapy, with an immediate intensification phase with cyclophosphamide, cytosine arabinoside, and 6-mercaptopurine together with CNS prophylaxis. A similar consolidation therapy followed after 3 months. A preliminary analysis of the separate trials revealed only small differences attributable to the regimens adopted, and the results presented are therefore pooled from all the trials concerned. Remission failures, which were somewhat rarer in common ALL (Table 10), were mainly caused by early deaths and less by nonresponse to therapy. The rate of relapses during the first year of remission was markedly lower in common ALL. Conversely, a substantial rise in the proportion of relapses was observed in the second year of remission for common ALL and pre-T-ALL, but not for T-ALL. The relapse rate after 2 years of remission was generally small, being somewhat lower in T-ALL than in common or null ALL. The distinct relapse patterns of common ALL and T-/pre-T-ALL become evident in the remission curves computed following life-table analysis (Fig. 2). The difference in relapse pattern remains the same even when the patients are analysed within different treatment groups (curves not shown). Since the WBC count is a major prognostic factor, and since there is an unequal distribution of patients with high WBC count in the different immunological subclasses (see Table 9), it is important to determine whether the prognostic significance of the cell type is an independent effect or merely reflects its correlation with WBC. There is a clear relation between the WBC count at presentation (grouped in 3 categories) and the remission duration of the patients in this study (see Fig. 3). For patients with CALLA-positive blasts, however, it made no difference whether they belonged to the low (0–10,000) or to the medium (10,000–50,000) WBC count category. Only common ALL patients with WBC count over 50,000 had a worse prognosis. In contrast, T/pre-T-ALL patients with low cell counts had an exceptionally good prognosis, whereas the same worse prognosis was noted for children with T-ALL in the medium WBC count group (10,000–50,000) as for those with high counts (over 50,000). Thus, the phenotype is of importance for children with leukocyte counts in the range of 10,000–50,000. This was valid for 28% of children with common or T-/pre-T-ALL in this study. In another study of children with ALL, there was a marked difference in remission duration for patients with T cell antigen-positive blasts versus children with Ia-positive blast cells [268]. HTA+ patients fared worse than Ia+ patients even when age and intitial WBC were taken into account for prognosis in this study [268]. In another large study there was a marked reduction of the prognostic importance of immunologic subtype, when adjustment for WBC was made in the common and T-ALL subclasses [277]. The immunologic phenotype had only a marginal independent significance [277]. Methodological differences in typing and in statistical analysis and different therapeutic protocols might be responsible for discrepancies between the various series reported.

In our study there were no differences in prognosis for patients with hemoglobin values less or more than 8 g/dl. The remission curves were somewhat better for patients with platelet counts over 50,000 than for patients with thrombocytopenia, irrespective of the cell type. Also, splenomegaly contributed to a worse prognosis to some extent (curves with a statistically significant difference in level of around 15%). A somewhat smaller but still visible difference (around 5%–10%, not significant) was recorded for hepatomegaly. The differences in prognosis caused by organomegalies (splenomegaly, hepatomegaly, lymphadenopathy) remained the same when analyses were done within common or T-/pre-T-ALL subclasses. The occurrence of mediastinal mass was a bad prognostic factor throughout the series of ALL patients (Fig. 4). Within the T-/pre-T-ALL group, however, there was no difference for the remission curves of children with or without mediastinal mass. Thus, the symptom of thymus tumor marks a subgroup of ALL patients in whom prognosis is no different from that of another group of children without thymus tumors, but with T cell markers. We can therefore conclude that mediastinal mass does not have any predictive value per se, but rather is an associative symptom for about 50% of patients with pre-T-/T-ALL. In contrast to our data, in another study prognostic significance was not recorded for T cell markers but was recorded for mediastinal mass [281]. Immunologic ALL classification, however, was performed solely by E rosetting and SIg staining in this study, and fewer patients with T cell markers ($n = 11$) were investigated [281].

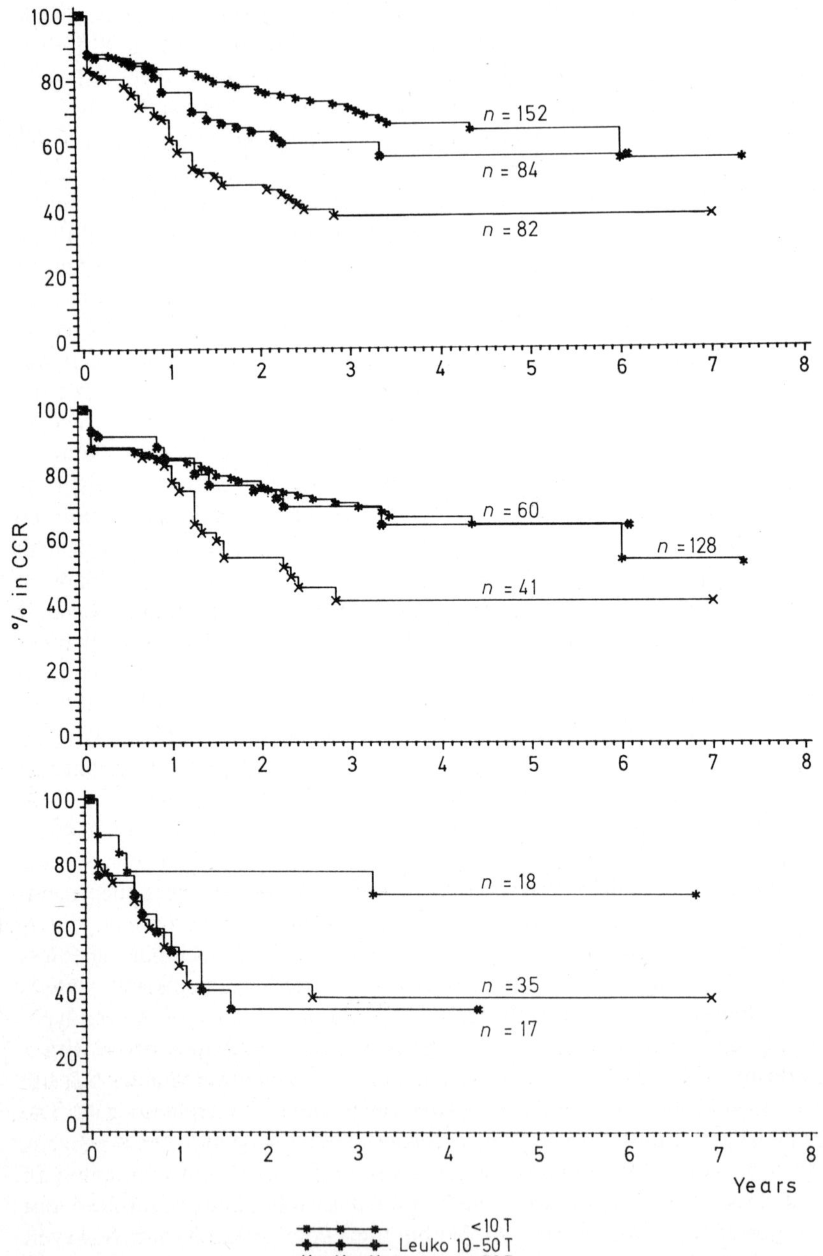

Fig. 3. Remission curves according to white cell count in all patients with ALL *(upper part),* in children with common ALL *(middle),* and in children with pre-T- or T-ALL *(lower part).* A grouping for three categories of WBC is performed: 0–10,000; 10,000–50,000; and over 50,000 leukocytes

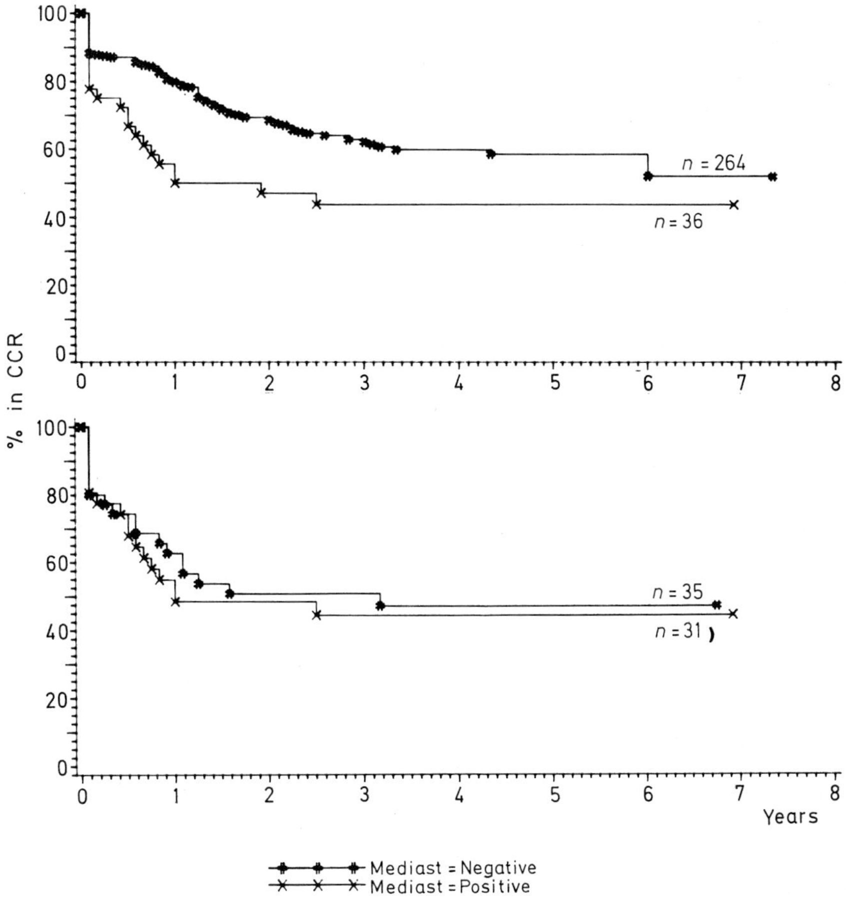

Fig. 4. Influence of mediastinal mass on remission duration. *Curves* all children with ALL *(upper part)* and of children with pre-T or T-ALL *(lower part)*

CNS involvement is also known to worsen the prognosis decisively and to have a relatively high incidence in T-ALL [276]. CNS leukemia was also strongly correlated with WBC [277]. In the study reported, the substantially higher incidence of CNS relapse (11/30) in T-ALL than in common ALL (18/270) was therefore analysed in relation to ALL subclass adjusted for WBC count [277]. The difference between T-ALL and other groups, although reduced, remained statistically significant. Accordingly in our study, in which we analysed the relation of primary CNS leukemia to subclass (see Table 9; rates significantly higher in T- and per-T-ALL) and prognosis, prognosis was poor for patients with primary CNS involvement (Fig. 5). Surprisingly, the unfavorable effect of CNS disease on prognosis was reduced when a CALLA-positive leukemia was involved. Thus, the immunologic phenotype appears to be of decisive importance in the clinical subgroup of ALL with CNS involvement.

Remission duration was longer for girls ($n = 155$) than for boys ($n = 174$) in our study (curves not shown). A difference was also recorded within the common ALL subclass (remission curve plateau is around 70% for girls and 55% for boys), which is a point against the suggestion that the difference for the whole ALL group might be caused solely by boys

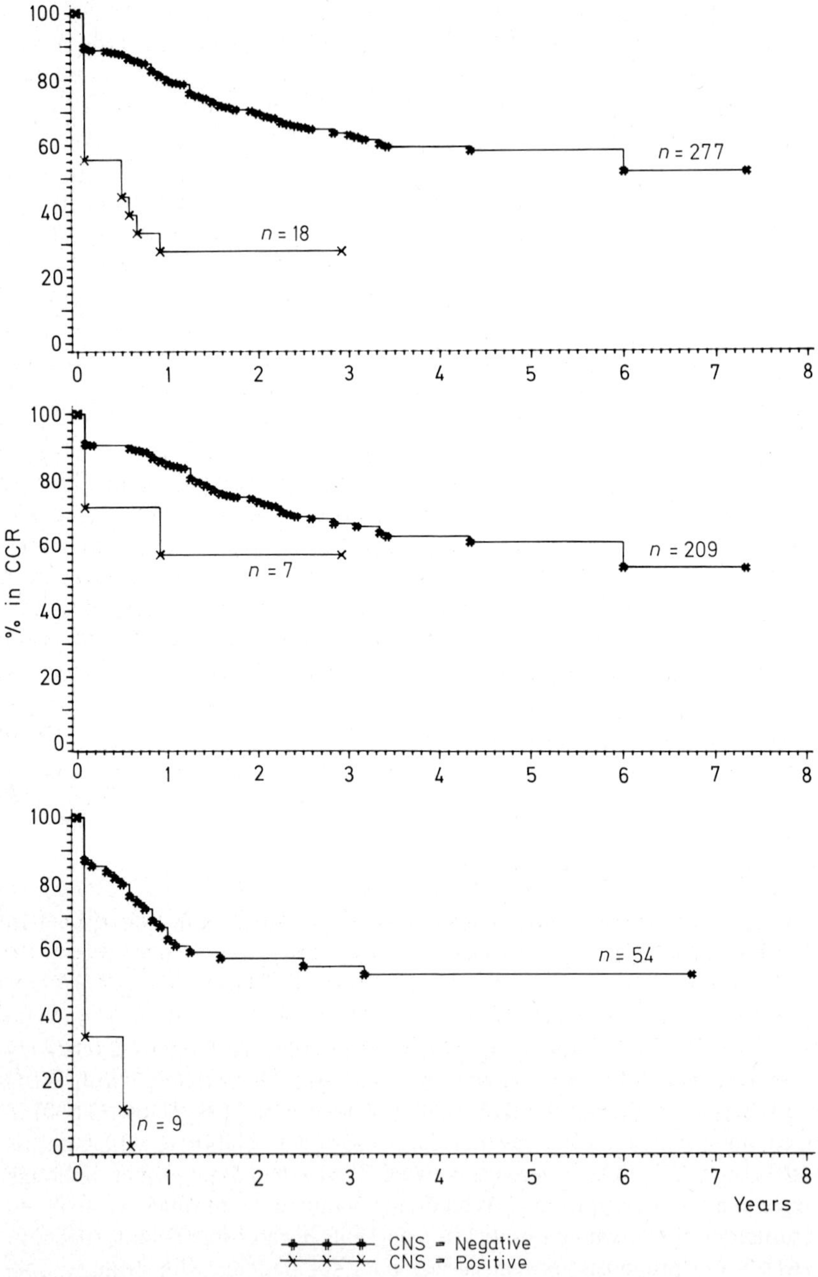

Fig. 5. Influence of primary CNS involvement on remission duration. *Curves* for all children with ALL *(upper part)*, of children with common ALL *(middle)*, and of children with pre-T or T-ALL *(lower part)*

with T-ALL. Also within the T-/pre-T-ALL group in our series, the remission curve plateau for girls ($n = 32$, plateau at 60% for continuous remission) was markedly higher than that (35%–40%) for boys ($n = 40$). This is in contrast to the other large study reported, where identical remission for boys and girls, both overall and in each ALL subclass, was recorded [277]. In another large study, however, as in our series there was a marked difference in the remission curves for boys and girls [282].

Age was also a predictive factor in our study, in which children under 2 years or over 10 years had a worse prognosis (curves not shown). Age-dependent differences were only marginally visible in common ALL and were more pronounced in pre-T-/T-ALL. Surprisingly, in the British study, age was hardly predictive, and there was no significant difference in remission between age groups [277]. From the data obtained in our study and other reported data recorded in children with ALL we can conclude that the immunologic phenotype of ALL blasts has a predictive value both for remission rate and remission duration. The prognostic value of the pre-T-/T-ALL phenotype can be explained largely by overlap with traditional clinical factors. In certain conditions, such as in a defined range of WBC count or in the case of primary CNS involvement, there is a strongly predictive value for the phenotype. In addition, the phenotype of the distinct subclasses is correlated with different age and sex distribution, distinct growth rate and sites of clonal expansion, and a different relapse pattern. Thus, various disease forms of the heterogeneous entity ALL appear to be caused by distinct biological features linked to the differentiation status of the blast cell phenotype. In this way, the immunologically detected phenotypic subtypes of leukemia cells may be the clue for definition of new subgroups of disease distinct in biology, incidence and probably etiology. The prognostic significance of the blast cell phenotype must be analysed and reanalysed in relation to the quality of therapy and of immunodiagnosis.

Prognostic Significance of Blast Cell Phenotype in Transformed Chronic Myelogenous Leukemia

Chronic myelogenous leukemia (CML) is a well defined myeloproliferative disorder associated in more than 90% of cases with a characteristic karyotypic marker, the Philadelphia chromosome (Ph^1) [283]. The chronic phase of CML is characterized by a marked overproduction of relatively mature granulocytes. Although most of the clinical manifestations of CML result from excessive clonal production and accumulation of myeloid cells, the Ph^1 chromosome can also be detected in megakaryocytes, erythroid cells, monocyte/macrophages, and B lymphocytes; this suggests that CML arises in a pluripotent stem cell [284–287]. The clonal nature of the disease has been further established by detailed analysis of X-linked glucose-6-phosphate dehydrogenase (G6PD) isoenzyme patterns in heterozygous patients with CML [288].

After a variable period of time (mean value around 3 years), the chronic phase undergoes transformation and evolves into an acute phase or "blast crisis" (CML-BC), which is characterized by decreasing cell maturity and superimposed additional chromosome abnormalities (e.g., trisomy 19 or 21, a second Ph^1, or isochromosome 17) [259]. The CML-BC cells often show evidence of partial differentiation along one or more hematopoietic pathways [289, 290]. The blasts of most patients are thought to resemble those seen in acute myeloblastic leukemia (myeloid CML-BC), although they are usually peroxidase negative and have no Auer rods [291]. About one-third of patients have blasts resembling the lymphoblasts of ALL (lymphoid CML-BC) in phenotype (Ia+, cALLA+, TdT+, and elevated 5′-N) [116, 125, 290]. Some cells also have cytoplasmic IgM, like pre-B ALL cells [292]. Recently, T cell surface antigens were reported in a case with CML-BC [293]. Since efforts to identify Ph^1 in T lymphocytes in the chronic phase have been largely unsuccessful [287], a common precursor cell for myeloid cells and some B, but not T cells has been suggested [294]. Although the occurrence of lymphoid CML-BC with T markers in Ph^1-positive blasts is a rare event, this finding points to the existence of a true omnipotent stem cell of the hematopoietic tissue.

The identification of a lymphoid type of CML-BC became important since dramatic responses to treatment with vincristine and prednisone – drugs that are useful in ALL therapy – were reported [295]. In some cases, hematologic and even cytogenetic remissions were observed, and the disease reverted to the chronic phase for up to 1 year. Since patients with myeloid CML-BC are generally unresponsive to chemotherapy, their survival being less than 6 months [291], an objective criterion for diagnosis of the lymphoid form appears to be important in view of the immature morphology of blasts in CML-BC. In this connection, TdT and cALLA have been shown to be highly significant predictors of initial responsiveness [117, 296]. In the last study cited, 14 of 15 cases with CALLA-positive blasts responded to therapy incorporating vincristine and prednisolone, while 21 of 25 patients who had no CALLA-positive blasts failed to respond [296]. Positivity with anti-ALL serum was the most sensitive and reliable marker, and TdT was an important aid [296]. Thus, the immunological phenotype proved to be an objective criterion for identification of a responsive blast cell type. This is noteworthy in the situation of CML-BC, where the allocation of blasts to the "lymphoid" or "myeloid" form is difficult by hematological methods.

Target Cell for Malignant Transformation and Leukemia Phenotype

Studies of the detailed phenotype of leukemic cells in recent years have provided evidence that consistent, composite phenotypes of different leukemia subclasses closely minic those of corresponding normal cells at equivalent levels of maturation. Soon after the establishment of two distinct differentiation pathways for nomal lymphoid development, it was recognized that lymphoid malignancies affect cells of either T or B lineage, but not both. Studies of leukemias in animal models revealed that malignant T and B cells, like their normal counterparts, have their origin in distinct, mostly central lymphoid tissues. Thus, removal of the thymus prevents certain T lymphoid malignancies in AKR mice, whereas thymus transplants restore susceptibility [297]. On the other hand, the bursa of Fabricius is the source of malignant B cells in avian lymphoid leukosis [298]. In the latter example, the virus-induced transformation only occurs at a very early stage in B-cell differentiation within the inductive bursal microenvironment [299]. Thus, the target cell susceptible for malignant transformation appears to play a critical role for the resulting leukemia type. Also, the risk of transformation of a given target cell may vary over the lifespan: malignancies of lymphocyte precursors occur predominantly in children and young patients, whereas malignancies of mature cells are almost exclusively adult diseases. One interpretation of this age association may be te risk through proliferative demand at various stages of early development or during prolonged function and turnover in the adult. One good example for a defined target cell has been given recently in human adult T cell leukemia-lymphoma, where an allocation to a peripheral T cell as target cell of the disease has been provided by transformation of cord blood T cells by leukemic cell-derived type C virus particles (see section: *Clinical Significance of T Cell Chronic Lymphatic Leukemia Cell Types*).

Target Cell and Maturation Arrest of the Clonogenic Cell Population

Chronic myelogenous leukemia (CML) is the best example illustrating that the dominant phenotype of leukemic cells (here mature granulocytes) cannot be similar to that of the leukemia target cell, here a Ph^1-positive pluripotent stem cell (see section: *Prognostic Significance of Blast Cell Phenotype in Transformed Myelogenous Leukemia)*. Thus, clonal production and accumulation of maturing leukemic cell elements are more pronounced in this disease during the chronic phase, whereas a maturation arrest such as occurs in acute leukemias is dominant in the acute phase of the same leukemic disease.

Obviously, the central lesion of this leukemic disease converts to a regulatory defect in the form of a maturation arrest, which occurs even in immature cell elements of the Ph^1-positive clone. Approximately one-third of patients with CML-BC have the common ALL phenotype and their condition is not immediately distinguishable from common ALL, although the target cells of CML-BC and common ALL are different. Since common ALL only very rarely transforms intraclonally to myeloid leukemia, and never to T-ALL, we conclude that common ALL probably results from the transformation of a B lineage-committed precursor cell, whereas the target cell of lymphoid CML-BC is still the Ph^1-positive pluripotential stem cell. Thus it is most likely that the occurrence of Ph^1-positive blasts with CALLA indicates maturation arrest, while the same phenotype in common ALL blasts gives information on the origin and commitment of the leukemic stem cells. Detailed and repeated analyses of the phenotype through the course of a leukemic disease may be important for the decision as to what to interpret as reflecting the imposed maturation arrest and what to take as an indicator of the target cell. In this field, the study of differentiation and clonal evolution in CML may provide a model for understanding the biology of malignancy [294]. It is important to note that whereas common ALL can be cured with current therapy, CML-BC cannot, although as expected short-term remissions and reversion to the chronic phase can be achieved. This underlines the importance of target cell biology for understanding of the clinical outcome and for the development of alternative therapeutic strategies, e.g., marrow transplants for Ph^1-positive leukemias. Two salient features of hematopoietic malignancies, i.e., the clonal origin, which provides a natural source of a large progeny of tumor cells derived from one single cloned cell, and the imposition of maturation arrest, which stabilizes the leukemic cell population with regard to differentiation, promise unique opportunities for analysis of hematopoietic cell differentiation. The assumption must therefore be correct that the phenotypic structures of leukemic cells are not altered, but only arrested at certain stages of cell differentiation. Since normal precursor cells are rare and are camouflaged by the vast heterogeneity of mature cell elements in hematopoietic tissue, information restricted to these cells is difficult to gain. The common ALL antigen first detected on leukemic cells helped to pinpoint rare lymphoid progenitor cells in normal bone marrow. The recent application of recombinant DNA technology to the study of immunoglobulin genes has demonstrated that rearranged *Ig* heavy chain genes can be detected in most of the CALLA-positive blast cells prior to the expression of cytoplasmic IgM (see section: *B Cell Leukemia/Lymphoma Phenotypes in Relation to the Framework of Normal B Cell Differentiation)* [180]. Thus it was possible to define a pre-pre-B cell phenotype with the aid of leukemia cell studies, and *Ig* gene rearrangement has been shown to be the first differentiation marker of the B cell system.

In many recent studies, the lymphoid phenotypes of ALL subclasses were arranged in a scheme of a putative sequence of differentiation, as suggested for normal lymphoid progenitors [10, 85, 158, 159, 236]. Nearly all leukemic phenotypes can be interpreted in a framework of sequential maturation stages versus B or T (see sections: *Comparative Phenotypic Characterization of Human Malignant T Cells* and *B Cell Leukemia/Lymphoma Phenotypes in Relation to the Framework of Normal B Cell Differentiation)*. Thus it is now clear that ALL consists of two broad subtypes: one is "precursor-T", or equivalent to thymic (and prethymic?) precursors of T cells; the other, more common, variant is "precursor-B", or equivalent to B cell progenitors in bone marrow. Only the unclassified or null-ALL phenotype cannot be allocated to T or B and is therefore interpreted as a lymphoid-committed, bipotential stem cell in some schemes [159]. The markers of this cell type, however, namely TdT, HLA-DR and, sometimes, PAS staining are per se not cell lineage specific. Thus, the true lymphocytic commitment of this null-ALL phenotype remains unsettled. Some qualifications should nevertheless be made for the simple interpretation of ALL phenotypes as faithful replicas for particular stages of normal cell differentiation in which the leukemic cells are frozen. Detailed scrutiny of ALL phenotypes sometimes reveals more heterogeneity of phenotype than can be accommodated within the framework of the supposed normal differentiation sequence; the consistent combination of strong staining for both HLA-ABC and TdT on most T-ALL is surprising, since normal thymic TdT-positive cells have very low levels of HLA until they mature to the TdT-negative stage [163]. Interestingly, TdT-positive HLA-ABC-negative leukemias have not yet been observed. These observations may reflect the existence of some minor alterations in gene expression, e.g., possible asynchrony.

Phenotypic Shifts of Leukemic Cell Phenotypes in Vivo

A confirmation of the above view that ALL phenotypes broadly reflect stages of maturation within the early compartments of B and T lineages was provided by the observation of altered phenotypes in relapsed ALL [235, 236, 300]. In around 20% of the patients monitored, changes such as acquisition or loss of the CALL antigen or loss of the E receptor with retention of T antigens were observed. Relapse affecting sites different than those at the original diagnosis did not affect the expression of surface markers. The altered phenotypes in second relapses were relatively close to the initial phenotype. Since widely different phenotypes, e.g., common ALL→T-ALL or T-ALL→B-ALL were not found, a random mutation process seems not to be very likely. A selection of pre-existing veriant cells under the selective pressure of therapy seems to be a good explanation for the observed phenotypic shifts. Detailed scrutiny of leukemic phenotypes reveals that not all blast cells of an individual patient are identical at diagnosis. Phenotypic categorization merely reflects the dominant phenotype, but in practice some diversity can always be detected with respect to quantity and even quality of antigens. These different but clearly related phenotypes yield information on preceding or subsequent maturation stages of the dominant leukemic cell phenotype. The interpretation favored for this intraclonal diversity is that in large part it reflects the variable stringency of maturation arrest, i.e., all cells do not appear to be arrested at precisely the same developmental position. Thus, the rules of "survival of the fittest" may be the explanation for the continuous emergence of successive clones of tumor cell variants gradually replacing one another, through the intervention of natural or artificial selection pressures [301].

Modulation of Leukemic Cell Phenotypes In Vitro

Since the phenotype of leukemic cells reflects the apparent imposition of maturation arrest it is of some interest to determine whether maturation is inducible. Extensive experimental studies with Friend virus erythroleukemia and rat myeloid leukemia cell lines indicated that leukemic cells may retain the competence for differentiation [187]. Recent in vitro experiments using a variety of maturation inducers (phorbol diester TPA, retinoids, butyric acid, DMSO) indicate that the maturation arrest can also be bypassed in some human leukemias (cell lines and fresh cells), entailing more differentiated cell phenotypes. Thus, some T-ALL cell lines can be induced by TPA to irreversibly modulate their composite phenotype from that of an immature or thymic variety to that of a mature T cell subset [302]. TPA- or PHA-conditioned leukocyte culture media were capable of inducing the expression of B1 (see section: *Lymphocyte Differentiation Antigens as Defined by Classic Meteroantisera)* on non-T ALL cell lines, and tumor cells of patients with common ALL lacking B1 and cytoplasmic IgM expressed these pre-B markers after in vitro treatment with TPA [182]. Also, the expression of receptors for mouse erythrocytes – a B-cell feature, observed in B-CLL – was inducible in common ALL blasts after culture in diffusion chambers implanted in irradiated mice [37]. Recently, phenotypic Ig synthesis was demonstrated in ALL cells where a genetic B commitment (pre-pre-B cell phenotype) was identified by gene probes before cultures [303]. The antigenic changes were accompanied by a decrease or slowing in cell cycling in all experiments in which this was investigated. This provides further support for the view that maturation arrest in leukemia may be a reversible regulatory defect which uncouples maturation and proliferation [187].

Leukemia Maturation Induction in Vivo – A New Approach to the Treatment

The experiments discussed above suggest a possible "reprogramming" of leukemic cells with normal differentiation under the influence of certain substances. The potential this offers would be exploited if a continuous treatment by such substances or biological factors could be organized for maintenance of normal differentiation of leukemic cells, as proposed in a recent annotation [304]. Accordingly, some pilot therapy trials with prolonged administration of small doses of cytostatic drugs such as cytosine arabinoside or aclacinomycin A have revealed surprising remissions of myeloid leukemias in the few patients treated so far [305–307]. The dosage of cytosine arabinoside used in these studies was lower than is needed for an antimitotic effect, and lay in a range in which interference with differentiation processes has been reported. Remarkably, a remission has been reported in a woman with a relatively long history of AML disease with recurrence and resistance to conventional, intensive cytotoxic treatment [306]. In another study of patients with cutaneous T cell lymphoma, dramatic responses of the skin infiltrates were reported after daily treatment with 13-*cis*-retinoic acid [308].

It is tempting to speculate that this new approach to treatment may be of broader relevance than shown so far in the few patients in the preliminary studies reported. This approach was born of exact and detailed observation of leukemic cell phenotypes under varying conditions in vivo and in vitro. Hereby, cell markers may not only be useful for monitoring of induced maturation, but also in identifying cell types that can be induced to differentiate.

References

1. Virchow R (1845) Weisses Blut. Froriep's Notizen 36: 151
2. Bennett JN (1845) Case of hypertrophy of the spleen and liver, in which death took place from supparation of the blood. Edinb Med Surg J 64: 400
3. Thierfelder S, Rodt H, Thiele E (1977) Immunological diagnosis of leukemias and lymphomas. Springer, Berlin Heidelberg New York
4. Koehler G, Milstein C (1977) Continous cultures of fuses and lymphomas. Springer, Berlin Heidelberg New York
5. Knapp W (1981) Leukemia markers. Academic Press, London
6. Kumagai K, Abo T, Sekizawa T, Sasaki M (1975) Studies of surface immunoglobulins on human B lymphocytes. I. Dissociation of cell-bound immunoglobulins with acid pH or at 37° C. J Immunol 155: 982
7. Reyes F, Lejong JL, Gourdin MF, Mannoni P, Dreyfus B (1975) Application de la méthode de l'immunoperoxidase à l'étude de la membrane des lymphocytes humains. Pathol Biol (Paris) 23: 479
8. Taylor CR (1978) Immunoperoxidase techniques: theoretical and practical aspects. Arch Pathol Lab Med 102: 113
9. Dighiero G, Bodega E, Mayzner R, Binet JL (1980) Individual cell-by-cell quantitation of lymphocyte surface membrane Ig in normal and CLL lymphocytes and during ontogeny of mouse B lymphocytes by immunoperoxidase assay. Blood 55: 93
10. Thiel E, Dörmer P, Rodt H, Huhn D, Bauchinger M, Kley HP, Thierfelder S (1977) Quantitation of T-antigenic sites and Ig-determinants on leukemic cells by microphotometric immunoautoradiography Proof of the clonal origin of thymus-derived lymphocytic leukemias. Haematol Bluttransfus 20: 131
11. Herzenberg LA, Herzenberg LA (1978) Analysis and separation using the fluorescence activated cell sorter (FACS). In: Weir DM (ed) Handbook of experimental immunology vol 2,1. Blackwell, Oxford
12. Raff MC, Megson M, Owen JJT, Cooper MD (1976) Early production of intracellular IgM by B-lymphocyte precursors in mouse. Nature 259: 224
13. Gahings WE, Lawton AR, Cooper MD (1977) Immunofluorescent studies of the development of pre-B cells, B lymphocytes and immunoglobulin isotype diversity in humans. Eur J Immunol 7: 804
14. Pearl ER, Vogler LB, Okos AJ, Crist WM, Lawton AR, Cooper MD (1978) B lymphocyte precursors in human bone marrow: an analysis of normal individuals and patients with antibody-defiency states. J Immunol 120: 1169
15. Holm G, Mellstedt H, Petterson D, Biberfeld P (1977) Idiotypic immunoglobulin structure on blood lymphocytes in human plasma cell myeloma. Immunol Rev 34: 139
16. Fu SM, Winchester RJ, Feizi T, Walzer PD, Kunkel HG (1974) Idiotypic specificity of surface immunoglobulin and the maturation of leukaemic bone marrow derived lymphocytes. Proc Natl Acad Sci USA 71: 4487
17. Canale D, Collins RD (1974) Use of bone marrow particle sections in the diagnosis of multiple myeloma. Am J Clin Pathol 61: 382
18. Bach JF, Dormont J, Dardenne M, Balner H (1969) In vitro rosette inhibition by antihuman antilymphocyte serum. Correlation with skin graft prolongation in subhuman primates. Transplantation 8: 265
19. Coombs RRA, Gurner BW, Wilson AB, Holm G, Lindgren B (1970) Rosette formation between human lymphocytes and sheep red cells not involving immunoglobulin receptors. Int Arch Allergy Appl Immunol 39: 658
20. Brain P, Gordon J, Willetts WA (1970) Rosette formation by peripheral lymphocytes. Clin Exp Immunol 6: 681
21. Lay HL, Mendes NF, Bianco C, Nussenzweig V (1971) Binding of sheep red blood cells to a large population of human lymphocytes. Nature 230: 531

22. Fröland SS (1972) Binding of sheep erythrocytes to human lymphocytes. A probable marker of T-lymphocytes. Scand J Immunol 1:269
23. Jondal M, Holm G, Wigzell H (1972) Surface markers on human T- and B-lymphocytes. I. A large population of lymphocytes forming non-immune rosettes with SRBC. J Exp Med 136:207
24. Silveira NPA, Mendes NF, Tolnai MEA (1972) Tissue localization of two populations of human lymphocytes distinguished by membrane receptors. J Immunol 108:1456
25. Aiuti F, Wigzell H (1973) Function and distribution of human lymphocytes. I. Production of anti-T lymphocyte specific sera as estimated by cytotoxicity and elimination of function of lymphocytes. Clin Exp Immunol 13:171
26. Wick G, Gattringer C (1977) Two antibodies in anti-human T-cell sera. In: Thierfelder S, Rodt H, Thiel E (eds) Immunological diagnosis of leukemias and lymphomas. Springer, Berlin Heidelberg New York, p 361
27. Blackstock R, Humphrey GB (1982) Cell surface markers in the characterization of leukemias. Methods Cancer Res 19:3
28. Woda BA, Fenaglio CM, Nette EG, King DW (1977) The lack of specificity of the sheep erythrocyte – T lymphocyte rosetting phenomenon. Am J Pathol 88:69
29. Rodt H, Thierfelder S, Thiel E, Götze D, Netzel B, Huhn D, Eulitz M (1975) Identification and quantification of human T-cell antigen by antisera purified from antibodies crossreacting with hemopoietic progenitors and other blood cells. Immunogeneics 2:411
30. Thiel E, Rodt H, Netzel B, Huhn D, Wündisch GF, Haas R, Bender B, Thierfelder S (1978) T antigen positive but E-rosette negative acute lymphatic leukemia. Blut 36:363
31. Stathopoulos G, Elliott EV (1974) Formation of mouse or sheep red blood cell rosettes by lymphocytes from normal and leukaemic individuals. Lancet 1:600
32. Dobozy A, Husz S, Hunyadi J, Simon N (1976) Formation of mouse erythrocyte rosettes by human lymphocytes. A B-cell marker. Clin Exp Immunol 23:382
33. Forbes IJ, Zalewski PD (1976) A subpopulation of human B-lymphocytes that rosette with mouse erythrocytes. Clin Exp Immunol 26:99
34. Bertoglio J, Thierry C, Flores G, Boucharel C, Dore JF (1977) Mouse red cell rosette formation by subpopulations of human lymphocytes. Clin Exp Immunol 27:172
35. Gupta S, Pahwa R, O'Reilly R, Good RA, Siegal FP (1976) Ontoheny of lymphocyte subpopulations in human fetal liver. Proc Natl Acad Sci USA 73:919
36. Bertoglio J, Peaud PY, Bryon PA, Treille D, Felman P, Dore JF (1976) Prognostic value of mouse re cell rosette formation in chronic lymphocytic leukemia. Biomedicine 25:227
37. Thiel E, Lau B, Rodt H, Jäger G, Pachmann K (1981) Appearance of B- or T-lymphocyte markers after diffusion chamber culture of acute lymphoblastic leukemia cells. Blut 42:315
38. Boyden SV, Sorkin E (1964) The absorption of antibody and antigen by spleen cells in vitro. Some further experiments. Immunology 4:244
39. Uhr JW, Philipps JM (1966) In vitro sensitization of phagocytes and lymphocytes by antigen-antibody complexes. Ann NY Acad Sci 129:792
40. Huber H, Fudenberg HH (1976) Receptor sites of human monocytes for IgG. Int Arch Allergy Appl Immune 34:18
41. Henson PM (1976) Membrane receptors on neutrophils. Immunol Commun 5:757
42. Dickler HB, Kunkel HG (1972) Interaction of aggregated-globulin with B lymphocytes. J Exp Med 136:191
43. Fröland SS, Natvig JB (1973) Identification of three different human lymphocyte populations by surface markers. Transplant Rev 16:114
44. Moretta L, Webb SR, Grossi CE, Lydyard PM, Cooper MC (1976) Functional analysis of two subpopulations of human T cells and their distribution in immunodeficient patients. Clin Res 24:488
45. Yodoi J, Miyama M, Masuda T (1978) Immunological properties of Fc receptors on lymphocytes. 2. Differentiation from FcR− to FcR cells and their functional differences in vitro antibody response. Cell Immunol 35:266

46. Bianco C, Patrick R, Nussenzweig V (1970) A population of lymphocytes bearing a membrane receptor of antigen-antibody complement complexes. I. Separation and characterization. J Exp Med 132: 702
47. Bianco C, Nussenzweig V (1971) Theta-bearing and complementreceptor lymphocytes are distinct populations of cells. Science 173: 154
48. Ross GD, Polley MJ, Rabellino EM, Grey HM (1973) Two different complement receptors on human lymphocytes. J Exp Med 138: 798
49. Bokisch VA, Sobel AT (1974) Receptor for the fourth component of complement on human B lymphocytes and cultured human lymphoblastoid cells. J Exp Med 140: 1336
50. Chiao JW, Good RA (1976) Studies of the presence of membrane receptors for complement, IgG and the sheep erythrocyte rosetting capacity on the same human lymphocytes Eur J Immunol 6: 157
51. Rabellino EM, Ross GD, Trang HTK, Williams N, Metcalf D (1978) Membrane receptors of mouse leukocytes. II. Sequential expression of membrane receptors and phagocytic capacity during leukocyte differentiation. J Exp Med 147: 434
52. Gelfand MC, Elfenbein GJ, Frank MM, Paul WE (1974) Ontogeny of B lymphocytes. II. Relative rates of appearance of lymphocytes bearing surface immunoglobulin and complement receptors. J Exp Med 139: 1125
53. Reif AE, Allen JV (1963) Specificity of isoantisera against leukemia and thymic lymphocytes. Nature 200: 1332
54. Raff MC (1969) Theta isoantigen as a marker of thymus-derived lymphocytes in mice. Nature 224: 378–379
55. Williams RC, De Board JR, Mellbye OJ, Messner RP, Lindstrom RF (1973) Studies of T- and B-lymphocytes in patients with connective tissue diseases. J Clin Invest 52: 283
56. Smith RW, Terry WD, Buell DN, Sell KW (1973) An antigeneic marker for human thymic lymphocytes. J Immunol 110: 884
57. Anderson LC, Karhi KK, Gahmberg CG, Rodt H (1980) Molecular identification of T cell-specific antigens on human T lymphocytes and thymocytes. Eur J Immunol 10: 359
58. Evans RL, Lazarus H, Penta AC, Schlossman SF (1978) Two functionally distinct subpopulations of human T cells that collaborate in the generation of cytotoxic cells responsible for cell-mediated lympholysis. J Immunol 120: 1423
59. Rodt H, Thiel E, Hoffmann-Fezer G, Netzel B, Thierfelder S (1980) Identification of two different T-cell antigens expressed on early and mature thymus-derived lymphocytes and leukemic cells. Exp Hematol [Suppl 7] 8: 15
60. Goodfellow P, Barnstable C, Jones E, Bodmer FW, Crumpton MJ, Snary D (1976) Production of specific antisera to human B-lymphocytes. Tissue Antigens 7: 105
61. Balch CM, Dougherty PA, Vogler LB, Ades EW, Ferrone S (1978) A new B-cell differentiation antigen (BDA) on normal and leukemic human B lymphocytes that is distinct from known DR (Ia-like) antigens. J Immunol 121: 2322
62. Wang CY, Fu SM, Kunkel HG (1979) Isolation and immunological characterization of a major surface glycoprotein (gp 54) preferentially expressed on certain human B cells. J Exp Med 149: 1424
63. Berntrop E, Turesson I, Zettervall O (1979) Heterologous B-cell antisera may detect non-Ig, non-HLA-DR antigens. Scand J Immunol 10: 17
64. McDevitt HO, Benacerraf B (1969) Genetic control of the immune response. Adv Immunol 11: 31
65. Benacerraf B, McDevitt HO (1972) Histocompatibility linked immune response genes. Science 175: 273
66. Dachs D, Cone JL (1973) A mouse "B" cell allo-antigen determined by gene(s) linked to the major histocompatibility complex. J Exp Med 138: 1289
67. Shreffler DC, David CS (1972) Studies on recombination within the mouse H-2 complex. I. Three recombinants which position the Sc locus within the complex. Tissue Antigens 2: 232

68. Götze D, Thiel E, Rodt H, Thierfelder S (1977) Heterologous group specific antiserum against Ia^K determinants. Haematol Bluttransfus 20: 341
69. Wernet P (1978) Human Ia-type alloantigens: methods of detection, aspects of chemistry and biology, markers for disease states. Transplant Rev 30: 271
70. Billing R, Rafizadeh B, Drew I, Hartmann G, Gale R, Terasaki P (1976) Human B-lymphocyte antigens expressed by lymphocytic and myelocytic leukemia cells. I. Detection by rabbit antisera. J Exp Med 144: 167
71. Schlossman SF, Chess L, Humphreys RE, Strominger JL (1976) Distribution of Ia-like molecules on the surface of normal and leukemic human cells. Proc Natl Acad Sci USA 73: 1288
72. Siphardt MJ, Kaufman JF, Fuks A, Albrechtsen D, Solheim BG, Brunning JW, Strominger JL (1977) HLA-d associated alloantisera react with molecules similar to Ia antigens. Proc Natl Acad Sci USA 74: 3533
73. Billing RJ, Safani M, Peterson P (1976) Isolation and characterization of human B cell alloantigens. J Immunol 117: 1589
74. Winchester RJ, Ross GD, Jarowski CJ, Wang CY, Halper J, Broxmeyer HE (1977) Expression of Ia-like antigens on human granulocytes during early phases of differentiation. Proc Natl Acad Sci USA 74: 4012
75. Cline MS, Billing R (1977) Antigens expressed by lymphocytes and myeloid stem cells. J Exp Med 146: 1143
76. Winchester RJ, Meyers PA, Broxmeyer HE, Wang CY, Moore MAS, Kunkel HG (1978) Inhibition of human erythropoietic colony formation in culture by treatment with Ia antisera. J Exp Med 148: 613–617
77. Belzer M, Fitchen JH, Ferrone S, Foon KA, Billing RJ, Golde D (1981) Expression of Ia-like antigens on human erythroid progenitor cells as determined by monoclonal antibodies and heteroantiserum to Ia-like antigens. Clin Immunol Immunopathol 20: 111–115
78. Evans RI, Faldetta TJ, Humphreys RE, Pratt DM, Yunis EJ, Schlossman SF (1978) Peripheral human T cells sensitized in mixed leukocyte culture synthesize and express Ia-like antigens. J Exp Med 148: 1440–1445
79. Fu SM, Chiorazzi N, Wang CY, Montazeri G, Kunkel HG, Ko HS, Gottlieb AB (1978) Ia-bearing T lymphocytes in man. Their identification and role in the generation of allogenic helper activity. J Exp Med 148: 1423–1428
80. Greaves MF, Brown G, Rapson N, Lister TA (1975) Antisera to acute lymphoblastic leukemia cells. Clin Immunol Immunopathol 4: 67
81. Rodt H, Netzel B, Thiel E, Jäger G, Huhn D, Haas R, Götze D, Thierfelder S (1977) Classification of leukemic cells with T- and O-ALL-specific antisera. Hematol Bluttransfus 20: 87–95
82. Borella L, Sen L, Casper JT (1977) Acute lymphoblastic leukemias (ALL) Antigens detected with antisera to E rosette-forming and non-E rosette-forming ALL blasts. J Immunol 188: 309–315
83. Billing R, Minowada J, Cline M, Clark B, Lee K (1978) Acute lymphocytic leukemia-associated cell membrane antigens. J Natl Cancer Inst 61: 423–429
84. Brown G, Hogg N, Greaves MF (1975) A candidate human leukemia antigen. Nature 258: 454
85. Greaves MF, Janossy G (1978) Patterns of gene expression and the cellular origins of human leukaemias. Biochim Biophys Acta 516: 193
86. Metzgar RS, Mohanakumar T (1977) Serologic studies of the diagnosis and nosology of human leukemia. Am J Clin Pathol 68: 699
87. Sutherland R, Smart J, Niaudet P, Greaves MF (1978) Acute lymphoblastic leukaemia associated antigen II. Isolation and partial characterization. Leuk Res 2: 115–216
88. Greaves MF, Hauri G, Newman RA, Sutherland DR, Ritter MA, Ritz J (1983) Selective expression of the common acute lymphoblastic leukemia (gp 100) antigen on immature lymphoid cells and their malignant counterparts. Blood 61: 628

89. Braun MP, Martin PJ, Ledbetter JA, Hansen JH (1983) Granulocytes and cultured human fibroblasts express common acute lymphoblastic leukemia-associated antigen. Blood 61: 718
90. Lippman ME, Yabro GK, Leventhal BG (1978) Clinical implications of glucocorticord receptors in human leukemia. Cancer Res 38: 4251
91. Nakao Y, Tsuboi S, Fujita T, Masaoka T, Morikawa I, Watanabe S (1981) Glucocorticord receptors and terminal deoxynucleotidyl transferase activities in leukemic cells. Cancer 47: 1812
92. Yabro GK, Lippman ME, Johnson GE, Leventhal BG (1977) Glucocorticord receptors in subpopulation of childhood acute lymphocyte leukemia. Cancer Res 37: 2688
93. Bloomfield CD, Peterson BA, Smith KA, Gajl-Peczalska KJ, Munck A (1980) In vitro glucocorticord studies for predicting response to glucocorticord therapy in adults with malignant lymphoma. Lancet 1: 952
94. Kontula K, Andersson LC, Paavonen T, Myllyla G, Teerenhovi L, Uuopro P (1980) Glucocorticoid receptors and glucocorticoid sensitivity of human leukemic cells. Int J Cancer 26: 177
95. Reisner Y, Biniaminov M, Rosenthal E, Sharon N, Ramot B (1979) Interaction of peanut agglutinin with normal lymphocytes and with leukemia cells. Proc Natl Acad Sci USA 76: 447
96. Kedar E, Bonavida B (1974) Histamine receptor-bearing Leukocytes (HRL). I. Detection of histamine receptor-bearing cells by rosette formation with histamin-coated erythrocytes. J Immunol 113: 1544
97. Plaut M, Lichtenstein LM, Henney CS (1975) Properties of a subpopulation of T cells bearing histamine receptors. J Clin Invest 55: 856–874
98. Ballet JJ, Merler E (1976) The separation and reactivity in vitro of a subpopulation of human lymphocytes which bind histamine: correlation of histamine reactivity with cellular maturation. Cell Immunol 24: 250–269
99. Rocklin RE (1976) Modulation of cellular-immune responses in vivo and in vitro by histamine receptor-bearing lymphocytes. J Clin Invest 57: 1051–1058
100. Roszkowski W, Plaut M, Lichtenstein LM (1977) Selective display of histamine receptors on lymphocytes. Science 195: 683–685
101. Helderman JH, Strom TB (1978) Specific insulin binding site on T and B lymphocytes as a marker of cell activation. Nature 274: 62
102. Esber EC, Buell DN, Leikin SC (1976) Insulin binding of acute lymphocytic leukemia cells Blood 49: 33
103. Pochet R, Delespesse G, Gausset PW, Collet H (1979) Distribution of beta-adrenergic receptors on human lymphocyte subpopulations. Clin Exp Immunol 38: 578
104. Marone G, Plaut M, Lichtenstein LM (1978) Characterization of a specific adenosine receptor on human lymphocytes. J Immunol 121: 2153
105. Goodwin JS, Wiik A, Lewis M, Bankhurst AD, Williams RC (1979) High-affinity binding sites for prostaglandin E on human lymphocytes. Cell Immunol 43: 150
106. Ruscetti FW, Gallo RC (1981) Human T-lymphocyte growth factor: Regulation of Growth and function of T-lymphocytes. Blood 57: 379
107. Jodal M, Klein G (1973) Surface markers on human B and T lymphocytes. II. Presence of Epstein-Barr virus receptors on B lymphocytes. J Exp Med 138: 1365
108. Jondal M, Klein G, Oldstone MBA, Bokisch V, Yefenot E (1976) Surface markers on human B and T lymphocytes. VIII. Association between complement and Epstein-Barr virus receptors on B lymphocytes. Scand J Immunol 5: 401
109. Vladimarsson H, Agnarsdottin G, Lachmann PJ (1975) Measles virus receptor on human T lymphocytes. Nature 255: 554
110. Teodorescu M, Bratescu A, Mayer EP (1979) The use of the natural T- and B-lymphocyte subpopulations in blood smears. Clin Immunol Immunopathol 13: 194
111. Nakahara K, Ohashi T, Oda T, Hirano T, Kasai M, Okumura G, Tada T (1980) Asialo GM_1, as a cell-surface marker detected in acute lymphoblastic leukemia. N Engl J Med 302: 674

112. Hildebrand J, Strychmans PA, Vanhouse J (1972) Gangliosides in leukemic and non-leukemic human leukocytes. Biochim Biophys Acta 260: 272
113. Geisen HP, Dorken D, Lenhard V, Roelckew D (1977) The autoantigen determinants I/i, Pr i-3 of normal and leukemic leukocytes, Haematol Bluttrans 20: 347
114. Revesz T, Greaves MF, Capellaro D, Murray RK (1976) Differential expression of cell surface binding sites for cholera toxin in acute and chronic leukaemias. Br J Haematol 34: 623
115. Blatt J, Reaman G, Poplack DG (1980) Biochemical markers in lymphoid malignancy. N Engl J Med 303: 918
116. Bollum FJ (1979) Terminal deoxynucleiotidyl transferase as a hematopoietic cell marker. Blood 54: 1203
117. Marks SM, Baltimore D, McCaffrey R (1978) Terminal transferase as a predictor of initial responsiveness to vincristine and prednisone in blastic chronic myelogenous leukemia: a co-operative study. N Engl J Med 298: 812
118. Hutton JJ, Coleman MS, Moffitt S, Greenwood MF, Holland P, Lampkin B, Kisher T, Krill C, Kastelic JE, Valdez L, Bollum FJ (1982) Prognostic significance of terminal transferase activity in childhood acute lymphoblastic leukemia: a prospective analysis in 164 patients. Blood 60: 1267
119. Bradstock KF, Hoffbrand AV, Ganeshaguru K, Llewelein P, Patterson K, Wonke B, Prentice AG, Benett M, Pizzolo G, Bollum FJ, Janossy G (1981) Terminal deoxynucleotidyl transferase expression in acute non-lymphoid leukemia: an analysis by immunofluorescence. Br J Haematol 47: 133
120. Gutensohn W, Thiel E, Emmerich B (1983) Evaluation of 5′-Nucleotidase as biochemical marker in leukemias and lymphomas. Klin Wochenschr 61: 57
121. Silber R, Conklyn M, Grusky G, Zucker-Franklin D (1975) Human lymphocytes: 5′Nucleotidase-positive and -negative subpopulations. J Clin Invest 56: 1324
122. Thompson LF, Boss GR, Spiegelberg HL et al. (1979) Ecto-5′nucleotidase activity in T and B lymphocytes from normal subjects and patients with congenital X-linked agammaglobulinemia. J Immunol 123: 2475
123. Kanter RJ, Freiberger IA, Rai KR, Sawitsky A (1979) Lymphocymphocyte populations with 5′-nucleotidase in chronic lymphocytic leukemia. Clin Immunol Immunopathol 12: 351
124. Reaman GH, Levin N, Muchmore A, Holiman BJ, Poplack DG (1979) Diminished lymphoblast 5′-nucleotidase activity in acute lymphoblastic leukemia with T-cell characteristics. N Engl J Med 300: 1374
125. Gutensohn W, Thiel E (1981) High levels of 5′nucleotidase activity in blastic chronic myelogenous leukemia with common ALL-antigen. Leuk Res 5: 505
126. Koya M, Kanoh T, Sawada H, Uchino H, Neda K (1981) Adenosine deaminase and ecto-5′-nucleotidase activities in various leukemias with special reference to blast crisis: significance of ecto-5′-nucleotidase in lymphoid blast crisis of chronic myeloid leukemia. Blood 58: 1107
127. Giblett ER, Anderson JE, Cohen F, Pollara B, Meuwissen HJ (1972) Adenosine deaminase deficiency in two patients with severely impaired cellular immunity. Lancet 2: 1067
128. Giblett ER, Ammann AJ, Wara DW, Sandman R, Diamond LK (1975) m-Nucleoside-phosphorylase deficiency in a child with severly defective T-cell immunity and normal B-cell immunity. Lancet 1: 1010
129. Biggar WD, Giblett ER, Ozere RL, Grover BD (1978) A new form of nucleoside phosphorylase deficiency in two brothers with defective T-cell function. J Pediatr 92: 354
130. Johnson SM, North ME, Asherson GL, Allsop J, Watts RWE, Webster ADB (1977) Lymphocyte purine 5′-nucleotidase deficiency in primary hypogammaglobulinaemia. Lancet 1: 168
131. Edwards NL, Magilavy DB, Cassidy JT, Fox IH (1978) Lymphocyte ecto-5′-nucleotidase deficiency in agammaglobulinemia. Science 201: 628
132. Tung R, Silber R, Quagliata F, Conklyn M, Gottesman J, Hirschhorn R (1976) Adenosine deaminase activity in chronic lymphocytic leukemia: relationship to B- and T-cell subpopulations. J Clin Invest 57: 756

133. Coleman MS, Greenwood MF, Hutton JJ et al. (1978) Adenosine deaminase, terminal deoxynucleotidyl transferase (TdT) and cell surface markers in childhood acute leukemia. Blood 52: 1125
134. Meier J, Coleman MS, Hutton JJ (1976) Adenosine deaminase activity in peripheral blood cells of patients with hematological malignancies. Br J Cancer 33: 312–319
135. Koller CA, Mitchell BS, Grever MR, Mejias E, Malspeis L, Metz EN (1979) Treatment of acute lymphoblastic leukemia with 2′-deoxycoformycin: clinical and biochemical consequences of adenosine deaminase inhibition. Cancer Treat Rep 63: 1949–1952
136. Borgers M, Verhaegen H, De Brabander M et al. (1978) Purine nucleoside phosphorylase in chronic lymphocytic leukemia (CLL). Blood 52: 886–894
137. Ellis RB, Rapson NT, Patrick AD, Greaves MF (1978) Expression of hexoaminidase isoenzymes in childhood leukemia. N Engl J Med 298: 476
138. Besley GTN, Broadhead DM, Bain AD, Dewar AE, Eden OB (1978) Enzyme markers in acute lymphoblastic leukemia. Lancet 2: 1311
139. Yam LT (1974) Clinical significance of the human acid phosphatase. Am J Med 56: 604
140. Catovsky D, Greaves MF, Pain C, Cherchi K, Janossy G, Kay HE (1978) Acid-phosphatase reaction in acute lymphoblastic leukaemia. Lancet 1: 749
141. Huhn D, Thiel E, Rodt H (1980) Classification of normal and malignant lymphatic cells using acid phosphatase and acid esterase. Klin Wochenschr 58: 65
142. Osserman EF, Lawlor DP (1966) Serum and urinary lysozyme (muramidase) in monocytic and myelomonocytic leukemia. J Exp Med 124: 921
143. Garson JA, Beverly PCL, Coakham HB, Harper ET (1982) Monoclonal antibodies against human T-lymphocytes label Purkinji neurones of many species. Nature 298: 375
144. Bach MA, Bach JF (1981) The use of monoclonal anti-T cell antibodies to study T cell imbalances in human diseases. Clin Exp Immunol 45: 449
145. Howard IC, Butcher GW, Galfre G, Milstein C, Milstein CP (1983) Monoclonal antibodies as tools to analyse the serological and genetic complexities of major transplantation antigens. Immunol Rev 47: 139
146. Reinherz EL, Kung PC, Goldstein G, Schlossman SF (1979) Separation of functional subsets of human T cells by a monoclonal antibody. Proc Natl Sci Acad USA 76: 4061
147. Reinherz EL, Kung PC, Goldstein G, Schlossman SF (1980) A monoclonal antibody reactive with the human cytotoxic/suppressor T cell subset previously defined by a heteroantiserum termed TH_2. J Immunol 124: 1301
148. Stutman O (1977) Two main features of T-cell development: Thymic traffic and post thymic maturation. Contemp Top Immunobiol 7: 1
149. Gatien JG, Schneeberger EE, Merler E (1945) Analysis of human thymocyte subpopulations using discontinous gradient of albumin: precursor lymphocytes in human thymus. Eur J Immunol 5: 312
150. Galili U, Polliack A, Ohon E, Gambel H, Izak G (1982) Human prothymocytes: membrane properties, differentiation patterns, glucocorticoid sensitivity and ultrastructural feature. J Exp Med 148: 1423
151. Reinherz EL, Kung PC, Goldstein G, Levey R, Schlossman SF (1980) Discrete stages of human intrathymic differentiation: analysis of normal thymocytes and leukemic lymphoblasts of T cell lineage. Proc Natl Acad Sci USA 77: 6152
152. Hoffmann-Fezer G, Knapp W, Thierfelder S (1983) Anatomical distribution of CALL antigen expressing cells in normal lymphatic tissue and in lymphomas. Leuk Res 6: 761
153. McMichael AJ, Pilch JR, Galfre G, Mason DY, Fabre JW, Milstein C (1979) A human thymocyte antigen defined by a hybrid myeloma monoclonal antibody. Eur J Immunol 9: 205
154. Munker R, Stünkel K, Thiel E, Thierfelder S (1983) Analysis with monoclonal antibodies of human lymphoid cells forming rossettes with rabbit red blood cells. Clin Exp Immunol 51: 479
155. Bhan AK, Reinherz EL, Poppema S, Cluskey RT, Schlossman SF (1980) Location of T cell and major histocompatibility complex antigens in the human thymus. J Exp Med 152: 771

156. Janossy G, Tidman N, Selby WS, Thomas JA, Granger S, Kung PC, Goldstein G (1980) Human T lymphocytes of inducer and suppressor type occupy different microenvironments. Nature 288:81
157. Abdou NL, Alavi JB, Abdou NI (1976) Human bone marrow lymphocytes: B and T cell precursors and subpopulations. Blood 47:423
158. Thiel E, Rodt H, Huhn D, Netzel B, Grosse-Wilde H, Ganeshaguru K, Thierfelder S (1980) Multimarker classification of acute lymphoblastic leukemia: evidence for further T subgroups and evaluation of their elinical significance. Blood 56:759
159. Foon KA, Schroff RW, Gale RP (1982) Surface markers on leukemia and lymphoma cells: recent advances. Blood 60:1
160. Bernard A, Boumsell L, Reinherz EL, Nadler LM, Ritz I, Coppin H, Richard Y, Valensi F, Dausset J, Flandrin G, Lemerle J, Schlossman SF (1981) Cell surface characterization of malignant T cells from lymphoblastic lymphomas using monoclonal antibodies: evidence for phenotypic differences between malignant T cells from patients with acute lymphoblastic leukemia and lymphoblastic lymphoma. Blood 57:1105
161. Findley HW, Cooper MD, Kim TH, Alvarado C, Ragab AH (1982) Two new acute lymphoblastic leukemia cell lines with early B-cell phenotypes. Blood 60:1
162. Greaves MF, Rao J, Hariri G, Verbi W, Catovsky D, Kung P, Goldstein G (1981) Phenotypic heterogeneity and cellular origins of T cell malignancies. Leuk Res 5:281
163. Brandstock KF, Janossy G, Bollum FJ, Milstein C (1980) Anomalous gene expression in human thymic acute lymphoblastic leukemia (Thy-LL). Nature 294:455
164. Boumsell L, Bernard A, Reinherz EL, Nadler LM, Ritz J, Coppin H, Richard Y, Dubertret L, Valensi F, Degos L, Lemerle J, Flandrin G, Dausset J, Schlossman SF (1981) Surface antigens on malignant Sézary and T-CLL cells correspond to those of mature T cells. Blood 57:526
165. Kung PC, Berger CL, Goldstein G, LoGerfo P, Edelson RL (1981) Cutaneous T cell lymphoma: characterization by monoclonal antibodies. Blood 57:261
166. Broder S, Edelson RL, Lutzner MA, Nelson DL, McDermott RP, Durm ME, Goldman CK, Meade BD,Waldmann TA (1976) The Sézary syndrome: a malignant proliferation of helper T cells. J Clin Invest 58:1297
167. Pandolfi F, Strong DM, Slease ML, Smith ML, Orfaldo JR, Herberman RB (1980) Characterization of a suppressor T-cell chronic lymphocyte leukemia with ADCC but not NK activity. Blood 56:653
168. Schlimok G, Thiel E, Rieber EP, Huhn D, Feucht H, Lohmeyer J, Riethmüller G (1982) Chronic leukemia with a hybrid surface phenotype (T lymphocytic/myelomonocytic): leukemic cells displaying natural killer activity and antibody-dependent cellular cytotoxicity. Blood 59:1157
169. Riethmüller G, Lohmeyer J, Rieber EP, Feucht H, Schlimok G, Thiel E (1982) Unique combination of surface markers on human NK cells: a phenotypic compromise at last. In: Hebermann R (ed) NK cells and other effector cells. Academic Press, London, p 53
170. Koniyama A, Kawai H, Miyagawa Y, Akabane T (1982) Childhood lymphoblastic leukemia cell lines retaining the activity. Blood 60:1429
171. Broder S, Uchiyama T, Muul LM, Goldman C, Sharrow S, Poplack DG, Waldmann TA (1981) Activation of leukemic pro-suppressor cells to become suppressor-effector cells. N Engl J Med 304:1382
172. Miyoshi I, Kubonishi I, Yoshimoto S (1981) Type C virus particles in a cord T-cell line derived by co-cultivating normal human cord leukocytes and human leukaemic cells. Nature 294:770
173. Poiesz BJ, Ruscetti FW, Gazdar AF, Bunn PA, Minna JD, Gallo RC (1981) Detection and isolation of type C retrovirus particles from fresh and cultured lymphocytes of a patient with cutaneous T-cell lymphoma. Proc Natl Acad Sci USA 77:7415
174. Stashenko P, Nadler LM, Hardy R, Schlossman SF (1980) Characterization of a human B lymphocyte-specific antigen. J Immunol 125:1678

175. Nadler LM, Stashenko P, Hardy R, Agthoven A, Terhost C, Schlossmann SF (1981) Characterization of a human B cell-specific antigen (B-2) distinct from B 1. J Immunol 120: 1941
176. Brooks DA, Beckman IG, Bradley J, McNamara PJ, Thomas ME, Zola H (1981) Human lymphocyte markers defined by antibodies derived from somatic cells hybrids. I. Hybridoma secreting antibody against a marker specific from human 5 lymphocytoes. Clin Exp Immunol 39: 477
177. Brooks DA, Beckman IG, Bradley J, McNamara PJ, Thomas ME, Zola H (1981) Human lymphocyte markers defined by antibody derived from somatic cell hybrids. IV. A monoclonal antibody reacting specifically with a subpopulation of human B lymphocytes. J Immunol 126: 1373
178. Catovsky D, Cherchi M, Brooks D, Bradley J, Zola H (1981) Heterogeneity of B-cell leukemias demonstrated by the monoclonal antibody FMC7. Blood 58: 406
179. Ziegler A, Stein H, Müller C, Wernet P (1981) Tü-1: a monoclonal antibody defining a B cell subpopulation – usefulness for the classification of non-Hodgkin's lymphomas. In: Knapp W (ed) Leukemia markers. Academic Press London, p 113
180. Abramson CS, Kersey JH, LeBien TW (1981) A monoclonal antibody (BA-1) reactive with cells of human B lymphocyte lineage. J Immunol 126: 83
181. Korsmeyer SJ, Hieter PA, Ravech JV, Poplack DG, Waldmann TA, Leder P (1981) Developmental hierarchy of immunoglobulin gene rearrangements in human leukemic pre-B-cells. Proc Natl Acad Sci USA 78: 7096
182. Nadler LM, Ritz J, Bates MP, Park EK, Andferson KC, Sallen SE, Schlossman SF (1982) Induction of human B cell antigens in non-T cell acute lymphoblastic leukemia. J Clin Invest 70: 433
183. Martin PJ, Hansen KA, Nowinski RC, Brown MA (1980) A new human T-cell differentiation antigen: unexpected expression on chronic lymphocytic leukemia cells. Immunogenetics 11: 429
184. Munker R, Thiel E, Kummer U, Rodt H, Thierfelder S (1983) Crossreaction of monoclonal anti-T-cell antibodies: implications for classifying B-cell leukemia. Blut 46: 95
185. Caligaris-Cappio F, Gobbi M, Bofill M, Janossy G (1982) Infrequent normal B lymphocytes express features of B-chronic lymphocyte leukemia. J Exp Med 155: 623
186. Greaves MF, Delia D, Robinson J, Sutherland R, Newman R (1981) Exploitation of monoclonal antibodies: a "Who's Who" of haemapoietic malignancy. Blood Cells 7: 257
187. Sachs L (1981) Constitutive uncoupling of pathways of gene expression that control growth and differentiation in myeloid leukemia: a model for the origin and progression of malignancy. Proc Natl Acad Sci USA 78: 4515
188. Thiel E, Kummer U, Rodt H, Stünkel K, Munker R, Majidic O, Knapp W, Thierfelder S (1982) Comparison of currently available monoclonal antibodies with conventional markers for phenotyping of one hundred acute leukemias. Blut 44: 95
189. Kersey J, Goldman A, Abrahamson C, Nesbit M, Perry G, Gajl-Peczalska K, LeBien TW (1982) Clinical usefulness of monoclonal-antibody phenotyping in childhood acute lymphoblastic leukemia. Lancet 2: 1419
190. Ritz J, Schlossman SF (1982) Utilization of monoclonal antibodies in the treatment of leukemia and lymphoma. Blood 59: 1
191. Reinherz EL, Kung PC, Pesando JM, Ritz J, Goldstein G, Schlossman SF (1979) Ia determinants on human T cell subsets defined by monoclonal antibodies: activation stimuli required for expression. J Exp Med 150: 1472
192. Beverly PCL, Callard RE (1981) Distinctive functional characteristics of human "T" lymphocytes defined by E rosetting or a monoclonal anti T cell antibody. Eur J Immunol 11: 329
193. Van Wauwe J, Goosens J, Decock W, Rung P, Goldstein G (1981) Suppression of human T cell mitogenesis and E rosette formation by the monoclonal antibody OKT11 A. Immunology 44: 865

194. Kamoun M, Martin PJ, Hansen JA, Brown MA, Siadack WA, Nowinski RC (1981) Identification of a human T lymphocyte surface protein associated with the E rosette receptor. J Exp Med 153: 207
195. Howard FD, Ledbetter JA, Wong J, Breber CP, Stinson EB, Herzenberg LA (1981) A human T lymphocyte differentiation marker defined by monoclonal antibodies that block E-rosette formation. J Immunol 126: 2117
196. Engleman EG, Warnke R, Fox RJ, Dilley C, Benike CJ, Levy R (1981) Studies of a human T lymphocyte antigen recognized by a monoclonal antibody. Proc Natl Acad Sci USA, 78: 1791
197. Engleman EG, Benike CJ, Glickman E, Evans RL (1981) Antibodies to membrane structures that distinguish suppressor cytotoxic and helper T lymphocyte subpopulations block the mixed leukocyte reaction in man. J Exp Med 154: 193–198
198. Ritz J, Pesando JM, Notis-McConarty J, Lazarus H, Schlossman SF (1980) A monoclonal antibody to human acute lymphoblastic leukemia antigen. Nature 283: 583
199. Knapp W, Majdz O, Bettelheim P, Liszka K (1980) VIL-A1, a monoclonal antibody reactive with common acute lymphatic leukemia cells. Leuk Res 6: 137
200. LeBien TW, Bone DR, Bradley JG, Kersey JH (1982) Antibody affinity may influence antigenic modulation of the common acute lymphoblastic leukemia antigen in vitro. J Immunol 129: 2287
201. Lampson LA, Levy R (1980) Two populations on Ia-like molecules on a human B-cell line. J Immunol 125: 293
202. Bennett JM, Catovsky D, Daniel MT, Flandrin G, Galton DAG, Gralnick HR, Sultan C (1976) Proposals for the classification of acute leukemias. Br J Haematol 33: 451
203. Jager G, Hoffmann-Fezer G, Rodt H, Huhn D, Thiel E, Thierfelder S (1977) Myeloid antigens and antigen densities in mice and men. Haematol Bluttransfus 20: 109
204. Roberts M, Greaves MF (1978) Maturation linked expression of a myeloid cell surface antigen. Br J Haematol 38: 439–452
205. Billing R, Clark B, Koeffler P, Foon KA, Terasaki PI (1980) Acute myelogenous leukemia heteroantisera. Clin Immunol Immunopathol 16: 202–210
206. Mohanakumar T, Baker MA, Roncari DAK, Taub RN (1981) Serologic characterization of a monkey antiserum to human leukemic myeloblasts. Blood 56: 934
207. Knapp W (1982) Monoclonal antibodies against differentiation antigens of myelopoiesis. Blut 45: 301
208. Civin CI, Mirro J, Banquerigo ML (1981) My-1, a new myeloid-specific antigen identified by a mouse monoclonal antibody. Blood 57: 842
209. Majdic O, Liszka K, Lutz D, Knapp W (1981) Myeloid differentiation antigen defined by a monoclonal antibody. Blood 58: 1127
210. Uchanska-Ziegler B, Wernet P, Ziegler A (1981) Myeloid differentiation antigen defined by a monoclonal antibody. Blood 58: 1127
210a. Uchanska-Ziegler B, Wernet P, Ziegler A (1981) Monoclonal antiboidies against human lymphoid and myeloid antigens = AMML cells as immunogen. In: Knapp W (ed) Leukemia markers. Academic Press, London, p 243
211. Ugolini V, Nunez G, Smith RG, Stastny P, Capra DJ (1980) Initial characterization of monoclonal antibodies against human monocytes. Proc Natl Acad Sci USA 77: 6764
212. Todd RF, Nadler LM, Schlossman SF (1981) Antigens on human monocytes identified by monoclonal antibodies. J Immunol 126: 1435
213. Griffin JD, Ritz J, Nadler LM, Schlossman SF (1981) Expression of myeloid differentiation antigens on normal and malignant myeloid cells. J Clin Invest 68: 932
214. Linker-Israeli M, Billing RJ, Foon KA, Terasaki PI (1981) Monoclonal antibodies reactive with acute myelogenous leukemia cells. J Immunol 127: 2473
215. Breard J, Reinherz EL, Kung PC, Goldstein G, Schlossman SF (1980) A monoclonal antibody reactive with human peripheral blood monocytes. J Immunol 124: 1943–1948

216. Marie JP, Perrot JY, Boucheix C, Zittoun J, Martyre MC, Kayibanda M, Rosenfeld C, Mishal Z, Zittoun R (1982) Determination of ultrastructural peroxidases and immunologic membrane markers in the diagnosis of acute leukemias. Blood 59:270
217. Andersson LC, Gahmberg CG, Teerenhovi L, Vuopio P (1979) Glycophorin A as a cell surface marker of early erythroid differentiation in acute leukemia. Int J Cancer 23:717
218. Edwards PAW (1980) Monoclonal antibodies that bind to the human erythrocyte membrane glycoproteins glycophorin A and band 3. Biochem Soc Trans 8:334
219. Robinson J, Sieff C, Delia D, Edwards P, Greaves MF (1981) Expression of cell surface HLA-DR, HLA-ABC and glycophorin during erythroid differentiation. Nature 289:68
220. Greaves MF (1981) Monoclonal antibodies as probes for leukemic heterogeneity and hemopoietic differentiation. In: Knapp W (ed) Leukemia markers. Academic Press, New York, p 19
221. Lozzio BB, Lozzio CB (1979) Properties and usefullness of the original K 562 human myelogenous leukemia cell line. Leuk Res 3:363
222. Andersson LC, Jokinen M, Gahmberg CG (1979) Induction of erythroid differentiation in the human leukaemia cell line K 562. Nature 278:364
223. Breton-Gorius J, Reyes F, Duhamel G, Najman A, Gorin NC (1978) Megakaryoblastic acute leukemia = identification by the ultrastructural demonstration of platelet peroxidase. Blood 51:45
224. McMichael AJ, Rust NA, Pilch JR, Solchynsky R, Morton J, Mason DY, Ruan C, Tobelem G, Caen J (1981) Monoclonal antibody to human platelet glycoprotein I:I. immunological studies. Br J Haematol 49:501
225. Brouet JC, Flandrin G, Sasportes M, Preud'homme JL, Seligmann M (1975) Chronic lymphocyte leukemia of T-cell origin. Immunological and clinical evaluation in eleven patients. Lancet II:890
226. Huhn D, Thiel E, Rodt H, Schlimok G, Theml H, Rieber P (1983) Subtypes of T-cell chronic lymphatic leukemia. Cancer 51:1434
227. Hattori T, Uchiyama T, Toibana T, Takatsuki K, Uchino H (1981) Surface phenotype of Japanese adult T-cell leukemia cells characterized by monoclonal antibodies. Blood 58:645
228. Uchiyama T, Yodoi J, Sagawa K, Takatsuki K, Uchino H (1977) Adult T-cell leukemia = clinical and haematologic features of 16 cases. Blood 50:481
229. Catovsky D, Greaves MF, Rose M (1982) Adult T-cell lymphoma-leukaemia in Blacks from the West Indies. Lancet 1:639
230. Grossman B, Schlechter GP, Horton JE, Pierce L, Jaffe E, Wahl L (1981) Hypercalcemia associated with T-cell lymphoma-leukemia. Am J Pathol 75:149
231. Popovic M, Reitz MS Jr, Sarngadharan MG (1982) The virus of Japanese adult T-cell leukaemia is a virus of the human T-cell leukaemia virus group. Nature 300:63
232. Bunn PA, Schechter GP, Jaffe E, Blayney D, Young RC, Matthews MJ, Blattner W, Broder S, Robert-Guroff M, Gallo RC (1983) Clinical course of retrovirus-associated adult T-cell lymphoma in the United States. N Engl J Med 309:257
233. Zielinski CC, Waksal SD, Tempelis LD, Khiroya RH, Schwartz KS (1980) Surface phenotypes in T-cell leukaemia are determinded by oncogenic retroviruses. Nature 288:489
234. Gallo RC, Wong-Staal F (1982) Retroviruses as etiologic agents of some animal and human leukemias and lymphomas as tools for elucidating the molecular mechanism of leukemogenesis. Blood 60:545
235. Greaves MF (1981) Analysis of the clinical and biological significance of lymphoid phenotypes in acute leukemia. Cancer Res 41:4752
236. Thiel E, Rodt H, Thierfelder S (1981) Leukemic cell phenotypes and the lymphoid differentiation pathway. Haematologica 66:389 (editorial)
237. Bessis M, Brecher G (eds) (1975) Unclassifiable leukemias. Springer, Berlin Heidelberg New York

238. Hoelzer D, Thiel E, Löffler H, Bodenstern H, Büchrer T, Messerer D (1983) Multicentre pilot study for therapy of acute lymphoblastic and acute undifferentiated leukemia in adults. Haematol Bluttransfus 28: 36
239. Sen L, Borella L (1975) Clinical importance of lymphoblasts with T markers in childhood acute leukemia. N Engl J Med 292: 828
240. Tsukimoto I, Wong KY, Lampkin BC (1976) Surface markers and prognostic factors in acute lymphoblastic leukemia. N Engl J Med 294: 245
241. Coccia PF, Kersey JH, Kazamiera J, Gajl-Peczalska KJ, Krist W, Nesbit ME (1976) Prognostic significance of surface marker analysis in childhood non-Hodgkin's lymphoproliferative malignancies. Am J Hematol 1: 405
242. Belpomme D, Mathé G, Davies AJS (1977) Clinical significance and prognostic value of the T-B immunological classification of human primary acute lymphoid leukaemias. Lancet 1: 555
243. Chessels JM, Hardisty RM, Rapson NT, Greaves MF (1977) Acute lymphoblastic leukemia in children: classification and prognosis. Lancet 2: 1307
244. Vogler LB, Crist WM, Bockman DE, Pearl ER, Lawton AR, Cooper MD (1978) Pre-B cell leukemia: a new phenotype of childhood lymphoblastic leukemia. N Engl J Med 298: 872
245. Bronet JC, Preud'homme JL, Penit C, Valensi F, Rouget P, Seligmann M (1979) Acute lymphoblastic leukemia with pre-B-cell characteristics. Blood 54: 269
246. Miller DR, Leikin S, Albo V, Hammond D (1979) Prognostic significance of lymphoblast morphology (FAB classification) in childhood leukemia (ALL). Proc Am Soc Clin Oncol 20: 345
247. Bennett JM, Catovsky D, Daniel MT, Flandrin G, Galton DAG, Gralnick HR, Sultan C (1981) The morphological classification of acute lymphoblastic leukaemia: concordance among abservers and clinical correlations. Br J Haematol 47: 553
248. Third Workshop on Chromosomes in Leukemia (1981) Clinical significance of chromosomal abnormalities in acute lymphoblastic leukemia. Cancer Genet Cytogenet 4: 111
249. Brearly RL, Johnson SAN, Lister TA (1975) Acute lymphoblastic leukemia in adults: clinico-pathological correlations with the French-American-British (FAB) co-operative group classification. Eur J Cancer 15: 905
250. Palmer MK, Hann IM, Jones PM, Ewans DIK (1980) A scoreat diagnosis for predicting length of remission in childhood acute lymphoblastic leukemia. Br J Cancer 42: 841
251. Koziner B, Mertelsmann R, Andreff M, Arlin Z, Hansen H, DeHarven E, McKenzie S, Gee T, Good RA, Clarkson B (1980) Heterogeneity of cell lineages in L3 leukemias. Blood 55: 694
252. Murphy SDB, Borella L, Sen L, Mauer A (1975) Lack of correlation of lymphoblast cellsize with presence of T-cell markers or with outcome in childhood acute lymphoblastic leukemia. Br J Haematol 31: 95
253. Huhn D, Thiel E, Rodt H, Andrewa P (1981) Cytochemistry and membrane markers in acute lymphatic leukaemia (ALL). Scand J Haematol 26: 311
254. Pullen DJ, Faletta JM, Crist WM, Vogler LB, Dowell B, Humphrey GB, Blackstock R, van Eys J, Cooper MD, Metzgar RS, Meydreck EF (1981) Southwest Oncology Group experience with immunologic phenotyping in acute lymphocytic leukemia of childhood. Cancer Res 41: 4802
255. McKenna RW, Brynes RK, Nesbit ME, Bloomfield CD, Kersey JH, Spanjers E, Brunning MD (1979) Cytochemical profiles in acute lymphoblastic leukemia Am J Pediatr Hematol Oncol 3: 263
256. Kulenkampff J, Janossy G, Greaves MF (1977) Acid esterase in human lymphoid cells and leukaemic blasts: a marker for T lymphocytes. Br J Haematol 36: 231
257. Williams DL, Tsiatis A, Brodeur GM, Look AT, Melvin SL, Bowman WP, Kalwinsky DK, Rivera G, Dahl GB (1982) Prognostic importance of chromosome number in 136 untreated children with acute lymphoblastic leukemia. Blood 60: 864
258. Bloomfield CD, Lindquist LL, Arthur D, McKenna RW, LeBien TW, Peterson BA, Nesbit ME (1981) Chromosomal abnormalities in acute lymphoblastic leukemia. Cancer Res 41: 4838

259. Oshimura M, Freeman AI, Sandberg AA (1977) Chromosomes and causation of human cancer and leukemia. Cancer 40: 1161
260. Roozendaal KJ, van der Reijden HJ, Geraedts JPM (1981) Philadelphia chromosome positive acute lymphoblastic leukaemia with T-cell characteristics. Br J Haematol 47: 145
261. Barlogic B, Drewinko B, Schumann J, Gohde W, Dosik G, Latreille J, Johnston DH, Freireich EJ (1980) Cellular DNA content as a marker of neoplasia in man. Am J Med 69: 195
262. Look AT, Melvin SL, Williams DL, Brodeur GM, Dahl GV, Kalwinsky DK, Murphy SB, Mauer AM (1982) Aneuploidy and percentage of S-phase cells determined by flow cytometry correlate with cell phenotype in childhood acute leukemia. Blood 60: 959
263. Dow LW, Chang LJA, Tsiatis AA, Melvin SL, Bowman WP (1982) Relationship of pretreatment lymphoblast proliferative activity, and prognosis in 97 children with acute lymphoblastic leukemia. Blood 59: 1197
264. Foadi M, Cooper E, Hardisty RM (1968) Proliferative activity of leukaemia cells at various stages of acute leukaemia in childhood. Br J Haematol 15: 269
265. Murphy SB, Aur RJA, Simone JV, George S, Mauer AM (1977) Pretreatment cytokinetic studies in 94 children with acute leukemia. Relationship to other variables at diagnosis and to outcome of standard treatment, Blood 49: 683
266. Thiel E, Rodt H, Huhn D, Stunkel K, Gutensohn W, Thierfelder S (1981) Evidence for further ALL-subsets of discrete T-cell maturation and evaluation of their clinical significance. In: Knapp W (ed) Leukemia markers. Academic Press, London, p 471
267. Bronet JL, Seligmann M (1978) The immunological classification of acute lymphoblastic leukemias. Cancer 42: 817
268. Sallan SE, Ritz J, Pesando J, Gelber R, O'Brien C, Hitchcock S, Coral F, Schlossman SF (1980) Cell surface antigens = prognostic implications in childhood acute lymphoblastic leukemia. Blood 55: 395
269. Preud'homme JL, Brouet JC, Danon F, Flandrin G, Schiaison G (1981) Acute lymphoblastic leukemia with Burkitt's lymphoma cells: membrane marker and serum immunoglobulin. J Natl Cancer Inst 66: 261
270. Magrath IT, Ziegler JL (1980) Bone marrow involvement in Burkitt's lymphoma and its relationship to acute B-cell leukemia. Leuk Res 4: 33
271. Anderson J, Buxbaum J, Citronbaum R, Douglas S, Forni L, Melchers F, Pernis B, Stott D (1974) IgM producing tumors in the balb/c mouse: a model for B-cell maturation. J Exp Med 140: 742
272. Pinkel D (1979) The ninth annual David Karnofsky lecture = treatment of acute lymphocyte leukemia. Cancer 43: 1128
273. Haghbin M, Murphy ML, Tans CC (1980) A long-term clinical follow-up of children with acute lymphoblastic leukemia treated with intensive chemotherapy regimens. Cancer 46: 242
274. Simone JV, Verzosa MS, Rudy JA (1975) Initial features and prognosis in 363 children with acute lymphocytic leukemia. Cancer 36: 2099
275. Lister TA, Roberts MM, Brearly RL, Woodruff RK, Greaves MF (1979) Prognostic significance of cell surface phenotype in adult acute lymphoblastic leukemia. Cancer Immunol Immunother 6: 227
276. Dow LW, Borella L, Sen L Aur RJA, George SL, Mauer AM, Simone JV (1977) Initial prognostic factors and lymphoblastic leukemia. Blood 50: 671
277. Greaves MF, Janossy G, Peto J, Kay H (1981) Immunologically defined subclasses of acute lymphoblastic leukemia in children = their relationship to presentation features and prognosis. Br J Haematol 48: 179
278. Riehm H, Gadner RH, Welte K (1977) Die West-Berliner Studie zur Behandlung der akuten lymphoblastoiden Leukämie des Kindes. Klin Paediatr 189: 89
279. Henze G, Langermann HJ, Fengler R, Schellong W, Riehm H (1982) Therapiestudie bei Kindern und Jugendlichen: intensivierte Reinduktionstherapie für Patientengruppen mit unterschiedlichem Rezidivrisiko. Klin Paediatr 194: 195

280. Haas RJ, Netzel B, Janka G, Rodt H, Thiel E, Thierfelder S (1978) Diagnostischer Einsatz spezifischer Antiseren bei der akuten lymphatischen Leukämie im Kindesalter. Klin Paediatr 191: 446
281. Hann HWL, Lustbader ED, Evans AE, Toledano SR, Lillie PD, Jasko LB (1981) Lack of influence of T-cell marker and importance of mediastinal mass on the prognosis of acute lymphocyte leukemias of childhood. J Natl Cancer Inst 66: 285
282. Sather H, Miller D, Nesbit M, Heyn R, Hammon D (1981) Differences in prognosis for boys and girls with acute lymphoblastic leukemia. Lancet 1: 739
283. Nowell PC, Hungerford DA (1960) Chromosome studies on normal and leukemic human leukocytes. J Natl Cancer Inst 25: 85
284. Whang J, Frei E, Tijo JH, Carbone PD, Brecher G (1963) The distribution of the Philadelphia chromosome in patients with chronic myelogenous leukemia. Blood 22: 664
285. Chervenick PA, Ellis LD, Pan SF, Lawson AL (1971) Human leukemic cells: in vitro growth of colonies containing the Philadelphia (Ph^1) chromosome. Science 174: 1134
286. Golde DW, Burgaleta C, Sparkes RS, Cline MJ (1977) The Philadelphia chromosome in human macrophages. Blood 49: 367
287. Fialkow PJ, Denman AM, Jacobson RJ, Lowenthal J (1978) Chronic myelocytic leukemia: origin of some lymphocytes from leukemic stem cells. J Clin Invest 62: 825
288. Fialkow PJ, Jacobson RJ, Papayannopoulou T (1977) Chronic myelocytic leukemia: clonal origin in a stem cell common to the granulocyte, erythrocyte, platelet and monocyte/macrophage. Am J Med 63: 125
289. Boggs DR (1976) The pathogenesis and clinical patterns of blastic crisis of chronic myeloid leukemia. Semin Oncol 3: 296
290. Janossy G, Roberts M, Greaves MF (1976) Target cell in chronic myeloid leukemia and its relationship to common ALL. Lancet 2: 1058
291. Rosenthal S, Canellos GP, Whang-Peng J, Gralnick HR (1977) Blast crisis of chronic granulocytic leukemia: morphologic variants and therapeutic implications. Am J Med 63: 542
292. LeBien TW, Hozier J, Minowada J, Kersey JH (1979) Origin of chronic myelocytic leukemia in a precursor of pre-B lymphocytes. N Engl J Med 301: 144
293. Griffin JD, Tantravahi R, Canellos GP, Wisch JS, Reinherz EL, Sherwood G, Beveridge RP, Daley JF, Lane H, Schlossman SF (1983) T-cell surface antigens in a patient with blast crisis of chronic myeloid leukemia. Blood 61: 640
294. Greaves MF (1982) "Target" cells, differentiation and clonal evolution in chronic granulocytic leukemia = a "model" for understanding the biology of malignancy. In: Shaw M (ed) Chronic granulocytic leukemia. Praeger, London, p 15
295. Canellos GP, DeVita WT, Whang-Peng J, Carbone PD (1971) Hematologic and cytogenetic remission of blastic transformation in chronic granulocytic leukemia. Blood 38: 671
296. Janossy G, Woodruff RK, Pippard MJ, Prentice G, Hoffbrand AV, Paxton A, Lister TA, Bunch C, Greaves MF (1979) Relation of "lymphoid" phenotype and response to chemotherapy incorporating uncristine-prednisolone in the acute phase of Ph^1 positive leukemia. Cancer 43: 426
297. Miller JFAP (1961) Etrology and pathogenesis of mouse leukemia. Adv Cancer Res 6: 291
298. Peterson RDA, Burmester BR, Frederickson G, Purchase HG, Good RA (1964) Effect of bursectomy and thymectomy on the development of visceral lymphomatosis in the chicken. J Natl Cancer Inst 32: 1343
299. Cooper MD, Purchase HG, Bockman DW, Gathings WE (1974) Studies on the nature of the abnormality of B cell differentiation in avian lymphoid leukosis: production of heterogeneous IgM by tumor cells. J Immunol 113: 1210
300. Borella L, Casper TL, Lauer SJ (1979) Shifts in expression of cell membrane phenotypes in childhood lymphoid malignancies at relapse. Blood 54: 64
301. Kerbel RS (1979) Implications of immunological heterogeneity of tumours. Nature 280: 358

302. Nagasawa K, Mark TW (1980) Phorbol esters induce differentiation in human malignant T lymphoblasts. Proc Natl Acad Sci USA 77: 2964
303. Cossman J, Neckers LM, Arnold A, Korsmeyer SJ (1982) Induction of differentiation in a case of common acute lymphoblastic leukemia. N Engl J Med 20: 1251
304. Sachs L (1978) The differentiation of myeloid leukemia cells: new possibilities for therapy. Br J Haematol 40: 509
305. Baccarini M, Tura S (1979) Differentiation of myeloid leukemia cells: new possibilities for therapy. Br J Haematol 42: 485
306. Housset M, Daniel MT, Degos L (1982) Small doses of ARA-C in the treatment of acute myeloid leukaemia: differentiation of myeloid leukaemia cells? Br J Haematol 51: 125
307. Sukurai M, Sampi K, Hozumi M (1983) Possible differentiation of human acute myeloblastic leukemia cells by daily and intermittent administration of aclacinomytin A. Leuk Res 7: 139
308. Kessler JF, Meyskens FR, Levine N, Lynch PJ, Jones SE (1983) Treatment of cutaneous T-cell lymphoma (myelosis fungoides) with 13-*cis*-retinoic acid. Lancet 1: 1345

Acute Lymphoblastic Leukemia: Current Status of Therapy in Children

F. Lampert, G. Henze, H.-J. Langermann, G. Schellong, H. Gadner, and H.-J. Riehm

Universitäts-Kinderpoliklinik, Feulgenstrasse 12, 6300 Giessen, FRG

Introduction

The symptoms of acute lymphoblastic leukemia (ALL) – pallor, bleeding, and infection or erythro-, thrombo-, and granulocytopenia – are due to the massive accumulation of undifferentiated cells in the bone marrow. The purpose of therapy, therefore, is to eradicate these leukemic cells in all body compartments. Prolonged disease-free survival (and subsequent cure) depends on the rapidity and thoroughness of cytoreduction. Thus, curative efforts have evolved to their present form as aggressive combination chemotherapy.

Thirty-five years – the time of a human generation – have passed since the first leukemic cell kiling agent, aminopterin, was introduced into clinical medicine [17]. Since then, ALL in childhood has changed from a 100% fatal disease to one that is curable in almost 70% of patients. Many factors have contributed to this success story.

One factor are the drugs: methotrexate (MTX), corticosteroids, and 6-mercaptopurine (6-MP), in the 1950s; and vincristine (VCR), cyclophosphamide (CP), cytosine arabinoside (Ara-C), daunorubicin (DR), adriamycin (ADR), and L-asparaginase (L-ASP) in the 1960s. The late 1950s witnessed the beginning of combination therapy [20] and the founding of cooperative groups (e.g., in 1956, Acute Leukemia Group B) which conducted multicentrer clinical trials "to treat and study a greater number of patients with rare diseases in a shorter period through a predetermined method."

Further factors were the researchers and therapeutic strategies. Only a few names will be given here. As early as 1949 W. Zuelzer demonstrated the inverse relationship between initial white blood cell count and length of survival in 38 untreated leukemic children [78]. He achieved long-term survival of up to 5 years – basically dependent on the duration of the first remission – in a few of 175 patients with "composite cyclic therapy" [79]. In 1965, in all 53 long-term survivors in childhood were collected [7]. In an update, the late C. Gasser described 11 children, diagnosed as early as 1952, surviving 10–28 years after a modified "monotherapy" given for 2–10 years [21]. In the late 1960s and early 1970s D. Pinkel and his group at St. Jude Children's Hospital in Memphis Tennessee claimed the first real "cures", i.e., leukemia-free continuous complete remissions for 6 years and longer. They combined all known effective agents for "total therapy" [55], giving this at a maximally tolerated dosage during remission [56], and introduced effective prophylaxis of central nervous system (CNS) leukemia by 24 Gy cranial irradiation plus intrathecal MTX [35]. The cure rate increased to about 50%. CNS prophylaxis was rapidly incorporated into ALL treatment protocols, and the incidence of CNS leukemia fell from about 50% [16, 75] to less than 10% of patients. This was also seen in Europe where cranial irradiation doses of 24 Gy and as little as 18 Gy were used in some institutions [39, 30].

Recent Results in Cancer Research. Vol. 93

The improved survival in children with ALL has been documented all over the world, in small and large patient series, at single hospitals or in multi-institution cancer study groups [14, 28, 37, 44, 47, 52, 77]. It is also reflected in the general population trend, as seen in the United States for example. The age-adjusted mortality rate for all childhood leukemias between 1950 and 1976 decreased from 4.4 per 100,000 to 2.4 per 100,000 children under 15 years of age [70]. The most dramatic increase in observed 5-year survival rates was seen between the 1965–1969 cohort (7%) and the 1970–1973 cohort (34%).

Despite improved survival rates the major obstacle to cure in ALL is still recurrent disease in the bone marrow. The relapse rate in the bone marrow is now considered to be the appropriate indicator of therapeutic effectiveness. For this purpose more aggressive combination chemotherapies were developed the L-2 protocol being an early example [26], culminating in the "maximally intensified induction therapy" of H. Riehm and the BFM group [59]. They administer eight drugs and include CNS irradiation within 8 weeks of the induction period. The "quality of remission" [66] was further improved in high-risk ALL by adding an intensive 6-week reinduction course in these patients within the first 6 months of remission [29]. This "risk-adapted induction and re-induction therapy" of the BFM group resulted in relapse-free survival for up to 70% of all patients.

The next concern, then, is quality of cure and incidence of late sequelae. How many toxic treatment elements can be eliminated without a drop in cure rate? It seems that once again MTX the oldest and most specific agent, in altered dosage and administration schedules [24, 49, 72], is leading the way, probably making cranial irradiation obsolete in patients with standard risk (unpublished results: BFM study 81/83).

Cellular Classification

In the mid-1970s, it became evident that ALL in childhood is not a uniform disease reacting in a consistent manner to the same therapy. Different leukemic cell features were related to prognosis, and could be recognized by different methods.

By examining cell surface properties, such as sheep erythrocyte receptors, surface membrane immunoglobulins, and antigens detected by heteroantisera, at least four subtypes of ALL can be distinguished [8, 19, 63] (Chap. 5): (a) T-cell (about 15%–20% of patients); (b) B cell (1%–3%); (c) non-T, non-B cell, either common antigen-positive (65%) or (d) negative (15%), the true null cell ALL. The closest correlation with a very poor response to treatment was seen in B cell ALL [76].

In recent years, besides immunological characterization of ALL a new classification relying upon morphological and cytochemical observations has become widely accepted: the French-American-British (FAB) classification [3]. With minor modifications (Table 1), the Children's Cancer Study Group found this purely morphological classification reproducible, useful, and of prognostic value in over 700 children with ALL [46]. L1 type leukemia accounted for 85.1%, L2 type 14.1%, and L3 type 0.8% of the studied patients. Children with over 25% L2 lymphoblasts had a higher relapse rate and poorer survival. This classification is now used by the Children's Cancer Study Group "to allocate patients into graded treatment protocols based upon clinical prognositc factors".

As to cytochemical methods, the myeloperoxidase reaction is important for the purpose of distinguishing between L2 ALL (scattered azurophilic granules in blasts are negative) and M1 myeloblastic leukemia (over 3% of the blasts are positive). In some cases, discrimination of L2 and M1 morphology and ALL versus AML is difficult or impossible.

Table 1. Modified FAB classification for childhood ALL [46]

Cytologic features	L1	L2	L3
% L1 cells	75–100	< 75	< 75
Cell size	Small cells predominate; occasionally mixed pattern	Large cells predominate; occasionally mixed pattern	Large, homogeneous
Nuclear chromatin	Fine or clumped, usually homogeneous, but occasionally mixed pattern	Fine, usually homogeneous	Fine, homogeneous
Nuclear shape	Regular with clefts; occasionally larger cells with fine chromatin and clefts or convolutions[a]	Regular, oval to round; occasionally with clefts or convolutions	Regular, oval to round[a]
Nucleoli	Indistinct or not visible[a]	One or more per cell, large, prominent[a]	One or more per cell, prominent
Amount of cytoplasm	Scanty[a]	Moderately abundant[a]	Moderately abundant
Basophilia of cytoplasm	Slight	Slight	Deep[a]
Vacuolization	Variable	Variable	Prominent[a]

[a] Distinguishing features of subgroups

Biochemical measurements of terminal deoxynucleotidyl transferase (TdT) activity in mononuclear cells from bone marrow has proved valuable in distinguishing between lymphoblastic and nonlymphoblastic acute leukemia [74], but does not have any prognostic significance according to an analysis in 164 children with ALL [36].
Whether determination of glucocorticoid receptor sites [73] or cellular DNA and RNA content [1] will be useful in clinical practice remains to be seen.
Cytogenetic methods have also demonstrated the heterogeneity of ALL, and are now becoming more and more clinical routine. Chromosomal analysis of the blast cell population in the bone marrow utilizing refined banding techniques has distinguished at least three subtypes [38, 42]: 8; 14 translocation or t (8;14) (q 24; q 32) in B-cell ALL [4]; 9; 22 translocation or t (9;22) (q 34; q 11) in Ph^1-positive acute leukemia [57]; 4; 11 translocation or t (4; 11) (q 13; q 22) in congenital and null cell ALL [51].
ALL karyotypes with these nonrandom translocations are usually associated with very high initial white blood count and a poor prognosis in clinical practice.

Results of Treatment

Progress in ALL treatment, i.e., improvement of prognosis by refinement of therapy, can only be proved convincingly by large-scale clinical trials with many hundreds of patients. This can be accomplished in a relatively short time when cooperative groups of several pediatric cancer centers carry out prospective treatment protocols under controlled

conditions. This protocol-based treatment in specialized centers is the best guarantee for better patient care and continued progress in science. Comparison of results of different clinical trials in the literature cannot be as accurate as analysis of the data supplied by national cooperative groups where background and resources are intimately known.
To demonstrate the striking progress in the quality and quantity of treatment in childhood ALL we will limit ourselves, therefore, to the presentation of results of four clinical trials in the Federal Republic of Germany involving over 1,000 patients in the last decade. The main points of difference in these studies were the mode of treatment during the first 6 months after diagnosis and the number of participating institutions.

Treatment Characteristics in over 1,000 Patients

In the Federal Republic of Germany, clinical trials in ALL were initiated in 1970, although a childhood leukemia work group founded 5 years earlier had provided an exchange of knowledge. The first two trials, DAL 71/74 and BFM 70/76, were nonrandomized studies with very different induction regimens. They also differed in the number of participating institutions and patients.
Treatment in DAL 71/74 [30, 39] was slightly adapted from the St. Jude protocol VII. In 1971 this protocol was thought to be effective, and because of its simplicity it could be used in many children nationwide in many, pediatric hospitals, even small ones. Remission induction was obtained with VCR and prednisone (4 weeks), occasionally reinforced by L-ASP, DR, or both; CNS prophylaxis with cranial irradiation and intrathecal MTX followed; and maintenance therapy with 6-MP and MTX was then given for 28 months. In addition, some patients were given CP or prednisone/VCR reinduction pulses during the first year.
Treatment in BFM 70/76 [31, 59] was characterized by an intensive 8-week multidrug regimen (for details see section: Antileukemic Chemotherapy under Current Management) and required a great deal of experience. Therefore, at first, this West Berlin induction protocol was confined to three pediatric centers (since 1974), i.e., *B*erlin, *F*rankfurt, and *M*ünster. Remission was induced with VCR, prednisone, L-ASP, and DR (given for 4 weeks); consolidated within the next 4 weeks with CP, 6-MP, Ara-C, craniospinal or cranial irradiation, and intrathecal MTX; and maintained with 6-MP and MTX and VCR/prednisone reinduction pulses. In addition, some patients were given CP. The total duration of therapy was 21–36 months.
In BFM study 76/79 [32], the number of participating institutions was increased to nine and the number of patients to 158. All patients received the above-mentioned Berlin induction regimen, now well known and named protocol I. A risk index, however, was established in the study for definition of high-risk patients. Children and adolescents with a risk index equal to or over three received, in addition to the former therapy, a reinforced reinduction protocol (II) within the first 6 months after diagnosis. This intensive reinduction treatment (Fig. 10) consisted of dexamethasone, VCR, ADR, ASP (given for 4 weeks); followed by CP, Ara-C, intrathecal MTX, and 6-thioguanine (given for an additional 2 weeks). The total duration of treatment was 104 weeks (2 years) in the standard risk group and 128 weeks ($2^1/_2$ years) in the high-risk group. The risk score was calculated by the sum of points given for initial total WBC ($\geq 25{,}000/\mu l = 3$), initial CNS involvement (= 2), a thymic mass (= 1), a positive acid phosphatase reaction and/or a positive E rosette test (= 1), a negative PAS reaction (= 1), age at diagnosis (< 2 and > 10 years = 1), and a significant extranodal tumor, e.g., in gonads, kidneys, bones (= 1).

In BFM study 79/81 [33], after a certain learning effect and nation wide communication of the results of risk-adapted induction and reinduction therapy, the number of institutions participating rose to 19, with a total of 325 patients enlisted in sequence from April 1979 to March 1981. In contrast to BFM study 76/79, patients with standard risk features (risk score below 3) received therapy intensification with protocoll III (similar to protocol II, but for only 4 weeks, without CP) early in remission. Therapy in high-risk patients (risk score equal to or over 3) was the same as in study BFM 76/79, except that the total duration of treatment was reduced to 24 months. In the standard-risk group, patients were randomized to receive or not receive reinduction pulses with prednisone/VCR during remission maintenance.

Clinical Characteristics in over 1,000 Patients

The pretreatment clinical features of 1,097 patients treated from 1970 to 1981 are presented in Table 2. In all four trials, diagnostic findings once considered of prognostic importance were distributed in a comparable range: male sex in about 56%; initial leukocyte count over 25,000/μl in about 30% and over 100,000/μl in almost 10%; presence of a mediastinal mass in about 10%; initial CNS involvement in up to 3%; and age over 10 years in about 20% of patients. In the last study (BFM 79/81) unfavorable factors were found in an even higher percentage than in the first study (DAL 71/74), particularly age over 10 years and very high white blood cell count. This is partly because adolescents were more frequently enrolled in this pediatric ALL trial. This has to be kept in mind when the outcome is considered; it means that the results can be attributed to the improvement of treatment strategy with even greater conviction than if the incidence of risk factors had been the same in all trials.

Table 2. Childhood ALL: Pretreatment characteristics in four cooperative German clinical trials

	Study groups				
	DAL 71/74	BFM 70/76	BFM 76/79	BFM 79/81	Total
	Participating hospitals				
	n (%)	*n* (%)	*n* (%)	*n* (%)	*n* (%)
Patients	495 (100)	119 (100)	158 (100)	325 (100)	1,097 (100)
Median age (years)	4 11/12	5 7/12	4 11/12	5 5/12	
Boys	264 (53.3)	78 (65.5)	89 (56.3)	189 (58.2)	620 (56.5)
Median age (years)	4 11/12	5 8/12	4 5/12	5 3/12	
Girls	231 (46.7)	41 (34.5)	69 (43.7)	136 (41.8)	477 (43.5)
Median age (years)	5 0/12	5 5/12	5 2/12	5 9/12	
WBC ≥ 25 000/μl	137 (27.7)	40 (33.6)	51 (32.3)	111 (34.2)	339 (30.9)
WBC ≥ 100,000/μl	41 (8.3)	13 (10.9)	10 (6.3)	37 (11.4)	101 (9.2
Initial CNS involvement	7 (1.4)	9 (7.6)	4 (2.5)	11 (3.4)	31 (2.8)
Thymic mass	47 (9.5)	15 (12.6)	14 (8.9)	29 (8.9)	105 (9.6)
Age < 2 years	40 (8.1)	10 (8.4)	15 (9.5)	39 (12.0)	104 (9.5)
Age ≥ 10 years	73 (14.8)	21 (17.6)	37 (23.4)	84 (25.8)	215 (19.6)

Table 3. Childhood ALL: Results of treatment in four cooperative German clinical trials

	Study groups			
	DAL 71/74	BFM 70/76	BFM 76/79	BFM 79/81
	Participating hospitals			
	40 *n* (%)	3 *n* (%)	9 *n* (%)	19 *n* (%)
Patients	495 (100)	119 (100)	158 (100)	325 (100)
Nonresponders	7 (1.4)	1 (0.8)	1 (0.6)	5 (1.5)
Died during remission induction	14 (2.8)	5 (4.2)	4 (2.5)	7 (2.2)
Achieved remission	474 (95.8)	113 (95.0)	153 (96.9)	313 (96.3)
Died in CCR	37 (7.5)	8 (6.7)	6 (3.8)	16 (4.9)
Relapses	268 (54.1)	39 (32.8)	39 (24.7)	53 (16.3)
BM (isolated)	175 (35.4)	26 (21.8)	13 (8.2)	24 (7.4)
CNS (isolated)	36 (7.3)	6 (5.0)	8 (5.1)	10 (3.1)
Testes (isolated)	20 (4.0)	6 (5.0)	5 (3.2)	4 (1.2)
BM/CNS	16 (3.2)	1 (0.8)	3 (1.9)	8 (2.5)
BM/testes	16 (3.2)	0 (0.0)	8 (5.1)	4 (1.2)
Others	5 (1.0)	0 (0.0)	2 (1.3)	3 (0.9)
In CCR	167 (33.7)	66 (55.5)	108 (68.4)	244 (75.1)

24 February 1983

Overall Results Within a Decade

Long-term results in these 1,097 patients treated from 1970 to 1981 can be expressed in actual numbers (Table 3). An initial complete remission, i.e., less than 5% blasts in the bone marrow, was achieved in about 95% of patients in all four studies, which is a common experience worldwide [44, 47]. But how many patients remained in complete remission? What was the "quality of remission"? The number of patients in continuous complete remission (CCR) including all patients from the beginning of therapy rose from 33.7% to 55.5%, and now to 68.4% (median observation 5 years) or 75.1% (median observation period $2^1/_2$ years). This improvement was mainly due to the reduced incidence of bone marrow relapses, which decreased from over 35% in the DAL study to 22% and now to 8% or 7% in the BFM studies. We are aware that the results of study BFM 79/81 are still preliminary, but it seems that the favorable figures obtained in the previous study will be confirmed in this much larger multicenter trial. CNS relapses were rare, with an incidence below 10%, in all studies (due to CNS prophylaxis in all trials). There was no increase in non-leukemia-related fatalities due to the intensification of chemotherapy, as the death rates in CCR (continuous complete remission) decreased from 7.5% in the DAL study to 6.7% and latterly to less than 5% in the BFM studies. The 16 fatalities in the BFM 79/81 study can be subdivided into eight patients (2.5%) lost during intensive consolidation and reinduction treatment and eight patients (2.5%) lost during maintenance therapy. Fatalities in CCR in DAL 71/74 were mainly due to interstitial pneumonia or varicella. These diseases have lost their deadly impact in recent years since cotrimoxazol was introduced into routine supportive care and varicella hyperimmune globulin and acyclovir

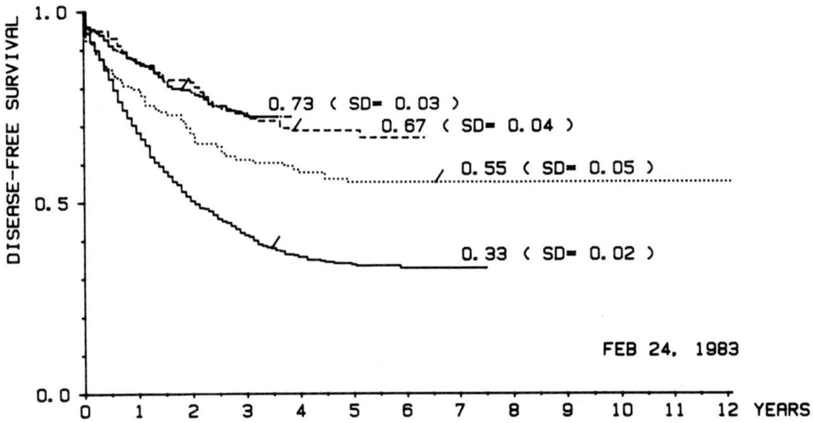

Fig. 1. Probability of disease-free survival in four German ALL therapy studies. ———, DAL 71/74 (n = 495; 167 in CCR) (evaluation date 31 July, 1978); · · · · ·, BFM 70/76 (n = 119; 66 in CCR); (– – –, BFM 76/79 (n = 158; 108 in CCR); – · –, BFM 79/81 (n = 325, 244 in CCR)

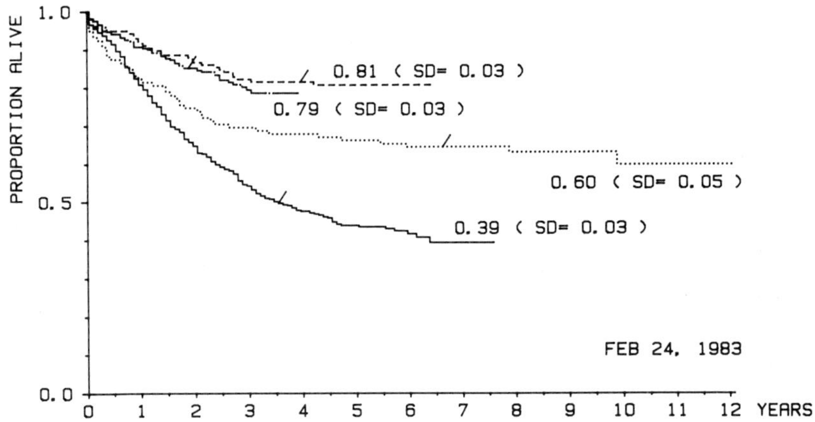

Fig. 2. Comparison of probability of survival in four German ALL therapy studies. ———, DAL 71/74 (n = 495; 215 alive) (evaluation date 31 July, 1978); · · ·, BFM 70/76 (n = 119; 75 alive); – – –, BFM 76/79 (n = 158; 128 alive); – · –, BFM 79/81 (n = 325; 264 alive)

became available. Treatment results can be even better demonstrated by life-table analysis: the probability of disease-free survival (Fig. 1) rose from 33% to 55%, and latterly to 67% (73%). This includes all patients from the start of treatment and with due consideration of all adverse events, i.e., no response, death during induction or CCR, all medullary and extramedullary relapses. As patients with ALL can now survive testicular, CNS, or even bone marrow relapse, overall survival rather than CCR will be a meaningful measure of success of treatment again in the future (Fig. 2).
Consideration of the preliminary results of BFM 79/81 shows that the results of study 76/79 probably will be repeated in a larger number of patients treated in more institutions.

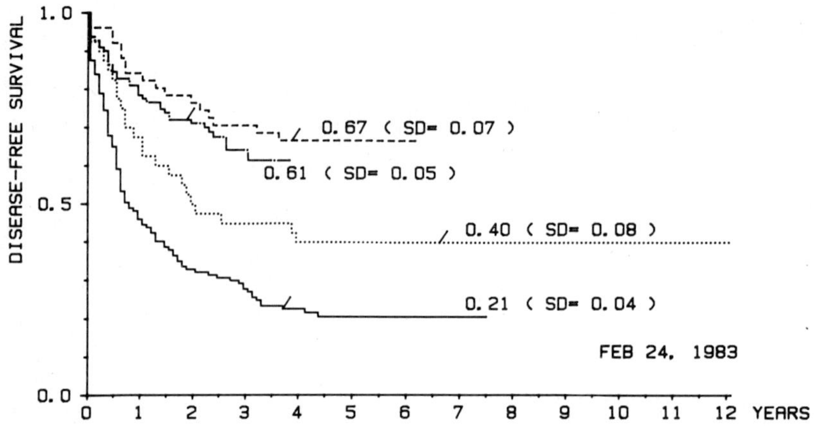

Fig. 3. Probability of disease-free survival in patients with WBC ≧ 25,000 (4 studies). ———, DAL 71/74 (*n* = 137; 29 in CCR) (evaluation date 31 July, 1978); · · · · ·, BFM 70/76 (*n* = 40; 16 in CCR); – – –, BFM 76/79 (*n* = 51; 34 in CCR); – · –, BFM 79/81 (*n* = 111; 73 in CCR)

Analysis of Prognostic Risk Factors

The effects of more aggressive induction therapy can be specifically analysed in these German trials with respect to factors considered to be associated with a poor prognosis.

High Initial White Blood Cell Count (WBC)

As seen in Fig. 3, the disease-free survival rate (proportion of patients surviving without any adverse event) in patients with WBC over 25,000/µl increased successively from 0.21 in the DAL study to 0.40, 0.67, and 0.61 in the BFM studies. Figure 4 shows even more clearly that the consideration of high initial WBC as an adverse prognostic factor can be completely eliminated through the concept of stratified, risk-adapted therapy (study BFM 76/79).

The significance of initial peripheral blood leukocyte count as a sign for bad survival prognosis was known from large clinical trials in the United States [22, 67], persisting as a factor for 24 months after onset of therapy [65]. Less aggressive attempts to wipe out this heavy initial burden by additive chemotherapy in the remission maintenance phase were unsuccessful in the early 1970s [48].

Mediastinal Mass

As seen in Fig. 5, the disease-free survival rate for patients with mediastinal masses at diagnosis increased from 0.13 in the DAL 71/74 study to 0.47 in the BFM 70/76 study and to 0.79 in the BFM 76/79 study. The currently projected proportion of 0.47 in the BFM 79/81 study is likely to be explained by four deaths in CCR (no death in CCR in BFM 76/79) and the different distribution of risk factors within the patient group with mediastinal mass compared with the previous study. Only in the DAL 71/74 study (with weak induction

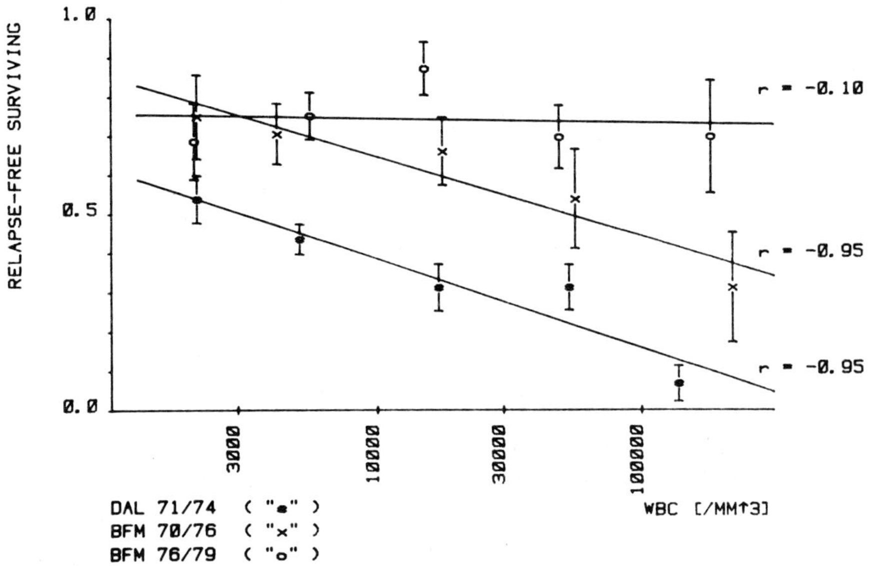

Fig. 4. Probability of relapse-free survival as a function of initial WBC in three ALL therapy studies after 5 years (DAL 71/74, BFM 70/76) and 4.5 years (BFM 76/79)

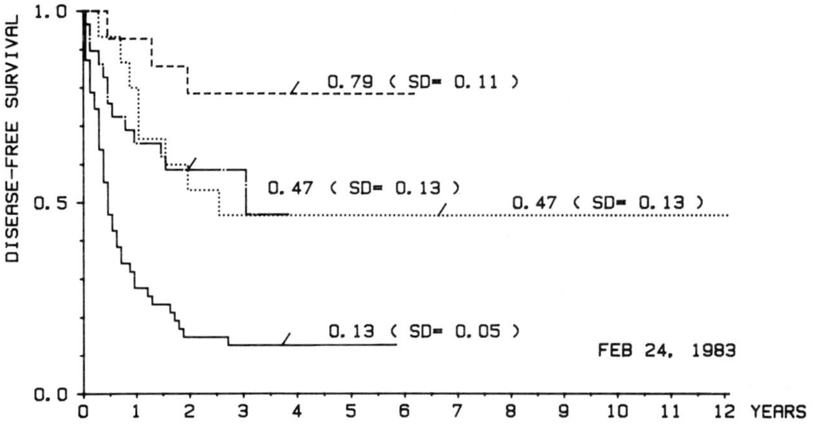

Fig. 5. Probability of disease-free survival in patients with mediastinal masses (4 studies). ———, DAL 71/74 ($n = 47$; 6 in CCR) (evaluation date 31 July, 1978); · · · · ·, BFM 70/76 ($n = 15$; 7 in CCR); – – –, BFM 76/79 ($n = 14$; 11 in CCR); – · –, BFM 79/81 ($n = 29$; 16 in CCR)

regimen) was a highly significant difference in outcome found between children with and those without mediastinal mass. In the BFM studies thymic involvement was not found to be an independent risk factor [31]. However, as also suggested by a study in Philadelphia [27], patients with mediastinal masses need special therapy. With more intensive induction and reinduction treatment, as experienced in BFM study 76/79, these patients do not have a poorer prognosis than patients without mediastinal masses.

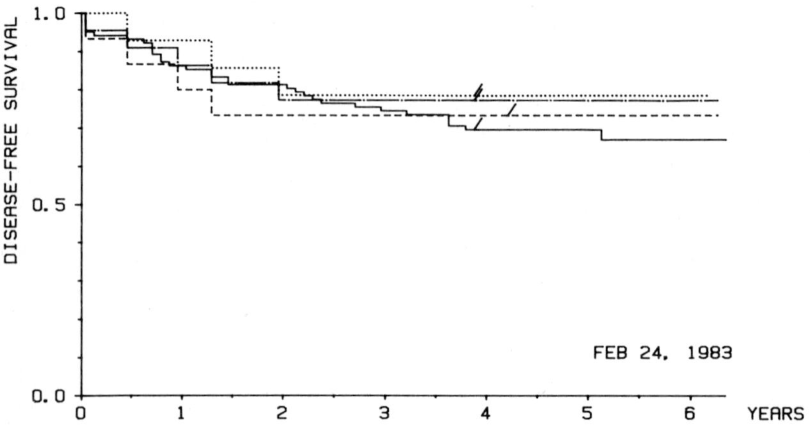

Fig. 6. Probability of disease-free survival in patients with and without T characteristics: BFM 76/79. ———, no thymic involvement. E negative (n = 102; 72 in CCR); · · · · ·, thymic involvement (n = 14; 11 in CCR); – – –, E-positive (n = 15; 11 in CCR); – · · –, thymic involvement and/or E positive (n = 22; 17 in CCR)

T Cell Characteristics

After elimination of the most pronounced clinical findings of T cell ALL, i.e., thymic involvement and initial high white blood count, as adverse prognostic factors by therapy adjustment, it was also possible in BFM 76/79 to analyse T cell markers that were thought to be clinically important [13].

As shown in Fig. 6, there was no difference in the probability of CCR (p-CCR) between children with and those without immunologically identifiable T-ALL characteristics when the former group was stratified to the more intensive treatment group (in most cases because of the high concomitant WBC).

Male Sex

Boys are thought to have more relapses, not only in the testicles, but also in the bone marrow [2]. A worse prognosis for boys was, indeed, found in a retrospektive analysis of over 3,000 children with ALL treated according to recent CCSG protocols, and this was partly explained by the higher frequency of T cell disease in males [64]. This sex-related difference in outcome, however, was seen only in our DAL study 71/74 [30]. The p-CCR for girls (0.39; n = 231) was better than that for boys (0.28, including testicular relapses; 0.33, excluding testicular relapses; n = 264). In contrast, the BFM studies showed no influence of sex outcome. The incidence of isolated testicular relapses was also low, being under 4% (15 of 405 boys treated according to BFM protocols) [18]. As seen with CNS relapse, intensified systemic chemotherapy did not influence the frequency of testicular relapse. Intermediate-dose MTX, however, seems to prevent testicular relapse [24, 49].

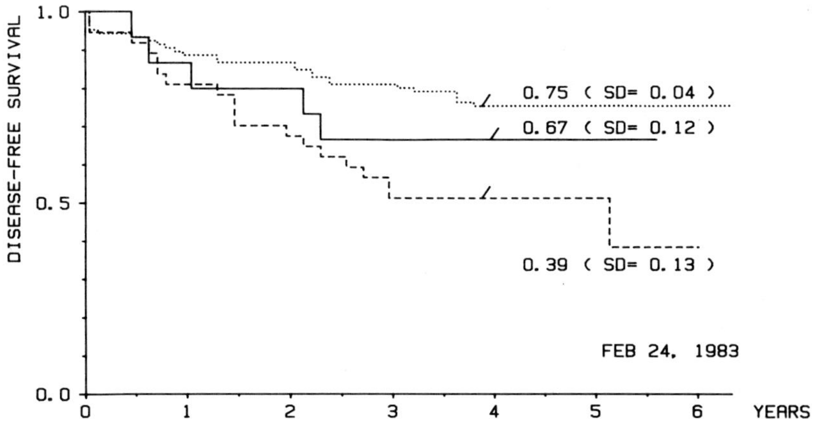

Fig. 7. Probability of disease-free survival in different age groups: BFM 76/79. ———, age < 2 years (n = 15; 10 in CCR); · · · · ·, age ⩾ 2 and < 10 years (n = 106; 80 in CCR); – – –, age ⩾ 10 years (n = 37; 18 in CCR)

Age

Analysis of large clinical trials [22, 62] suggested that age at diagnosis which deviates from the usual age peak for ALL manifestation was a factor associated with poorer prognosis. In neither DAL 71/74 nor BFM 70/76 were significant differences found among the groups (younger vs older than 2 vs older than 10 years at diagnosis). However, in the BFM 76/79 study (Fig. 7), a lower p-CCR was found in the age group older than 10 years than in younger age groups. On the other hand, infants also had more frequent relapses. The preliminary results of BFM 79/81 follow the same trend as seen in BFM 76/79. The influence of age on prognosis probably is independent of the initial risk features. More recent results (BFM 81/83) suggest that the poorer prognosis in patients over 10 years of age might be due to the consequence of inappropriate dosage of anthracycline (Henze et al.: Adriblastin Symposium, Frankfurt, 1981).

Significance of Initial Leukemic Cell Mass

A risk index based on initial clinical findings was introduced in BFM 76/79, and has been found to be very useful for therapy adaptation. But it is reasonable to postulate that more sensitive methods can provide an even better indication of individual risk of relapse at diagnosis.

A retrospective analysis of commonly reported risk factors was made by Cox regression in BFM 70/76 [25]. Both one-parametric and multiparametric analysis revealed only the peripheral blast cell count and enlargement of liver and spleen as significant ($P < 0.001$). A method was then developed to calculate the "total tumor burden" in the patient [41]. The estimated blast cell mass related to patient's body weight proved to be highly significant ($P \ll 0.001$) in BFM 70/76: p-CCR for patients with an initial leukemic cell mass of less than 3% of body weight was 0.75; when leukemic cell mass was 3%–6% of body weight p-CCR was 0.55; and when it was more than 6% of body weight p-CCR was only 0.34. This method of initial leukemic cell mass determination has been simplified and is now being used in

BFM 81/83 to define the "risk factor." According to the risk factor (< 1.2; $\geqslant 1.2 - < 1.7$; $\geqslant 1.7$), patients can be separated into three groups with different risks of relapse, and therefore allocated to different intensive treatment regimens. These three groups (SR, standard risk; MR, medium risk; HR, high risk) account for 65%, 25%, and 10%, respectively, of all children with ALL (of non-B cell type). The practical application will be described in the next section.

Current Management

It may seem presumptuous in a review article to give a detailed account of the therapeutic management of children with ALL as currently practiced by the BFM group in Germany. On the other hand, "generalizations" from the literature have not been of much help in clinical practice.

Calculation of Risk Factor and Patient Stratification

Before starting cytostatic treatment, the individual risk factor for the patient is determined with the aid of a diagram (Fig. 8): the absolute number of leukemic blast cells in the peripheral blood (total leukocyte count times percentage of blasts in the differential) is marked in the first scale of the diagram and a line drawn to the mark of liver size (centimeters below costal margin in medioclavicular line, patient lying supine). A line is then drawn from the point of intersection with the intermediate sum to the mark of spleen size (centimeters below costal margin in longitudinal axis). This will cross the number of the risk factor (RF) in the middle scale.
Patients with $RF < 1.2$ are considered to have a standard risk; those with $RF \geq 1.2$ and < 1.7 to have a medium risk; and those with $RF \geq 1.7$ to have a high risk.
Patients with confirmed B cell features are treated completely differently than others. Children who still have more than 5% blasts in the bone marrow after 4 weeks of induction treatment (after phase 1 of protocol I) are considered to be at high risk for relapse and are treated according to the corresponding protocol.

Antileukemic Chemotherapy

Remission Induction

All patients with non-B cell ALL, regardless of risk, receive treatment according to induction protocol I. This 8-drug, 8-week induction regimen [59] has been used for over a decade in many institutions all over Germany. Only minor modifications (omission of one CP dose, increase of DR dose, age adjustment of IT (intrathecal) MTX dose) [6] have recently been made for BFM 81/83 (Fig. 9).
A prerequisite for the administration of this induction regimen is careful daily evaluation of the patients to detect side-effects early and to fulfill the protocol up to the limits of the patients' tolerance. One must particularly look für early signs of sepsis. With well trained physicians and nurses, standardized supportive care and good blood banking and hospital facilities, this induction protocol is generally realized in all patients (100% of dosage given within time schedule). Early mortality in the BFM trials, which have become progressively

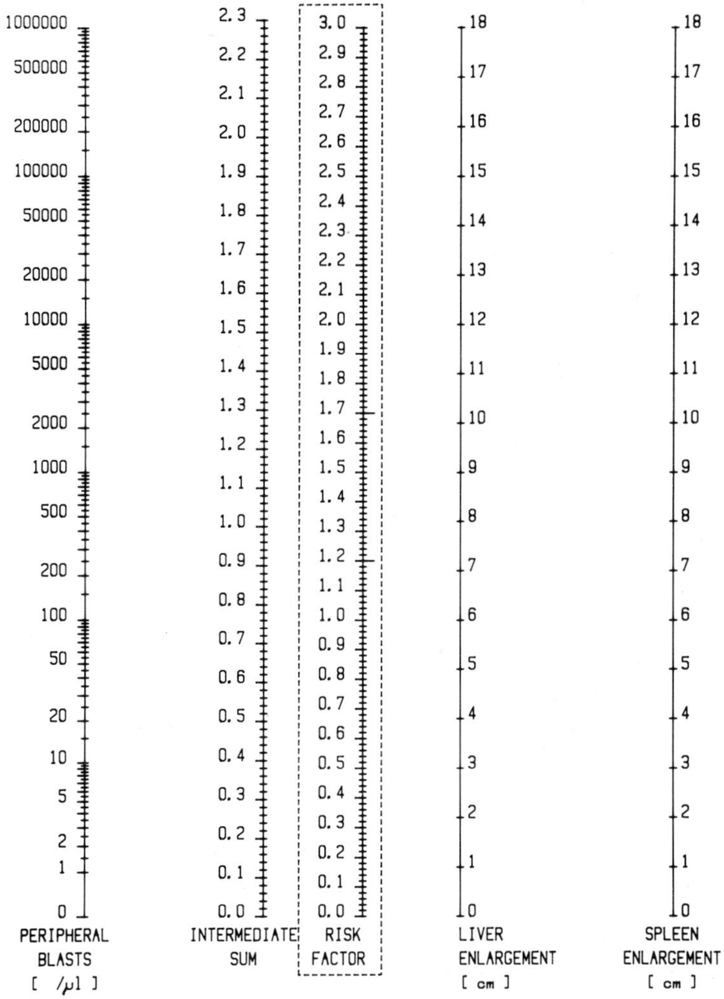

Fig. 8. Diagram for determination of risk factor according to $RF = 0.2^{*}\log(Bl + 1) + 0.06^{*} Li + 0.04^{*} Sp$. Its use is described in the text

larger as well as involving increasing numbers of institutions, is below 5% (2% early and disease-related, and 2% induction therapy-related mortality).

CNS Prophylaxis

High-risk and medium-risk patients receive cranial irradiation in phase 2 of protocol I in an age-adjusted dosage (age over 2 years: 24 Gy for high-risk; 18 Gy fo medium-risk patients). Standard-risk patients, as justified by observations in Norway [49] and also by preliminary results of randomization in BFM 81/83 (irradiation vs IT/IV intermediate-dose MTX), do not need cranial irradiation. After completion of protocol I (without IT MTX and cranial irradiation) and a 2-week rest period, these patients receive, at intervals of 2 weeks, four 24-hour infusions of 500 mg/m^2 MTX ($^1/_{10}$th of dose as IV push; $^9/_{10}$ths of dose as IV

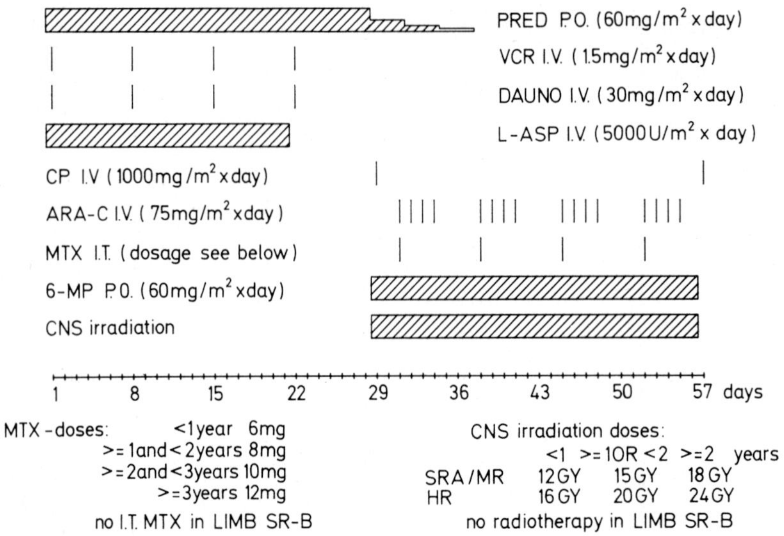

Fig. 9. Eight-week, 8-drug induction therapy: Protocol I. *PRED,* predinisone; *VCR,* vincristine; *DAUNO,* daunorubicin; *L-ASP,* L-asparaginase; *CP,* cyclophosphamide; *ARA-C,* cytosine arabinoside; *MTX,* intrathecal methotrexate; *6-MP,* 6-mercaptopurine

infusion) followed by two doses of Leucovorin 48 and 54 h after the start of infusion. During this 8-week period of MTX therapy the dose of oral 6-MP given for continuation therapy is reduced (usually to 25 mg/m^2 per day).

Intensified Reinduction

As has been shown by BFM 76/79, patients at an increased risk of relapse benefit dramatically from 6-week intensified reinduction course (Fig. 10, protocol II) administered either directly after (more toxic, now abandoned) or, preferably, 3 months after protocol I. In high-risk patients (risk factor $\geq$ 1.7) this reinduction protocol is even more intensified and is prolonged by a 2-week course of four doses of VM-26 (165 mg/m^2) and Ara-C (300 mg/m^2) before protocol II. This combined VM-26 and Ara-C regimen has been found to be effective in refractory childhood lymphocytic leukemia [60].

Continuation Therapy

After the first 7 months of intensive induction, prophylactic CNS, and reinduction therapy, all patients – regardless of risk – receive maintenance therapy with 6 MP PO daily and MTX PO weekly. The initial doses (50 mg/m^2 and 20 mg/m^2, respectively) are adjusted for the tolerance of the host (range of permissible leukocyte count 1,500–3,500/μl).
The necessary total duration of treatment for all patients with non-B ALL is currently being examined in a randomized fashion in BFM 81/83: 2 years vs 1$^1/_2$ years. Shortening of the total treatment time to 2 years for both standard-risk patients (BFM 76/79) [32] and high-risk patients (BFM 79/81) [33] did not have any deleterious effect on outcome.

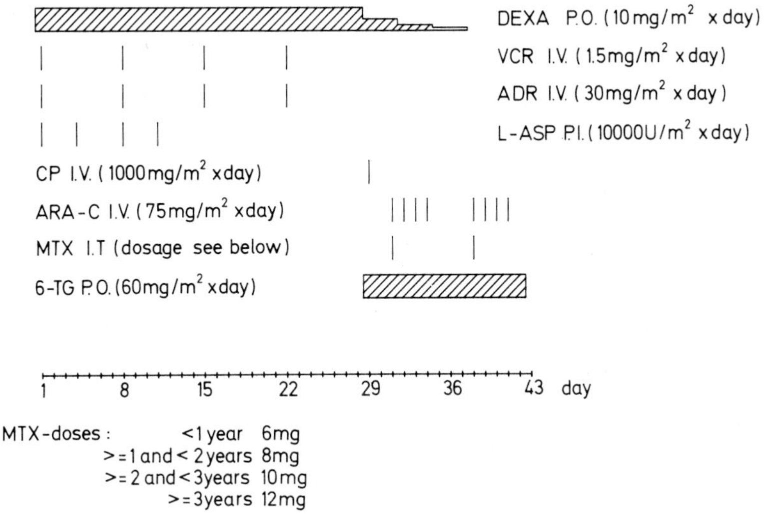

Fig. 10. Intensified reinduction therapy: Protocol II. *DEXA,* dexamethasone; *VCR,* vincristine; *ADR,* adriamycin; *L-ASP,* L-asparaginase; *CP,* cyclophosphamide; *ARA-C,* cytosine arabinoside; *MTX,* intrathecal methotrexate; *6-TG,* 6-thioguanine

The value of added prednisone-VCR "pulses" during the continuation phase was tested in a randomized fashion in BFM 79/81 [33], but no difference in prognosis was found (p-CCR 0.83 in both groups, with or without pulses). Thus, pulses may be omitted without any adverse effect.

Relapsed Leukemia

After completion of the $2^1/_2$-year therapy course in 278 of 639 children enrolled in eight consecutive "total therapy" (Memphis) studies, life-table estimates of the 4-year relapse rate were 0.24 for all patients and 0.22 for patients receiving adequate CNS prophylaxis [23]. This rate was higher than expected, although none of the 79 patients who remained in complete remission for at least 4 years after discontinuation of therapy have relapsed.

Rates for late relapses were lower in the BFM studies. The most likely explanation for this is that the intensity of treatment in the prolonged induction period eliminates more leukemic cells and reduces the chance that persistent leukemic cells will develop drug resistance. The introduction of an additional intensified reinduction therapy (protocol II) for high-risk patients shortened the risk period for relapse [29]. The probability of any first event (induction deaths, deaths in remission, all medullary and extramedullary relapses) dropped to zero $3^1/_2$ years after the start of treatment.

The time and site of first relapse are important for a child with ALL. If marrow relapse occurs during chemotherapy the prognosis is considered to be poor. If, however, children relapse after cessation of therapy [61] or after a long-term remission induced by nonaggressive chemotherapy, not all is lost. Ten to thirty percent of these children can achieve long-term disease-free remission by means of intensive multiple-drug chemotherapy, including repeated CNS prophylaxis [10, 61].

If relapsed patients have an appropriately matched sibling, bone marrow transplantation should be considered early in second remission. Long-term survival in patients who receive transplants is around 10%–20%, and in some series even better. Of 22 patients with acute lymphoblastic leukemia who had two or more relapses and who received transplants, seven are surviving in remission 3–5 years later [71].

Central nervous system relapse, either during or after therapy, should be treated with IT and IV MTX. Infusion of MTX (500 mg/m^2) over 24 h combined with IT administration of MTX was found to be very powerful not only in prevention but also in treatment of CNS relapse [49] (BFM 81/83). These four-dose courses (8 weeks) can be repeated at intervals of 3 months. Other systemic chemotherapy should also be given, as there might also be some occult spreading to the marrow. Patients cured after CNS relapse are now encountered more frequently (personal experience).

Testicular relapse probably is due to a persistent local disease with danger of systemic spread. Treatment, therefore, should not only be local in the form of irradiation (24 Gy), but should also include intensive multiple-agent chemotherapy. Treatment results are then favorable [18]: In BFM studies 70/76, 76/79 and 79/81, in all 29 boys experienced testicular relapse, usually occurring after cessation of maintenance therapy, 3–4 years after diagnosis of ALL; 15 of them had an isolated testicular relapse. After local and systemic therapy, 70% of these patients now enjoy disease-free survival. During the observation time (median 2 years), no difference in prognosis was found between combined and isolated testicular relapses.

Supportive Care

Needless to say, no greater susceptibility to infection is found than in the child with leukemia who is treated with extensive immunosuppressive chemotherapy, including irradiation. A strict supportive care regimen has been found to be very important in the realization of the 8-drug, 8-week induction protocol I.

Skin and mucosa: The oral mucosa is particularly vulnerable and is treated prophytreated with pyoctanin (brilliant green) dye solutions, nystatin suspensions, or miconazol jelly. The skin of the whole body, including the anogenital region, is inspected daily for injection sites, scratches, nodules, and abscesses (if possible tape and urine bags should not be attached to skin or mucosa). Patients are washed daily with soap and water. Hand washing before and after touching patients is obligatory for physicians, nurses, and relatives.

Blood components: Liberal use of packed erythrocytes (if Hb below 8–10 g/dl), thrombocytes (in thrombocytopenic bleeding), and plasma protein (if serum protein below 5 g/dl) is encouraged, as is immunoglobulin G substitution in phase 2 of protocols I and II.

Bowel movements: To prevent koprostasis mild laxatives or enemas are given (if no spontaneous bowel movements within 48 h).

Physical activity: This should be encouraged. Patients with intravenous microcatheters are quite mobile.

Prevention of hyperuricema (day 0–5 or longer in phase 1 of protocol I): Allopurinol 250 mg/m^2 PO daily in two doses; sodium bicarbonate (up to 3–4 g/m^2) daily PO or IV if urinary pH under 6.5; force fluids (2,500 ml/m^2 glucose saline IV or tea PO).

Prevention of *Pneumocystis carinii* pneumonia [34]: Co-trimoxazole (30 mg/kg sulfamethoxazole) daily PO in the first 4 months of therapy, starting in phase 2 of protocol I, and also in protocol II. In manifest *Pneumocystis* pneumonitis, a five-fold dose is given, reinforced by pentamidine.

Prevention of cyclophosphamide-induced hematuria: Force fluids (2,500 ml/m^2 daily IV or PO) and (recently) the specific uroprotector uromitexan (Mesna) is given.

Treatment of varicella [58]: Acyclovir (500 mg/m^2 per dose) IV in 1-h infusions every 8 h for 7 days; Zoster immunoglobulin is given in addition.

Treatment of septicemia: Liberal use of antibiotics in combination (e.g., gentamicin + cephalosporin derivative + piperacillin).

Reduction of bowel bacteria: Polymyxin E (Colistin) 3×10^6 U/m^2 daily PO in three doses is given (optional) in phase 1 of protocol I to prevent enterocolitis.

Treatment of hyperglycemia: Urine glucose should be checked daily during L-asparaginase therapy. Insulin is given for marked hyperglycemia (blood sugar over 400 mg/dl). Risk hypoglycemia means insulin administration must be monitored carefully.

Late Sequelae

The number of cures in children with ALL has increased dramatically since 1970. Careful observation over at least a 10-year period has allowed examination of the "quality of cure". Are there undesirable late effects of the eradicated disease or of the treatment which has long been discontinued?

CNS Disorders

Pediatricians are always concerned about giving ionizing irradiation in high doses to young, growing children. On the other hand, cranial irradiation was a decisive step forward in achieving cures in ALL.
The first alarm signal came from abnormalities seen at computed tomography (CT) of the brains of children with ALL that had been treated with cranial irradiation [54]. These findings have recently been disputed as controls before therapy were lacking.
The greatest concern of any parents, however, is the child's intellectual development. Both retrospective [15] and prospective studies have revealed dysfunctions in neuropsychological tests, particularly in children who were very young at the time of irradiation. Interestingly, patients who experienced a somnolence syndrome – a reversible, "harmless" disorder appearing 6–8 weeks after cranial irradiation – were more likely to develop neuropsychological complications later [3]. Whether or not the doses of cranial irradiation (18 vs 24 Gy) and of MTX given IV and/or IT during irradiation are decisive factors in the development of later complications remains to be clarified. At least on the basis of CT brain scans, MTX alone in the absence of CNS leukemia or cranial irradiation was found highly unlikely to produce structural CNS abnormalities [53].

Second Malignancies

Due to rigorous application of therapeutic modalities (surgery, irradiation, combination chemotherapy), it can be assumed that by the late 1980s, one of every 1,000 individuals 20 years of age will be a cured childhood cancer patient [68]. Compared with their age-peers, these patients who have been cured of one cancer will have a higher risk of developing a (second) malignant tumor. A probable hazard rate of 3% for developing a second malignancy after 11 years was calculated for 1,301 children with ALL who were admitted to St Jude Children's Research Hospital, Memphis, Tennessee, USA [68]. Interestingly, at St Jude's two of nine patients with a second malignancy after ALL developed Hodgkin's disease, an observation also made in Germany [40]. Besides carcinogenic radiation therapy (and chemotherapy?) genetic susceptibility is probably decisive in the risk of developing a second cancer. Surprisingly, added chemotherapy, such as actinomycin D in irradiated children, did not increase (and even decreased) the risk of developing a second cancer [11]. In the BFM studies (1970–1981) no second malignancy has so far been reported. This may provide further support for the assumption that increased intensive combination chemotherapy does not increase the risk of a second cancer.

Reproductive Function

After intellectual capability, parents are concerned with the fertility of their child once a cure is expected. So far, no large-scale systematic studies have been performed in survivors of ALL, but the few reports available are optimistic: aggressive multiple-agent chemotherapy did not adversely effect normal puberty or hypothalamic-pituitary-ovarian function in 35 girls and women [69]. Normal testicular development after antileukemic chemotherapy was also found in 14 boys [5], the majority of whom were treated before puberty. The ultimate proof of fertility has been provided by the offspring of several male and female ALL survivors [21, 50]. No malformations have been observed in the progeny of these treated individuals.

Monetary Cost

Thanks to the German health system (compulsory or private health insurance for all), hospitalization even for quite a long period does not mean a financial burden for the family. Nonetheless, the total cost in relation to effectiveness has to be considered for the total population of any country.

Treatment of acute leukemia in adults by bone marrow transplantation in the first complete remission was estimated in 1981 to cost about $ 70,000 per patient in the United States, the largest items being antibiotics, intensive care ($ 600 per day), and granulocytes.

A thorough analysis of total treatment costs in childhood ALL was carried out by the German pharmaceutical industry [12] in 1981, taking the BFM regimen as an example. Total ALL treatment costs were calculated to be DM 48,700 in the "normal," and DM 105,400 in the complicated case. Personnel costs during in- and outpatient care accounted for over 40% of total expenses, whereas, surprisingly, antileukemic drugs accounted for only 10% in most cases, and only 6% in complicated case. On the other hand, drugs for supportive care, including blood components, accounted for 4% of the total cost in relatively straightforward cases, and an astounding 27% in complicated cases.

Laboratory and technical examinations and x-ray diagnosis and treatment amounted to 6% in straightforward and 14% in complicated cases and so on. If ALL frequency and actual cure rates are considered in the Federal Republic of Germany, the total cost for treatment of ALL in childhood was DM 23 million per year, saving per year a total of 15,250 years of life in these patients. Thus, the efficiency of treatment in ALL was DM 1,515 per 1 year of life saved. This is low compared with regular dialysis treatment in chronic renal insufficiency, where the cost per patient-year of life is over US $ 11,000.

Conclusion

Due to the advent of intensive combination chemotherapy, childhood ALL has become a curable disease for the majority of patients. It is, however, a heterogenous disease characterized by various risk factors which influence prognosis under any uniform therapy. Reinforcement of chemotherapy by prolongation of induction, addition of more drugs, consolidation, and reintensification can overcome the influence of these risk factors and improve the quality of remission. The initial leukemic cell mass (burden) is the most important single determinant for treatment strategy. Current experience suggests that it may eventually be possible to shorten the duration of therapy to 1–2 years. Multicenter trials have demonstrated that patients can tolerate the necessary aggressive chemotherapy provided that appropriate support facilities are available. Careful long-term observation of the growing group of cured ALL patients and their offspring is necessary to determine whether an increased genetic risk exists.

References

1. Andreeff M, Darzynkiewiez Z, Sharpless TK, Clarkson BD, Melamed MR (1980) Discrimination of human leukemia subtypes by flow cytometric analysis of cellular DNA and RNA. Blood 55: 282–292
2. Baumer JH, Mott MG (1978) Sex and prognosis in childhood acute lymphoblastic leukaemia. Lancet 2: 128–129
3. Bennett JM, Catovsky D, Daniel MT, Flandrin G, Galto DAG, Gralnick HR, Sultan C (1976) Proposals for the classification of the acute leukaemias. French-American-British (FAB) co-operative group. Br J Haematol 33: 451–458
4. Berger R, Bernheim A, Flandrin G, Daniel M-T, Schaison G, Brovet J-C, Bernard J (1979) Translocation t (8; 14) dans la leucémie lymphoblastique de type Burkitt. Nouv Presse Med 8: 181–183
5. Blatt J, Poplack DG, Sherins RJ (1981) Testicular function in boys after chemotherapy for acute lymphoblastic leukemia. N Engl J Med 304: 1121–1124
6. Bleyer WA (1977) Clinical pharmacology of intrathecal methotrexate. II. An improved dosage regimen derived from age-related pharmacokinetics. Cancer Treat Rep 61: 1419–1425
7. Burchenal JH, Murphy ML (1965) Long-term survivors in acute leukemia. Cancer Res 25: 1491–1494
8. Chessels JM, Hardisty RM, Rapson NT, Greaves MF (1977) Acute lymphoblastic leukaemia in children: classification and prognosis. Lancet 2: 1307–1309
9. Ch'ien LT, Aur RJA, Stagner S, Cavallo K, Wood A, Goff J, Pitner S, Hustu HO, Seifert MJ, Simone JV (1980) Long-term neurological implications of somnolence syndrome in children with acute lymphocytic leukemia. Am Neurol 8: 273–277

10. Creutzig U, Schellong G (1980) Rezidivbehandlung bei akuter lymphoblastischer Leukämie im Kindesalter. Langzeitremissionen nach erstem Knochenmarksrezidiv. Dtsch Med Wochenschr 105: 1109–1112
11. D'Angio GJ (1982) The child cured of cancer: a problem for the internist. Semin Oncol 9: 143–149
12. Dinkel R, Schulze-Röbbecke T (1982) Kosten-Effektivitäs-Analyse der Zytostatikatherapie von akuter Leukämie im Kindesalter. Pharma Dialog 73
13. Dow LW, Borella L, Sen L, Aur RJA, George SL, Mauer AM, Simone JV (1977) Initial prognostic factors and lymphoblast-erythrocyte rosette formation in 109 children with acute lymphoblastic leukemia. Blood 50: 671–682
14. Ekert H, Waters KD, Smith PJ, Ellis WM (1978) Treatment of childhood lymphocytic leukemia with high white cellcounts. Br J Cancer 38: 619–623
15. Eser C, Lansdown R (1977) Retrospective study of inetellectual development in children treated for acute lymphoblastic leukemia. Arch Dis Child 52: 525–529
16. Evans AE, Gilbert E, Zandstra R (1970) The increasing incidence of central nervous system leukemia in children (Children's cancer study group A). Cancer 26: 404–409
17. Farber S, Diamond LK, Mercer RS, Sylvester RF, Wolff JA (1978) Temporary remissions in acute leukemia in children produced by folic acid antagonist, 4-aminopteroyl-glutamic acid (Aminopterin). N Eng J Med 238: 787–793
18. Fengler R, Henze G, Langermann H-J, Brämswig J, Jobke A, Kornhuber B, Ludwig R, Ritter J, Riehm H (1982) Häufigkeit und Behandlungsergebnisse testikulärer Rezidive bei der akuten lymphoblastischen Leukämie im Kindesalter. Klin Pädiat 194: 204–208
19. Foon KA, Herzog P, Billing RJ, Terasaki PI, Feig SA (1981) Immunologic classification of childhood acute lymphocytic leukemia. Cancer 47: 280–284
20. Frei E III, Holland JE, Schneiderman MA, Pinkel D, Selkirk G, Freireich EJ, Silver RT, Gold GL, Regelson W (1958) A comparative study of two regimens of combination chemotherapie in acute leukemia. Blood 13: 1126–1148
21. Gasser C (1980) Long-term survival (cures) in childhood acute leukemia. Paediatrician 9: 344–357
22. George SL, Fernbach DJ, Vietti TJ, Sullivan MP, Lane DM, Haggard ME, Berry DH, Lonsdale D, Komp D (1973) Factors influencing survival in pediatric acute leukemia. The SWCCSG experience, 1958–1970. Cancer 32: 1542–1553
23. George SL, Aur RJA, Mauer SM, Simone JV (1979) A reappraisal of the results of stopping therapy in childhood leukemia. N Engl J Med 300: 269–273
24. Green DM, Brecher ML, Blumenson LE, Grossi M, Freeman AJ (1982) The use of intermediate dose methotrexate in increased risk childhood acute lymphoblastic leukemia. Cancer 50: 2722–2727
25. Grosch-Wörner I, Langermann H-J, Brämswig J, Henze G, Odenwald E, Ritter J, Schellong G, Riehm H (1983) Behandlungsergebnisse mit Kindern mit akuter lymphoblastischer Leukämie nach isoliertem Knochenmarksrezidiv. Klin Pädiatr 196
26. Haghbin M, Tan CC, Clarkson BD, Mike V, Burchenal JH, Murphy ML (1974) Intensive chemotherapy in children with acute lymphoblastic leukemia (L-2 protocol). Cancer 33: 1491–1498
27. Hann HWL, Lustbader ED, Evans AE, Toledano SR, Lillie PD, Jasko LB (1981) Lack of influence of T-cell marker and importance of mediastinal mass on the prognosis of acute lymphocytic leukemias of childhood. J Natl Cancer Inst 66: 285–290
28. Hardisty RM, Till MM, Peto J (1981) Acute lymphoblastic leukaemia: four year survivals old and new. J Clin Pathol 34: 249–253
29. Henze G, Langermann H-J, Ritter J, Schellong G, Riehm H (1981) Treatment strategy for different risk groups in childhood acute lymphoblastic leukemia: a report from the BFM study group. Haematol Bluttransfus 26: 87–93 In: Neth et al. (eds) Modern trends in human leukemia 4. Springer, Berlin Heidelberg New York

30. Henze G, Langermann H-J, Lampert F, Neidhardt M, Riehm H (1979) Die Studie zur Behandlung der akuten lymphoblastischen Leukämie 1971–1974 der Deutschen Arbeitsgemeinschaft für Leukämie-Forschung und -Behandlung im Kindesalter e. V.: Analyse der prognostischen Bedeutung von Initialbefunden und Therapievarianten. Klin Pädiat 191: 114–126
31. Henze G, Langermann H-J, Kaufmann U, Ludwig R, Schellong G, Stollmann B, Riehm H (1981) Thymic involvement and initial white blood count in childhood acute lymphoblastic leukemia. Am J Pediatr Hematol Oncol 3: 369–376
32. Henze G, Langermann H-J, Gadner H, Schellong G, Welte K, Riehm H (1981) Ergebnisse der Studie BFM 76/79 zur Behandlung der akuten lymphoblastischen Leukämie bei Kindern und Jugendlichen. Klin Pädiat 193: 145–154
33. Henze G, Langermann H-J, Fengler R, Brandeis M, Evers KG, Gadner H, Hinderfeld L, Jobke A, Kornhuber B, Lampert F, Lasson U, Ludwig R, Müller-Weihrich S, Neidhardt M, Nessler G, Niethammer D, Rister M, Ritter J, Schaaff A, Schellong G, Stollmann B, Treuner J, Wahlen W, Weinel P, Wehinger H, Riehm H (1982) Therapiestudie BFM 79/81 zur Behandlung der akuten lymphoblastischen Leukämie bei Kindern und Jugendlichen: intensivierte Reinduktionstherapie für Patientengruppen mit unterschiedlichem Rezidivrisiko. Klin Pädiat 194: 195–203
34. Hughes WT, Kuhn S, Caudhary S, Feldman S, Verzosa M, Aur RJA, Pratt C, George SL (1977) Successful chemoprophylaxis for Pneumocystis Carinii pneumonitis. N Engl J Med 297: 1419–1426
35. Hustu HO, Aur RJA, Verzosa MS, Simone JV, Pinkel D (1973) Prevention of central nervous system leukemia by irradiation. Cancer 32: 585–597
36. Hutton JJ, Coleman MS, Mofi HS, Greenwood MF, Holland P, Lampkin B, Kisker T, Krill C, Kastelic JE, Valdez L, Bollum FJ (1982) Prognostic significance of terminal transferase activity in childhood acute lymphoblastic leukemia; a prospective analysis of 164 patients. Blood 60: 1267–1276
37. Jacquillat C, Weil M, Auclerc MF et al. (1978) Prognosis and treatment of acute lymphoblastic leukemia. Study of 650 patients. Cancer Chemother Pharmacol 1: 113–122
38. Kaneko Y, Rowley JD (1982) Clinical significance of chromosome abnormalities in childhood and adult leukemia. In: Humphrey GB et al (eds) Pankreatic tumors in children. Nijhoff, The Hague, pp 57–78
39. Lampert F (1977) Kombinations-Chemotherapie und Hirnschädelbestrahlung bei 530 Kindern mit akuter lymphoblastischer Leukämie. Dtsch Med Wochenschr 102: 917–921
40. Lampert F, Boosen K (1977) Morbus Hodgkin in der Remission einer akuten lymphoblastischen Leukämie. Klin Pädiat 189: 292–294
41. Langermann H-J, Henze G, Wulf M, Riehm H (1982) Abschätzung der Tumorzellmasse bei der akuten lymphoblastischen Leukämie im Kindesalter: prognostische Bedeutung und praktische Anwendung. Klin Pädiat 194: 209–213
42. Lawler SD (1982) Significance of chromosome abnormalities in leukemia. Semin Hematol 19: 257–272
43. Leukemia Committee and Working Party on Leukaemia in Childhood (1973) Treatment of acute lymphoblastic leukaemia. Effect of "prophylactic" therapy against central nervous system leukaemia. Br Med J 2: 381–384
44. Mauer AM (1980) Therapy of acute lymphoblastic leukemia in childhood. Blood 56: 1–10
45. Meadows AT, Massari DJ, Fergusson J, Gordon J, Littmann P, Moss K (1981) Declines in IQ scores and cognitive dysfunctions in children with acute lymphocytic leukaemia treated with cranial irradiation. Lancet 2: 1015–1018
46. Miller DR, Leikin S, Albo V, Sather H, Hammond D (1981) Prognostic importance of morphology (FAB classification) in childhood acute lymphoblastic leukemia (ALL). Br J Haematol 48: 199–206
47. Miller DR (1980) Acute lymphoblastic leukemia. Prediatr Clin North Am 27: 269–291
48. Miller DR, Sonley M, Karon M, Breslow N, Hammond D (1974) Additive therapy in the maintenance of remission in acute lymphoblastic leukemia of childhood: the effect of the initial leukocyte count. Cancer 34: 508–517

49. Moe PF, Seip M, Finne PH (1981) Intermediate dose methotrexate (IDM) in childhood acute lymphocytic leukemia in Norway. Acta Paediatr Scand 70: 73–79
50. Moe PF, Lethinen M, Wegelius R, Friman S, Kreuger A, Berg A (1979) Progeny of survivors of acute lymphocytic leukemia. Acta Paediatr Scand 68: 301–303
51. Morse HG, Heideman R, Hays T, Robinson A (1982) 4;11 translocation in acute lymphoblastic leukemia: a specific syndrome. Cancer Genet Cytogenet 7: 165–172
52. Muriel FS, Bustelo P, Pavlovsky S, Eppinger-Helft M, Svarch E, Braier JL, Garay G, Vergara B, Birman V, Peñalver J, Kvicala R, Divito J, Failace R, Dibar E (1981) Tratamiento de la leucemia linfoblastica aguda. Resultados en 1192 enfermos. Medicina (B Aires) [Suppl] 41: 5–14
53. Ochs JJ, Berger P, Brecher ML, Sinks LF, Kinkel W, Freeman AI (1980) Computed tomography brain scans in children with acute lymphocytic leukemia receiving methotrexate alone as central nervous system prophylaxis. Cancer 45: 2274–2278
54. Peylan-Ramu N, Poplack DG, Pizzo PA, Adornato BT, DiChiro G (1978) Abnormal CT scans of the brain in asymptomatic children with acute lymphocytic leukemia after prophylactic treatment of the central nervous system with radiation and intrathecal chemotherapy. N Engl J Med 298: 815–818
55. Pinkel D (1971) Five year follow-up of "total therapy" of childhood lymphocytic leukemia. JAMA 216: 648–652
56. Pinkel D, Hernandez K, Borella L, Holton C, Aur R, Samoy G, Pratt C (1971) Drug dosage and remission duration in childhood lymphocytic leukemia. Cancer 27: 247–256
57. Priest JR, Robison LL, McKenna RW, Lindquist LL, Warkentin PI, LeBien TW, Woods WG, Kersey JH, Coccia PF, Nesbit ME Jr (1980) Philadelphia chromosome positive childhood acute lymphoblastic leukemia. Blood 56: 15–22
58. Prober CG, Kirk LE, Keeney RE (1982) Acyclovir therapy of chickenpox in immunosuppressed children – a collaborative study. J Pediat 101: 622–625
59. Riehm H, Gadner H, Henze G, Langermann H-J, Odenwald E (1980) The Berlin childhood lymphoblastic leukemia therapy study, 1970–1976. Am J Pediatr Hematol Oncol 2: 299–306
60. Rivera G, Aur RJA, Dahl GV, Pratt CB, Wood A, Avery TL (1980) Combined VM-26 and cytosine arabinoside in treatment of refractory childhood lymphocytic leukemia. Cancer 45: 1284–1288
61. Rivera G, Aur RJA, Dahl GV, Pratt CB, Hustu HO, George SL, Maurer AM (1979) Second cessation of therapy in childhood lymphocytic leukemia. Blood 53: 1114–1120
62. Robison LL, Sather HN, Coccia PF, Nesbit ME, Hammond GD (1980) Assessment of the interrelationship of prognostic factors in childhood acute lymphoblastic leukemia. A report from childrens cancer study group. Am J Pediatr Hematol Oncol 2: 5–13
63. Rodt H, Netzel B, Thiel J, Huhn D, Haas R, Götze D, Thierfelder S (1977) Classification of leukemic cells with T- and 0-ALL-specific antisera. Hematol Bluttransfus 20: 87–95
64. Sather H, Coccia P, Nesbit M, Level C, Hammond D (1981) Disappearance of the predictive value of prognostic variables in childhood acute lymphoblastic leukemia: A report from childrens cancer study group. Cancer 48: 370–376
65. Sather H, Miller D, Nesbit M, Heyn R, Hammond D (1981) Differences in prognosis for boys and girls with acute lymphoblastic leukemia. Lancet 1: 739–743
66. Simone JV (1976) Annotation: factors that influence haematological remission duration in acute lymphocytic leukaemia. Br J Haematol 32: 465–472
67. Simone JV, Verzosa MS, Rudy JA (1975) Initial features and prognosis in 363 children with acute lymphocytic leukemia. Cancer 36: 2099–2108
68. Simone JV (1982) Late complications of treatment of children with leukemia and lymphoma. In: Malignant lymphomas. Academic Press, New York, pp 663–673
69. Siris ES, Leventhal BG, Vaitukaitis JL (1976) Effects of childhood leukemia and chemotherapy on puberty and reproductive function in girls. N Engl J Med 294: 1143–1146
70. Steinhorn SC, Myers MH (1981) Progress in the treatment of childhood acute leukemia: a review. Med Pediatr Oncol 9: 333–346

71. Thomas ED (1982) The use and potential of bone marrow allograft and whole body irradiation in the treatment of leukemia. Cancer 50: 1443–1454
72. Wang JJ, Freeman AI, Sinks LF (1976) Treatment of acute lymphocytic leukemia by high-dose intravenous methotexate. Cancer Res 36: 1441–1444
73. Wells RJ, Mascaro K, Young PCM, Cleary RE, Baehner RL (1981) Glucocorticoid receptors in the lymphoblasts of patients with glucocorticoid-resistant childhood acute lymphocytic leukemia. Am J Pediatr Heamtol Oncol 3: 259–264
74. Welte K, Ebener U, Hinderfeld L, Ritter J, Henze G, Kornhuber B (1981) Die Bedeutung der Terminalen desoxynukleotidyl Transferase in der Diagnostik der akuten Leukämie des Kindes – Ergebnisse von 63 Patienten. Klin Pädiat 193–171
75. West RJ, Graham-Pole J, Hardisty RM, Pike MC (1972) Factors in pathogenesis of central-nervous-system leukaemia. Br Med J 2: 311–314
76. Wolff LJ, Richardson ST, Neiburger JB, Neiburger RG, Irwin DS, Baehner RL (1976) Poor prognosis of children with acute lymphocytic leukemia and increased B cell markers. J Pediatr 89: 956–958
77. Zintl F, Plenert W, Hermann J (1981) Different therapy protocols for high risk and standard risk ALL in childhood. In: Neth R, Gallo RC, Graf T, Mannweiler K, Winker K (eds) Modern trends in human leukemia 4. Springer, Berlin Heidelberg New York (Hämatologie und Bluttransfusion, vol 26)
78. Zuelzer WW (1949) Current trends in hematology. Pediatrics 4: 269–276
79. Zuelzer WW (1964) Implications of long-term survival in acute stem cell leukemia treated with composite cyclic therapy. Blood 24: 477–494

Current Status of ALL/AUL Therapy in Adults

D. Hoelzer

Abteilung Hämatologie, Zentrum Innere Medizin, Universität Ulm,
Steinhövelstrasse 9, 7900 Ulm, FRG

Introduction

Results of treatment in acute lymphocytic leukemia (ALL) in children have improved progressively over recent years, reaching complete remission (CR) rates of over 90% and 5-year disease-free survival in 50% or more of the patients [43, 68, 79]. The results in childhood ALL are an ideal for adult ALL, but similar rates have not been attained with equivalent treatment regimens [38, 86]. The situation now seems to be changing in several respects. With intensified therapeutic regimens, long-term results in adults have improved and in a number of quite large therapeutic trials it is predicted that 21%–58% of the patients [24, 37, 45, 50, 63] will be disease-free at 2–9 years. This might be because treatment modalities that, have been optimized in childhood ALL, e.g., intensification of induction therapy, prophylaxis against central nervous system (CNS) leukemia and prolongation of maintenance therapy, are now also showing benefit in adult ALL therapy.
Further, progress is also due to the classification of acute lymphocytic leukemia by means of immunlogical and biochemical markers, which has greatly advanced the definition of prognostic factors in adult ALL, so that it may be possible to recognize risk groups requiring different forms of therapy. For high-risk patients, for example, an alternative approach could be allogeneic or autologous bone marrow transplantation in first remission, and in low-risk groups an attenuation of the intensive and aggressive treatment could be considered to avoid overtreatment, as in childhood ALL.

Diagnosis and Immunological Classification

Classification by means of morphology, cytochemistry, and immunological markers is covered elsewhere in this volume (see pp. 102–158), and in this chapter only acute undifferentiated leukemia (AUL) is of interest because of its variable allocation in ALL/AUL trials. More than 60% of the morphologically and cytochemically undefined acute leukemias, being negative for Sudan black, myeloperoxidase, fluoride esterase, and PAS, can be classified with immunological markers as subtypes of ALL (c-ALL, T-ALL or B-ALL) [94]. The remaining null ALL group (c-ALL−, nonT-ALL, non-B-ALL) is heterogeneous, being mostly positive for the enzyme terminal deoxynucleotidyl transferase (TdT), and has therefore to be included in the lymphatic cell lineage; but the TdT-negative ALL (or rather TdT-negative acute leukemia) may represent true stem-cell leukemias or even be early megakaryocytically or erythropoietically determined leukemias. The outcome for null ALL in adults is poor [50, 61]. Since null-ALL accounts for 20%–38% of

Recent Results in Cancer Research. Vol. 93

all cases of adult ALL [41, 94], its varying allocation in, and even complete exclusion from ALL studies may well affect the reported results in such trials.

Single Drugs in the Treatment of Adult ALL

The use of single drugs and the results of combination chemotherapy of ALL have recently been extensively reviewed by Henderson [46]. The efficacy of chemotherapy has been

Table 1. Single agents for remission induction

Drug	*n*	CR rate	References
Prednisone	11	36%	[78]
	22	36%	[18]
	26	42%	[89]
Vinca alkaloids			
Vincristine	5	20%	[25]
Vindesine	8	0%	[106]
	19[a]	37%	[9]
	14[a]	14%	[66]
Folic acid metabolites			
Methotrexate	7	14%	[34]
Purine antimetabolites			
6-Mercaptopurine	12	8%	[10]
	11	9%	[34]
Pyrimidine antimetabolites			
Cytosine arabinoside	43	43%	[16]
	22	50%	[30]
5-Azacytidine	10	10%	[70]
Anthracyclines			
Daunorubicin	38[a]	58%	[11]
Adriamycin	30	20%	[101]
	25[a]	36%	[67]
L-Asparaginase	21[a]	67%	[75]
	23[a]	68%	[21]
Alkylating agents			
Cyclophosphamide	61[a]	0–8%	[52]
Isophosphamide	12	33%	[83]
Epidodophyllotoxins			
VM 26	15[a]	7%	[14]
VP 16-213	10[a]	0%	[14]
Acridine derivatives			
m-AMSA	5	40%	[102]
	9	0%	[59]
	3	0%	[57]
	11	27%	[3]

[a] Includes children

mainly established in childhood ALL studies, but the limited number of results in adult ALL confirm the data obtained in childhood studies. The results are summarized in Table 1.

The drugs first found effective for remission induction were prednisone (P) and vincristine (V), and these are still the main drugs used (Table 1). Later the anthracyclines daunorubicin (D) and adriamycin (A), and also L-asparaginase (L-asp.) proved efficient in ALL. However, the data for L-asparaginase as a single drug for remission induction are all derived from work with groups including children, and its real effectiveness for adults may not be as high as the 67%–68% complete remission rate reported.

Cytosine arabinoside (Ara-C) has also proved to be a highly competent cytostatic agent in adult ALL, with CR rates of 43% and 50% (Table 1). Several possible reasons for this can be put forward but are only partly substantiated. Ara-C has been demonstrated to be active against T-ALL cells in vitro, and T-ALL makes up an appreciable proportion of about 20% [15] of all cases of adult ALL. Furthermore, since this agent is also the most effective in acute nonlymphoblastic leukemia (ANLL) it might be assumed that it is also active in null ALL and probably also in the small fraction of true mixed ALL, i.e., the types positive for c-ALLA and myeloid markers. These explanations are somewhat speculative, but in recent large trials which included Ara-C [24, 50] good overall results, especially improved remission duration, have been demonstrated in T-ALL.

There are too few data available to allow appraise of the true value of *cyclophosphamide* (C) as a single agent for remission induction in adult ALL, where CR rates of 0%–8% (Table 1) have been found. The CR rates of 18%–40% achieved in large childhood ALL studies with C as single agent [33, 51, 93] may be more realistic. Moreover, with a similar alkylating agent, isophosphamide, a CR rate of 33% was obtained in 12 adult patients (Table 1). Thus, although its efficiency as a single drug in adult ALL has not been established, C forms part of several consolidation regimens in adult ALL [24, 49, 63, 85, 86].

Combination Chemotherapy for Remission Induction

Vincristine and Prednisone

With the most widely used drug combination of vincristine and prednisone (VP), complete remission rates of 85%–95% can be obtained in childhood ALL [68] and about 50% in adult ALL, with a wide range from 33%–93%, as listed in Table 2. In early and also in current trials where the combination VP is used as induction regimen, the remission duration obtained varies from only 3–12 months, in spite of the variable maintenance and consolidation schedules used in these studies. This relatively short remission duration might mean that the quality of remission provided by VP induction treatment is unsatisfactory. Therefore, the VP therapy was escalated by addition of various other drugs. It should be mentioned, however, that a variety of other two-drug combinations (reviewed by Henderson [46]), including 6-mercaptopurine (6-MP), methotrexate (MTX), C, and Ara-C, also yielded similar but not superior CR rates in childhood ALL to those achieved with VP induction therapy.

Escalation of Vincristine/Prednisone Therapy

Vincristine and prednisone therapy intensified with either L-asparaginase and/or anthracyclines increases the CR rate to 70% and more, and also extends remission

Table 2. Vincristine and prednisone combination as induction therapy in adult ALL

Authors	*n*	CR rate	Median remission duration
Bernard et al. [12]	11	87%	
Henderson [44]	24	50%	12 months
Atkinson et al. [5]	31	39%	
Curtis et al. [27]	17	82%	
Einhorn et al. [28]	6	67%	3 months
Scavino et al. [88]	14	93%	9 months
Armitage and Burns [4]	5	60%	
Jacquillat et al. [54]	39	79%	
Lister et al. [62]	32	47%	
Sackmann-Muriel et al. [86]	27	33%	
Gottlieb and Weinberg [39]	50	50%	
Amadori et al. [2]	18	67%	
Willemze et al. [99]	84	51%	
Hess and Zirkle [47]	43	58%	8 months
deVries et al. [96]	25	36%	

duration; however, the improvement in remission duration is difficult to assess, especially when the drugs are given in sequence rather than simultaneously (Table 3). Thus Willemze improved the CR rate from 41% to a total of 83% by giving D in addition to VP, but D was only required by patients who had not achieved CR with VP alone, and the more severe disease might be reflected in the shorter median remission duration (MRD) in this group. The further addition of L-asp. or Ara-C brought no response in the severest cases. In the analysis made by Sackmann-Muriel et al. [86] a similar increase in CR rate was obtained by adding D, and results were even better when the combination VPD was given simultaneously. When L-asp. was included in the intial induction therapy [45] the improvement obtained in CR rate by the addition of D was not so marked. The simultaneous administration of L-asp. with VP and intrathecal MTX led to increased toxicity, which could be avoided by postponing the L-asp. [45] or, in another study where V, P, D, and L-asp. were used as induction agents [62], by increasing the intervals between drug administration from 1 to 2 weeks. That the toxicity caused by L-asp. is dose dependent is apparent from a childhood study [79], and a similar adult study [48] where the same drugs were used simultaneously for induction therapy but with a lower dose of L-asp. (5,000 U/m^2), in which no particularly severe toxicity was observed.

Early Intensification or Consolidation Therapy

After complete remission has been achieved by induction therapy, leukemic cells still persist and are responsible for the high relapse rates that occur later. Therefore additional therapy is required for their eradication. Whereas the purpose of maintenance therapy is the continuous suppression of persisting blast cells, that of early intensification or consolidation therapy is maximal leukemic cytoreduction with the object of simultaneously preventing the emergence of drug-resistant cells. This can be achieved either by adding new

Table 3. Escalation of VP therapy with D or L-asparaginase in adult ALL

Authors	Number of patients			CR rate	Median remission duration
	Total entered	Treated initially	Treated further		
Willemze et al. [98]					
Total entered	41				
V, P		41		19 (46%)	17 months
V, P + D			21	15 (71%)	11 months
V, P + D + L-asp./Ara-C			5	0	
Overall results				34/41 (83%)	
Sackmann-Muriel et al. [86]					
Total entered	75				
V, P		27		9 (33%)	
V, P + D			10	5 (50%)	
V, P, D		48		32 (67%)	
Overall results				46/75 (61%)	24 months
Henderson et al. [45]					
Total entered	149				
V, P, L-asp.		27		14 (52%)	
V, P, L-asp. + D			3	2 (67%)	
V, P + L-asp.		122		73 (60%)	14 months
V, P + L-asp. + D			30	18 (60%)	17 months
Overall results				107/149 (72%)	
Amadori et al. [2]					
Total entered	82				
V, P		18		12 (67%)	
V, P, D		27		16 (59%)	
V, P, L-asp.		37		27 (73%)	
Overall results				55/82 (67%)	25 months

drugs to the therapy schedule or by giving the same drugs as were successful in induction therapy. Such consolidation or early intensification therapies now form part of several adult ALL trials.

Overall Results of Multidrug Chemotherapy

Table 4 summarizes the results achieved in recent years with various combination therapy regimens and lists the drugs used. As can be seen, the induction therapy in most studies consists of the drugs V, P, D or A, L-asp., and sometimes Ara-C or C. Consolidation or early intensification therapy involves re-administration of the drugs used in induction therapy, or else other cytostatics such as Ara-C, C, 6-TG, BCNU, and occasionally MD-MTX may be introduced. The introduction of Ara-C and/or C in early intensification or consolidation therapy has shown promising results in some recent trials [24, 49, 63]. The strategy for further treatment differs considerably in these studies, from 6-MP, C, and PO MTX maintenance [62] to continuous reinduction and multiple-drug maintenance [24] or one intensified consolidation course after 3 months and a fairly simple maintenance therapy with 6-MP and MTX [48]. Thus it is difficult to distinguish the improvement affected by Ara-C and C alone.

Overall CR rates between 61% and 85% have been attained (Table 4), and a figure of 70% for CR in adult ALL is realistic. The duration of first CR varies; some reports give a duration of 8 months and in some studies the median has not yet been reached after an observation period of 2–5 years. A more informative parameter is the fraction of patients in continuous complete remission after 2 years or more. Such figures show that distinct improvements have been made during the last decade in adult ALL. In several studies [20, 31, 37, 63, 86], 25% or more patients are in CCR 3–6.5 years after remission induction. In some more recent studies with intensified therapy [24, 50] the CCR rates at 2 years are 44%–58%; in these studies a substantial cure rate may have been achieved.

Maintenance Therapy

The duration of unmaintained remission after successful remission induction is only about 2–4 months. The benefit of maintenance therapy for prolongation of remission duration was first demonstrated by Freireich, who used 6-MP [35]. The data for childhood ALL suggest that even when early intensification or consolidation therapy is given further maintenance therapy should not be omitted, at least at present. This also holds true for adult ALL. However, the optimal drugs, their sequence, and the duration of maintenance therapy are not yet established.

Although remission duration in children can be improved up to 1 year after CR by single drugs, e.g., by administration of MTX every 1 or 2 weeks, a combination of drugs is also of advantage in maintenance therapy [46]. The main drugs in current use for maintenance therapy are MTX and 6-MP with or without C, and with or without intermittent reinforcement courses of V and P.

There have also been attempts to intensify consolidation and maintenance therapy further by including a variety of other drugs such as BCNU [45, 98], adriamycin, and actinomycin D [24]. Such a multiple-drug maintenance and consolidation regimen repeated in sequence over 3 years seems to be very effective, and has yielded the best results reported to date in adult ALL [24].

The optimal duration of maintenance therapy has not been established, although a large number of childhood ALL studies have addressed the problem. Thus, in the UKALL II and UKALL III trials [23], periods of 2 years for girls and 3 years for boys were found satisfactory. It was concluded from another randomized study [65] that 2.25 years was the optimal duration. The U.S. Children's Cancer Study Group found in a randomized trial that 5 years of maintenance therapy had no advantage over 3 years [73]. From these results it seems that maintenance therapy should be continued for about 2.5–3 years. For adult ALL there are no data from randomized prospective studies. Schedules of childhood maintenance therapy are usually continued for about 2–3 years.

The increasing availability of surface markers should allow better characterization of leukemic cells and therefore detection of minimal residual leukemia in "remission" bone

Table 4. Combination chemotherapy for induction remission in untreated adult ALL/AUL

Authors	Year	*n*	Induction	Consolidation	Maintenance	CNS prophylaxis	CR rate	MRD (months)	Continuous complete remission
Jacquillat et al. [55]	1973	30	V, P, D	± V, P, D	± 6-MP, MTX	IT-MTX	73%	11	5% at 4 years
Sackmann-Muriel et al. [86]	1978	75	V, P, D	± Ara-C, C	6-MP, MTX	IT-MTX, CI IT-DXM	61%	24	39% at 3 years
Henderson et al. [45]	1979	149	V, P, D, L-asp.	MTX, 6-MP	MTX, 6-MP, V, P	IT-MTX, CI	72%	15	
Omura et al. [76]	1980	99	V, P, MTX	Ara-C, 6-TG, L-asp. V, P	MTX, 6-MP, C, V, P	IT-MTX, CI	80%	17	
Amadori et al. [2]	1980	82	V, P V, P, D V, P, L-asp.		6-MP, MTX, V, P	IT-MTX, IT-P	67%	25	
Brun et al. [19]	1980	92	V, P, D, L-asp. Ara-C		6-MP, MTX, V, P Ara-C, L-asp.	IT-MTX, CI	71%	10–14	
Willemze et al. [99]	1980	86	V, P, A/D		MTX, 6-MP, V, P	IT-MTX, CI	85%	15	
Clarkson et al. [24]	1981	29	V, P, D, Ara-C 6-TG	Ara-C, 6-TG, L-asp. V, BCNU	6-TG, C, D, HU, MTX BCNU, Ara-C, V	IT-MTX	79%	~ 24	21% at 9 years
		34	V, P, A, Ara-C 6-TG, MTX	Ara-C, 6-TG, MTX L-asp.	V, P, A, 6-MP, MTX BCNU, C, Dact.	IT-MTX, OM	85%	m.n.r.	44% at 5 years

		38	V, P, C, A	MTX, Ara-C, 6-TG, C, L-asp.	V, P, A, 6-MP, MTX BCNU, C, Dact.	IT-MTX, OM	84%	m.n.r.	58% at 2 years
Burns et al. [20]	1981	23	V, P, A, L-asp.		V, P, A, 6-MP, MTX BCNU, C, Dact.	IT-MTX, CI	74%	16	37% at 3 years
Esterhay et al. [31]	1982	24	MD-MTX, V, DXM, L-asp.	MD-MTX, L-asp./ HD-MTX, V, DXM	MTX, V, DXM, 6-MP	HD-MTX	75%	11	38% at 5 years
Hess and Zirkle [47]	1982	43	V, P	V, P	6-MP/C/MTX	± IT-MTX	66%	8	8% at ~ 6 years
Garay et al. [37]	1982	241	V, D, P				72%		25% at 5 years
Lister et al. [63]	1983	112	V, P, A, L-asp./C	V, P, A, L-asp./C	6-MP, MTX, C	IT-MTX, CI	66%	~ 24	28% at 6.5 years
Hoelzer et al. [50]	1984	162	V, D, P, L-asp., Ara-C, C, 6-MP	DXM, V, A, C, Ara-C 6-TG	6-MP, MTX	IT-MTX, CI	78%	20	44% at 2 years

V, vincristine; *P*, prednisone; *D*, daunorubicin; *L-asp.*, L-asparaginase; *MTX*, methotrexate; *MD-MTX*, moderate-dose MTX; *HD-MTX*, high-dose MTX; *Ara-C*, cytosine arabinoside; *A*, adriamycin; *C*, cyclophosphamide; *DXM*, dexamethasone; *6-MP*, 6-mercaptopurine; *6-TG*, 6-thioguanine; *BCNU*, 1,3-bis-(2-chloroethyl)-1-nitrosourea; *HU*, hydroxyurea; *Dact.*, actinomycin D; *CI*, cranial irradiation; *IT*, intrathecal; *m.n.r.*, median not reached; *OM*, Ommaya reservoir marrow aspirates. This would give an objective criterion for discontinuation or continuation of chemotherapy, or for the use of alternative therapeutic approaches such as bone marrow transplantation.

CNS Prophylaxis

In adults, an incidence of 39% [103] has been observed for CNS leukemia at autopsy, but clinical examination and examination of CSF give a much lower incidence of detectable CNS manifestations, with an average of 10.9% in 13 studies (summarized by Esterhay [31]); in a recent trial with 162 adult ALL/AUL patients [50] initial CNS leukemia could be detected in only 4.3%. The major problem, however, is not the treatment of initial CNS disease but the prevention of CNS relapse. With the increased disease-free survival in childhood CNS leukemia becomes apparent as a major obstacle, and CNS prophylaxis is now a mandatory part of the treatment programs in ALL. The essential data for therapeutic CNS regimens were established in controlled trials at St Jude's Children's Hospital [53]. It was demonstrated that the most effective CNS prophylaxis for prevention of CNS leukemia was the combination of cranial irradiation (CI) with 24 Gy and intrathecal (IT) MTX injections.

In several adult ALL trials without any prophylactic treatment of the CNS, a short remission duration of only 4–9 months has been observed (Table 5a), but to what extent CNS relapses contributed to the short remission duration is not stated. The CNS prophylactic regimen for childhood ALL was later adopted for adults and the standard therapy of CI with 24 Gy and IT-MTX was then widely used (Table 5b). With this form of CNS prophylaxis, CNS relapse occurred in 10%–29% of the patients with generally prolonged remission durations (Table 5b). However, as in childhood ALL, with the improvement of therapy and resultant increase in remission duration the CNS relapse rate becomes more evident when CNS prophylaxis is not given, as seen in a randomized study in which CNS irradiation with IT-MTX was compared with no CNS prophylaxis (see Table 5d). A clear decrease from 32.3%–10.7% for the CNS relapse rate was observed [76] when patients received CNS prophylaxis.

The neurotoxicity caused in some cases by the combination of CI and IT-MTX with CNS relapse rates still over 20% provoked a search for alternative measures. To avoid CNS irradiation several therapeutic modalities with chemotherapy alone were tried, consisting mainly of IT-MTX, intraventricular MTX by Ommaya reservoir, high-dose MTX IV, IT-Ara-C or high-dose Ara-C IV. MTX alone proved useful [99], with a CNS relapse rate of 6% as against 20% in the group receiving CI plus IT-MTX. Intraventricular MTX prophylaxis via an Ommaya reservoir was also beneficial, with only 8% CNS relapses [24], but CNS relapses could still not be entirely avoided and this method involves the risk of infection. High-dose IV MTX without prophylactic CNS irradiation and without IT-MTX seems to be similarly practical in preventing CNS leukemia, with a CNS relapse rate of 8.3% [31]. To what extent Ara-C is suitable for CNS prophylaxis in adult ALL remains to be proved. The addition of IT-Ara-C and hydrocortisone to IT-MTX did not reduce the CNS relapse rate in children [42, 92]. High-dose Ara-C is now under trial for ALL consolidation therapy, and it might be of value for CNS prophylaxis. Pyrimethamine PO has proved unsuccessful in CNS prophylaxis, with a frequency of 33% CNS leukemias [91]. A completely different approach in a childhood ALL study is the use of IT colloidal gold (Au^{198}) [107].

Table 5. CNS prophylaxis

Authors	*n*	Cranial irradiation	IT-MTX	Other drugs	CR rate	MRD (months)	CNS relapse rate
a. No CNS prophylaxis							
Whitecar et al. [97]	21	–	–	–	69%	5	
Gahrton et al. [36]	19	–	–	–	42%	4–7	
Rodriguez et al. [82]	38	–	–	–	61%	6	
Noon and Hess [74]	20	–	–	–	60%	7	
b. CNS prophylaxis with cranial irradiation and intrathecal treatment							
Cavalli et al. [22]	22	24 Gy	12 mg/m^2	–	64%	14	~20%
Lister et al. [62]	51	24 Gy	12.5 mg/m^2	IT Ara-C, 50 mg	71%	19	~10%
Sackmann-Muriel et al. [86]	75	24 Gy	12 mg/m^2	IT dexamethasone	61%	24	5%
Henderson et al. [45]	73	24 Gy	12 mg/m^2		76%	15	11%
	76	24 Gy	12 mg/m^2		73%		
AIL Study Group [1]	46	24 Gy	6 mg/m^2		72%	21	13%
Hoelzer et al. [50]	162	24 Gy	10 mg/m^2	–	78%	20	14%
c. CNS prophylaxis without cranial irradiation							
Smyth and Wiernik [91]	17	–	–	Pyrimethamine 1.5 mg/kg PO	53%	15	33%
Amadori [2]	82	–	12 mg/m^2	IT-P, 20 mg/m^2	67%	25	11%
Clarkson [24]	29 (L 2)	–	6.25 mg/m^2		79%	~24	
	34 (L 10)	–	6.25 mg/m^2 OM		85%	m.n.r.	8%
	38 (L 10 M)	–	6 mg/m^2 OM		84%	m.n.r.	
Esterhay [31]	38	–	–	HD-MTX IV, 100 mg/m^2	76%	11	8%
deVries [96]	25	–	15 mg OM		100%	19	13%
d. Comparative studies, with or without CNS prophylaxis							
Willemze et al. [99]	35	24 Gy	12 mg/m^2	–		15	20%
	29	–	12 mg/m^2	–	85%	17	6%
	9	–	–	–		6	50%
Omura et al. [76]	28	24 Gy	10 mg/m^2	–	80%	21	11%
	34	–	–	–		25	32%

Thus, some methods of CNS chemoprophylaxis in adult ALL seem to be at least equal to cranial irradiation and IT-MTX, with CNS relapse rates under 10%. However, at present the standard CNS prophylaxis with 24 Gy cranial irradiation and IT-MTX can still be recommended. In further trials the optimal chemotherapeutic procedures to replace CI should be evaluated.

Relapse Therapy

More than 50% of adult ALL patients still relapse during the course of their disease. The main causes are resistant disease and suboptimal therapy. The further outcome for such patients is very poor. In most cases, remission can be induced again but the remission durations are usually very short, only 4 months on average (Table 6).

In a first relapse of adult ALL, CR can be obtained in about 60% of the cases with the drugs already used for the first remission induction, which are generally prednisone, vincristine, daunorubicin/adriamycin and L-asparaginase. Similar results are reached with a combination of MTX and L-asparaginase, with a CR rate of about 60% in both childhood [64] and adult ALL (62%) [105]. Ara-C has also proved effective in the treatment of adult ALL in relapse. Thus, with the combination of Ara-C and daunorubicin, a CR rate of 67% in relapsed adult ALL was achieved by Early et al. [cited in ref. 46]. High-dose Ara-C might also be of value in relapsed ALL, since it has been used successfully in refractory ALL, but case numbers are still too low to judge its real efficiency [32, 100]. In a combination that introduces the new drug epipodophyllotoxin VM-26 together with Ara-C for refractory ALL in children Rivera et al. [81] reported a CR rate of 64%. This schedule is now being tested in adult ALL for consolidation and maintenance therapy.

In children with relapsed ALL, a second remission with long-term disease-free survival can be achieved in a substantial proportion of patients, especially when relapse occurs after completion of maintenance therapy [26, 56, 80]. Similar experience in adult ALL is lacking, since in most studies the proportion of long-term disease-free survivors has been too small to permit systematic analysis. The situation may change in the near future with larger prospective trials and a higher proportion of responders and long-term survivors.

Up to now, second or further remission obtained in adult ALL have lasted only a few months, and long-term remissions have not been reported. Therefore these relapsing patients should be considered for bone marrow transplantation (BMT) if suitable donors

Table 6. Chemotherapy of adult ALL in relapse

Authors	*n*	Drug combination	CR rate	Median remission duration (months)
Rodriguez et al. [82]	21	V, P, 6-MP, MTX	62%	4
Bodey et al. [17]	34	D, L-asp.	38%	3
Woodruff et al. [104]	23	V, P, A, ± L-asp.	69%	4
Yap et al. [105]	28	MTX, L-asp.	57%	5
Elias et al. [29]	10	V, P, A	50%	4
Esterhay et al. [31]	14	MD-MTX, V, L-asp., DXM	79%	7.5

are available, since at this stage results with BMT are superior to those obtained with chemotherapy. If no suitable donor is available autologous BMT with selective eradication of remaining leukemic cells in the autograft might be an alternative therapeutic approach for specific subtypes of ALL.

Relapse Sites

The recurrence of leukemia is most frequently observed in the bone marrow. CNS relapse is still a major obstacle but can now be reduced to about 10%, as already discussed. Of the other known extramedullary sites, the testis is of note in childhood ALL, where relapses mostly occur within 1 year after cessation of treatment [23]. Observations of testicular relapse in adult ALL are rare. In one study [63] with the relatively long median observation time of 2 years, extramedullary relapses were found in the testis in four and in the skin in one out of 45 cases. Extramedullary relapses outside the CNS were not, however, seen in a recent trial [24] with intensive induction, consolidation, and maintenance treatment. In another recent large study [50], only one of 70 relapsed patients had a testicular relapse. In both these last studies results for T-ALL, in which the tendency to extramedullary relapse is increased, are improved, and this may be related to the low incidence of relapse in the testis. Thus, relapse at this site may depend on the therapeutic schedule and the drugs used. The low incidence of testicular relapse in adult ALL therefore does not warrant prophylactic treatment of the testis or other extramedullary sites except the CNS.

Prognostic Factors

In adult ALL there is an urgent need for the evaluation of prognostic factors and consequent definition of risk groups. The recognition of high-risk groups could give reliable indications for the application of alternative therapeutic approaches such as BMT or intensification of chemotherapy in such cases. In low-risk patients the intention would be to avoid possible overtreatment, e.g., by omitting CNS irradiation, and thereby reducing toxicity. That such risk groups are not well defined in adult ALL is mainly due to the small number of patients in prospective trials and the nonuniform chemotherapy.

Age

In some childhood studies older children have a poorer prognosis [71, 90], and increased age has also had an adverse influence on the CR rate in most adult ALL studies (Table 7). However, this was largely evident when the extremes of age were compared, and the difference is statistically significant in only a few studies [2, 45, 85]. Evidence for an adverse effect of more advanced age on remission duration or survival was only suggestive in some studies [45, 85], but could be clearly shown in two recent trials, with a MRD of 23 months for patients below 35 years and of 13 months for patients of 35–65 years in one [50], while in the other 25% of patients aged 16–45 years were in continuous CR at 5 years versus no patients over 60 years [37]. The reasons for the poorer results in older patients are not yet clear. One possibility is that the therapy was suboptimal because doses were reduced for older patients on the grounds of toxicity. Attempts to improve therapeutic results for older ALL patients are limited at present, because both the intensification of chemotherapy and its alternative, BMT, carry increased risks for older patients.

Table 7. Age as a prognostic factor

Author	n	Age	CR rate		Median remission duration		Median survival time (months)	
Sackmann-Muriel et al. [86]	75	< 16	84%					
		> 16	61%					
Ruggero et al. [85]	138[a]	< 40	83%	$P < 0.02$			29	$P < 0.0002$
		> 40	65%				5	
Henderson et al. [45]	149	< 30	81%		20.3 months		30	
		> 60	45%		2.5 months		2	
Amadori et al. [2]	82	< 20	85%	$P = 0.05$				
		> 55	43%					
Omura et al. [76]	99	15–20	92%					
		> 20–50	73%					
		> 50	60%					
Garay et al. [37]	241	< 30	77%	$P < 0.001$	25% CCR at 5 years	$P < 0.0005$		
		> 60	36%		0% CCR at 5 years			
Hoelzer et al. [50]	162	< 35	81%	n.s.	23 months	$P = 0.006$		
		> 35	68%		13 months			

[a] Including children from 11 years

White Blood Cell Count

A factor that has proved to be of high prognostic significance in children is the white blood cell (WBC) count at diagnosis, which indicates the extent or progression of the disease [71, 79, 90]. An elevated WBC count had only a weakly adverse influence on the achievement of complete remission, as was also found in adult ALL (Table 8). However, for duration of remission the adverse influence is clear. In childhood ALL, a significant leukocyte level in a large trial was found at 25,000 cells/μl [79] but in adult trials the levels range from 10,000 to 30,000 cells/μl (Table 8), owing to the variation in treatment schedules. It has not been possible to set a uniform limit for the definition of risk, although it would be desirable, for instance, in the selection of patients requiring BMT.

Other Pretreatment Features

Hepato- or splenomegaly as a further expression of tumor mass and extramedullary infiltration has been found to be adversely correlated to the outcome of disease [62] and hepatomegaly, to have a slightly unfavorable influence on the achievement of CR but not on the duration of remission [50]. In children, the mediastinal mass was found to indicate a poor outcome but this could not be demonstrated in recent adult studies with improved remission duration [24, 50], probably because of the favorable outcome often associated with mediastinal mass in patients with T-ALL.

Other features at presentation, such as low platelet count [85], normal as opposed to low hemoglobin [24], infection [60], peripheral neuropathy [19], and high serum LDH [24], have been reported to be associated with poor prognosis but were not noted in most other studies. Although sex is a factor of major prognostic value in some childhood ALL studies, where superior long-term results have been shown in girls, up to now it has not been found to have any significance in adult ALL. Perhaps longer observation periods will reveal some influence. Workers are unanimous in accepting the adverse prognosis for L3 morphology as defined by FAB [7, 60, 63], but that of L2 morphology is controversial; the prognostic value of cytogenetic markers such as the Ph^1 chromosome is discussed elsewhere in this book (pp. 29).

Time to Achieve CR

Another factor that has been found to be of prognostic value in recent adult ALL studies is the duration and amount of treatment required to achieve CR, i.e., the number of weeks/courses needed. In four large trials with total CR rates of over 70% (Table 9) it was found that only about 50% of the adult patients achieved CR within 4 weeks. The remaining 20% of remitting patients required more than the first 4 weeks/courses to reach CR, whereby in two studies several new drugs were introduced after 4 weeks/courses [45, 50]. This parameter seems merely to reflect a more resistant leukemic cell population, since these patients were not spared chemotherapy for any reason during the first 4 weeks. In children, also, late response to therapy is correlated with poor prognosis but the proportion of such patients in childhood ALL is much lower, since 77.9%–100% achieve CR within 4 weeks [6, 77, 79, 87]. Interestingly enough, even in the favorable subtype c-ALL, only 52.3% of adults achieve CR within 4 weeks [50], which differs markedly from results known in children with the same subtype.

Table 8. Initial leukocyte count as a prognostic factor

Authors	n	Leukocytes per µl	CR rate	Median remission duration	Median survival time (months)
Rodriguez et al. [82]	38	< 35,000	92%		
		> 35,000	79%		
Gee et al. [38]	23	< 25,000		28 months	
		> 25,000		15 months	
Ruggero et al. [85]	138[a]	< 25,000			42 $P < 0.0002$
		> 25,000			20
Amadori et al. [2]	82	< 10,000	77%		42
		10,000–50,000	55%		Median not reached
		> 50,000	70%		9
Brun et al. [19]	92	< 25,000		24 months	
		> 25,000		7 months	
Garay et al. [37]	241	< 50,000		28% CCR at 5 years $P < 0.01$	
		> 50,000		9% CCR at 5 years	
Hoelzer et al. [50]	162	< 10,000	81%	29 months	
		10,000–50,000	77%	17 months $P = 0.03$	
		> 50,000	73%	10 months	

[a] Including children from 11 years

Table 9. Time to achieve complete remission

	Chemotherapy		n	CR within 4 weeks/courses	CR after 4 weeks/courses	CR total
	First 4 weeks/courses	After 4 weeks/courses				
Lister et al. [62]	V, P, A, L-asp.	V, P, A	51	47% (24/51)	24% (12/51)	71% (36/51)
Henderson et al. [45]	V, P, L-asp.	D	149	58.4% (87/149)	13.4% (20/149)	71.8% (107/149)
Lazzarino et al. [58]	V, P, D	V, P, D	62	43.5% (27/62)	29% (18/62)	72.5% (45/62)
Hoelzer et al. [50]	V, P, D, L-asp.	C, Ara-C, 6-MP	162	58.6% (95/162)	19.1% (31/162)	77.8% (126/162)

Table 10. Reasons for the inferior outcome of adult ALL compared with childhood ALL

		Adults (%)	References	Children (%)	References
1. Lower "primary" response to chemotherapy	CR within 4 weeks/courses	51.0	[62]	77.9	[77]
		58.7	[45]	78.1	[87]
		43.5	[58]	91.8	[6]
		58.6	[49]	100	[79]
2. Higher proportion of unfavorable immunological subtype	Null-ALL	27.8	[61]	4	[94]
		37.8	[41]	12.1	[41]
		25.6	[49]	16.6	[95]
		27.0	[50]		
Lower proportion of favorable immunological subtype	c-ALL	57.5	[61]	69	[94]
		50.5	[41]	75.6	[41]
		56.4	[49]	62.5	[95]
		52.0	[50]		
3. Lower CR rate within a particular immunological subtype	Null ALL	82.0	[61]	84	[40]
		67.0	[20]		
		75.0	[49]		
	c-ALL	78.0	[61]	89–97	[94]
		70.5	[50]	93	[40]

Differences in Outcome Between Childhood and Adult ALL

Surface marker analysis has revealed factors which may largely explain the differences in response to treatment between children and adults with ALL (Table 10). These are the different distribution of subtypes with varying prognosis in adults and children and the differences in response rates within a particular subtype. It is agreed that the subtype c-ALL is associated with the best prognosis in both children and adults [50, 63, 69]. However, results in c-ALL in adults differ from those obtained in childhood ALL in several respects (Table 10). First, it has been found that in a substantial proportion of adults with c-ALL, response to therapy is delayed until after 4 weeks of therapy. Furthermore, the c-ALL subtype was found in several studies to have a lower frequency in adults than in children, whereas the subtype null ALL, which so far is correlated with poor outcome [50, 63], is more frequent, up to 37%, in adults [41]. A third factor is the CR rate achievable within a defined subtype, which both for c-ALL and for null ALL is clearly lower in adults than in children (Table 10).

These results might not only explain differences in outcome between childhood and adult ALL, but also form a basis for comparison of different therapeutic strategies. Since the main subtype in childhood ALL is c-ALL and in children CR is usually obtained within 4 weeks, results in the subgroup of adult patients who fulfill the same criteria should be compared with the total results in children. In one study [50] with immunologically defined adult ALL patients the results were encouraging and comparable to those in children, with 63% of such early-responding c-ALL patients in continuous CR (CCR). When high-risk patients (WBC > 30,000/μl and age > 35 years) were excluded, the percentage in CCR rose to 79%. In another trial [63] 52% of adult c-ALL patients in the low-risk group (WBC < 25,000/μl) are in CCR at 6.5 years and further results in c-ALL, with 39% adults in CCR versus 73% in children [69], are reported.

For T-ALL, the situation has changed dramatically. This subtype was regarded in the past as having a bad prognosis in children as well as in adults [13, 20, 61]. The results are currently improving in childhood studies and also in some adult studies. In adult patients Clarkson [24] found no difference in CCR between patients with T-ALL and the whole group. In another trial, T-ALL is the subgroup with the best prognosis, having 58% in CCR [50]. These improved remission durations in T-ALL might be related to the use of Ara-C and C in the treatment regimens. The improved results in T-ALL are probably one of the main recent achievements in childhood and in adult ALL.

Indications for Bone Marrow Transplantation

The place of bone marrow transplantation (BMT) in ALL is controversial. In childhood ALL a second or subsequent remission is regarded as an indication for BMT, but this is not generally accepted [72] since reasonable long-term results can be achieved with chemotherapy alone in a substantial proportion of cases. The situation is even more debatable in adult ALL, with assertions at one extreme that all ALL patients over 15 years are high-risk patients and therefore candidates for BMT [8], and at the other that there is no place for BMT in first remission because chemotherapy results are good enough to make exposure of patients to the risks associated with BMT unnecessary [24].

One way of resolving this controversy would be by better definition of risk groups in adults, to characterize a low-risk group of patients who are sufficiently well cared for with cytostatic treatment and a high-risk group where BMT is at present the better approach. Although the prognostic factors so far established are somewhat dependent on the therapeutic schedules used, present estimation of risk as deduced from different ALL regimens can be generalized to some extent.

Age certainly plays a role, since in several adult ALL studies increased age had an adverse influence on CR rate, MRD, and survival. It was seen as a definitely poor prognostic factor only in older patients. Since the age limitation for BMT is about 40 years, poor-risk patients according to this criterion cannot profit from BMT. For the *white blood cell* count at presentation, the risk level is variably defined. In general, clearly inferior results are seen in most studies with 25,000–30,000/μl upwards. The *length of treatment required to achieve CR* is of relevance for the long-term results in adult ALL, and patients with delayed response to therapy have a poor prognosis. Regarding *immunological subtypes,* patients with null ALL or B-ALL still have a poor outcome. Thus, patients with one of these bad prognostic factors should be candidates for BMT in first remission. Conversely, patients with a low initial WBC count, early response to therapy, and c-ALL should not receive transplants in first remission. According to recent results in T-ALL the same holds true for this subgroup.

Such a definition of risk groups is certainly open to criticism, but forms a basis on which future therapeutic trials should be analysed. In an adult ALL/AUL trial [50] these factors have now been confirmed in more than 350 patients, and candidates for BMT in first remission are defined according to these criteria. However, the changing strategies in both chemotherapy and BMT entail continual re-evaluation of the risk group definitions and comparison of results with the various therapeutic approaches.

References

1. The A.I.L. Study Group (1979) A cooperative study on the therapy of acute lymphoblastic Leukemia. Results of the Italian Association against leukemia. Haematologica 64: 119
2. Amadori S, Montuoro A, Meloni G, Spiriti MAA, Pacilli L, Mandelli F (1980) Combination chemotherapy for acute lymphocytic leukemia in adults: results of a retrospective study in 82 patients. Am J Hematol 8: 175
3. Arlin ZA, Fanucchi MP, Gee TS et al. (1982) Treatment of refractory adult lymphoblastic leukemia (ALL) with 4′(9-acridinylamino)methanesulfon-M-anisidide (AMSA). Blood 60: 1224
4. Armitage JO, Burns CP (1977) Remission maintenance of adult acute lymphoblastic leukemia. Med Pediatr Oncol 3: 53
5. Atkinson K, Wells DG, Clink HMcD, Kay HEM, Powles R, McElwain TJ (1974) Adult acute leukaemia. Br J Cancer 30: 272
6. Aur RJA, Simone JV, Versoza MS et al. (1978) Childhood acute lymphocytic leukemia. Study VIII. Cancer 42: 2123
7. Baccarani M, Corbelli G, Amadori S et al. (1982) Adolescent and adult acute lymphoblastic leukemia: prognostic features and outcome of therapy. A study of 293 patients. Blood 60: 677
8. Barrett AJ, Kendra JR, Lucas CF et al. (1982) Bone marrow transplantation for acute lymphoblastic leukemia. Br J Haematol 51: 181
9. Baysass M, Gouveia J, Ribaud P et al. (1979) Phase II trial with vindesine for regression induction in patients with leukemias and hematosarcomas. Cancer Chemother Pharmacol 2: 247
10. Bernard J, Boiron M, Weil M et al. (1962) Etude de la rémission complète des leucémies aigues. Nouv Rev Fr Hematol 2: 195
11. Bernard J (1964) Acute leukemia treatment. Cancer Res 27: 2565
12. Bernard J, Boiron M, Jacquillat C et al. (1966) Traitement actuels des leucémies aigues. Presse Med 74: 1241
13. Bitran JD (1978) Prognostic value of immunologic markers in adults with acute lymphoblastic leukemia. N Engl J Med 299: 1317
14. Bleyer WA, Chard RL, Krivit W et al. (1978) Epipodophyllotoxin therapy of childhood neoplasia: a comparative phase 2 analysis of VM 26 and VP 16-213. Proc AACR/ASCO 19: 373 (abstract)
15. Bloomfield CF (1982) The clinical relevance of lymphocyte surface markers in adult acute lymphoblastic leukemia. In: Bloomfield CD (ed) Adult leukemias 1. Nijhoff, The Hague, pp 265–308
16. Bodey GP, Freireich EJ, Monto RW, Hewlett IT (1969) Cytosine arabinoside (NSC-63878) therapy for acute leukemia in adults. Cancer Chemother Rep 53: 59
17. Bodey GP, Hewlett JS, Coltmann CA, Rodriguez V, Freireich EJ (1974) Therapy of adult acute leukemia with daunorubicin and L-asparaginase. Cancer 33: 626
18. Boggs DR, Wintrobe MM, Cartwright GE (1962) The acute leukemias. Medicine 41: 163
19. Brun B, Vernant JP, Tulliez M et al. (1980) Acute non myeloid leukaemia in adults. Prognostic factors in 92 patients. Scand J Haematol 24: 29
20. Burns CP, Armitage JO, Aunan SB et al. (1981) Therapy of adult acute lymphoblastic leukemia: superior results of null vs. T-cell disease. Proc Am Assoc Cancer Res 22: 485
21. Capizzi RL, Bertino JR, Skeel RT et al. (1971) L-asparaginase: clinical, biochemical, pharmacological, and immunological studies. Ann Intern Med 74: 893
22. Cavalli F, Hartmann H, Tschopp L, Sauter C, Alberto P (1977) Therapieresultate und prognostische Faktoren bei der akuten lymphatischen Leukämie des Erwachsenen. Schweiz Med Wochenschr 107: 1361
23. Chessells JM (1982) Acute lymphoblastic leukemia. Semin Hematol 19: 155

24. Clarkson B, Schauer P, Mertelsmann R et al. (1981) Results of intensive treatment of acute lymphoblastic leukemia in adults. In: Burchenal JH, Oettgen HF (eds) Cancer. Achievements, challenges and prospects for the 1980s, vol 2. Grune and Stratton, New York, p 301
25. Cline MJ, Rosenbaum E (1968) Prediction of in vitro cytotoxicity of chemotherapeutic agents by their in vitro effect on leukocytes from patients with acute leukemia. Cancer Res 28: 2516
26. Creutzig U, Schellong G (1980) Rezidivbehandlung bei akuter lymphoblastischer Leukämie im Kindesalter. Dtsch Med Wochenschr 105: 1109
27. Curtis JE, Cowan DH, Bergsagel DE, Hasselback R, McCulloch EA (1975) Acute leukemia in adults: assessment of remission induction with combination chemotherapy by clinical and cell-culture criteria. Can Med Assoc J 113: 289
28. Einhorn LH, Meyer S, Bond WH, Rohn RJ (1975) Results of therapy in adult acute lymphocytic leukemia. Oncology 32: 214
29. Elias L, Shaw MT, Raab SO (1979) Reinduction therapy for adult acute leukemia with adriamycin, vincristine and prednisone: a southwest oncology group study. Cancer Treat Rep 63: 1413
30. Ellison RR, Holland JF, Weil M et al. (1968) Arabinosyl cytosine: a useful agent in the treatment of acute leukemia in adults. Blood 32: 507
31. Esterhay RJ, Wiernik PH, Grove WR, Markus SD, Wesley MN (1982) Moderate dose methotrexate, vincristine, asparaginase and dexamethasone for treatment of adult acute lymphocytic leukemia. Blood 59: 334
32. Febres R, Flessa C, Martelo OJ (1982) Efficacy of high dose cytosine arabinoside in refractory adult leukemia. Proc Am Soc Clin Oncol 1: 128 (abstract C-498)
33. Fernbach DJ, Griffith KM, Haggard ME (1966) Chemotherapy of acute leukemia in childhood: comparison of cyclophosphamide and mercaptopurine. N Engl J Med 275: 451
34. Frei III E, Freireich EJ, Gehan E (1961) Studies of sequential and combination antimetabolite therapy in acute leukemia: 6-mercaptopurine and methotrexate. Blood 18: 431
35. Freireich EJ, Gehan E, Frei III E et al (1963) The effect of 6-mercaptopurine on the duration of steroid-induced remissions in acute leukemia: a model for evaluation of other potentially useful therapies. Blood 21: 699
36. Gahrton G, Engstedt L, Franzen S et al. (1974) Induction of remission with L-asparaginas cyclophosphamide, cytosine arabinoside, and prednisolone in adult patients with acute leukemia. Cancer 34: 472
37. Garay G, Pavlovsky S, Eppinger-Helft M, Cavagnaro F, Saslavsky J, Dupont J (GATLA) (1982) Long term survival in adult lymphoblastic leukemia (ALL). Evaluation of prognositc factors. Proc Am Soc Clin Oncol 1: 237 (abstract C-531)
38. Gee TS, Haghbin M, Dowling MD, Cunningham I, Middleman MP, Clarkson BD (1976) Acute lymphoblastic leukemia in adults and children. Differences in response with similar therapeutic regimens. Cancer 37: 1256
39. Gottlieb AJ, Weinberg V (1979) Efficacy of daunorubicin in induction therapy of adult acute lymphocytic leukemia (ALL). A controlled phase III study (CALGB 7612). Blood [Suppl 1] 54: 188a (abstract)
40. Greaves MF, Janossy G, Peto J, Kay H (1981) Immunologically defined subclasses of acute lymphoblastic leukaemia in children: their relationship to presentation features and prognosis. Br J Haematol 48: 179
41. Greaves MF, Lister TA (1981) Prognostic importance of immunologic markers in adults with acute lymphoblastic leukemia. N Engl J Med 304: 119
42. Haghbin M (1977) Antimetabolites in the prophylaxis and treatment of central nervous system leukemia. Cancer Treat Rep 61: 661
43. Haghbin M, Murphy ML, Tan CC et al. (1980) A long term clinical follow-up of children with acute lymphoblastic leukemia treated with intensive chemotherapy regimens. Cancer 46: 241
44. Henderson ES (1973) Acute lymphoblastic leukemia. In: Holland JF, Frei E (eds) Cancer medicine, chapter XIX-1. Lea and Febiger, Philadelphia, p 1173

45. Henderson ES, Scharlau C, Cooper MR (1979) Combination chemotherapy and radiotherapy for acute lymphocytic leukemia in adults: results of CALGB protocol 7113. Leuk Res 3: 395
46. Henderson ES (1983) Acute lymphocytic leukemia. In: Gunz FW, Henderson ES (eds) Leukemia 4th ed, chapter 25. Grune and Stratton, New York, p 575
47. Hess CE, Zirkle JW (1982) Results of induction therapy with vincristine and prednisone alone in adult acute lymphoblastic leukemia: report of 43 patients and review of the literature. Am J Hematol 13: 63
48. Hoelzer D, Thiel E, Löffler H et al. (1983) Multizentrische Therapiestudie. Akute lymphatische Leukämie (ALL) und akute undifferenzierte Leukämie (AUL) des Erwachsenen. Verh Dtsch Krebsges 4: 723
49. Hoelzer D, Thiel E, Löffler H Bodenstein H, Büchner T, Messerer D (German Multicentre ALL/AUL Study Group) (1983) Multicentre pilot study for therapy of acute lymphoblastic and acute undifferentiated leukemia in adults. In: Neth R, Gallo RC, Greaves M, Moore R, Winkler K (eds) Modern trends in human leukemia 5. Springer, Berlin Heidelberg New York, p 36 (Hämatologie und Bluttransfusion, vol 28)
50. Hoelzer D, Thiel E, Löffler H et al. (1984) Intensified therapy in acute lymphoblastic and acute undifferentiated leukemia in adults. Blood (in press)
51. Holcomb TM (1979) Cyclophosphamide (NSC 26271 in the treatment of acute leukemia in children. Cancer Chemother Rep 51: 137
52. Hoogstraten B (1962) Cyclophosphamide (Cytoxan) in acute leukemia. Cancer Chemother Rep 16: 167
53. Hustu HO, Aur RJA (1978) Extramedullary leukemia. Clin Haematol 7: 313
54. Jacquillat C, Weil M, Auclerc MF et al. (1978) Prognosis and treatment of acute lymphoblastic leukemia. A study of 650 patients. Cancer Chemother Pharmacol 1: 113
55. Jacquillat C, Weil M, Gemon MF et al. (1973) Combination therapy in 130 patients with acute lymphoblastic leukemia (protocol 06 LA 66-Paris). Cancer Res 33: 3278
56. Kimball JC, Herson J, Sullivan MP (1980) Favourable response to maintenance therapy of second or subsequent remissions in childhood acute lymphocytic leukemia. Cancer 46: 1093
57. Lawrence JH, Ries CA, Reynolds RD et al. (1980) A promising new agent in refractory acute leukemia. Proc AACR/ACSO 21: 438 (abstract)
58. Lazzarino M, Morra E, Alessandrino EP et al. (1982) Adult acute lymphoblastic leukemia. Response to therapy according to presenting features in 62 patients. Eur J Cancer Clin Oncol 18: 813
59. Legha SS, Keating MJ, Zander AR (1980) 4′(9-Acridinylamino)methansulfan-M-anisidide (AMSA): a new drug effective in the treatment of adult acute leukemia. Ann Intern Med 93: 17
60. Leimert JT, Burns CP, Wiltse CG, Armitage JO, Clarke WR (1980) Prognostic influence of pretreatment characteristics in adult acute lymphoblastic leukemia. Blood 56: 510
61. Lister RA, Roberts MM, Brearly RL, Woodruff RK, Greaves MF (1979) Prognostic significance of cell surface phenotype in adult acute lymphoblastic leukemia. Cancer Immunol Immunother 6: 227
62. Lister TA, Whitehouse JMA, Beard MEJ et al. (1978) Combination chemotherapy for acute lymphoblastic leukaemia in adults. Br Med J 1: 199
63. Lister TA, Amess JAL, Rohatiner AZS, Henry G, Greaves MF (1983) The treatment of adult acute lymphoblastic leukaemia (ALL). Proc Am Soc Clin Oncol 2: 170 (abstract C-661)
64. Lobel JS, O'Brien RT, McIntosh S et al. (1979) Methotrexate and asparaginase combination chemotherapy in refractory ALL of childhood. Cancer 43: 1089
65. Mandelli F, Amadori S, Rajnoldi AC et al. (1980) Discontinuing therapy in childhood acute lymphocytic leukemia. Cancer 46: 1319
66. Mandelli F, Amadori S, Giona F et al. (1982) Vindesine in the treatment of refractory hematologic malignancies: a phase II study. Leuk Res 6: 649

67. Mathé G, Amiel J-L, Hayat M et al. (1970) L'adriamycin dans le traitement des leucémies aigues. Presse Med 79: 1997
68. Mauer AM (1980) Therapy of acute lymphoblastic leukemia in childhood. Blood 56: 1
69. Mayer RJ, Coral FS, Rosenthal DS, Sallan SE, Frei III E (1982) Treatment on non-T, non-B cell acute lymphocytic leukemia (ALL) in adults. Proc Am Soc Clin Oncol 1: 126 (abstract C-487)
70. McCredie KB, Bodey GP, Burgess MA et al (1973) Treatment of acute leukemia with 5-azacytidine (NSC 1028976). Cancer Chemother Rep 57: 319
71. Miller DR, Leikin S, Albo V et al. (1980) Use of prognostic factors in improving the design and efficiency of clinical trials in childhood leukemia: children cancer study group report. Cancer Treat Rep 64: 381
72. Nathan DG, Sallan SE, Weinstein HJ (1982) Bone marrow transplantation for acute lymphoblastic leukemia. N Engl J Med 306: 610
73. Nesbit ME, Sather HN, Robison LL, Ortega JA, Hammond GD (1983) Randomized study of 3 years versus 5 years of chemotherapy in childhood acute lymphoblastic leukemia. J Clin Oncol 1: 308
74. Noon MA, Hess CE (1976) Acute leukemia in adults: comparison of survival between a treated and an untreated group. South Med J 69: 1157
75. Oettgen HE, Old LJ, Boyse EA et al. (1967) Inhibition of leukemia in man by L-asparaginase. Cancer 27: 2619
76. Omura GA, Moffitt S, Vogler WR, Salter MM (1980) Combination chemotherapy of adult acute lymphoblastic leukemia with randomized central nervous system prophylaxis. Blood 55: 199
77. Ortega JA, Nesbit ME, Donaldson MH et al. (1977) L-asparaginase, vincristine, and prednisone for induction of first remission in acute lymphocytic leukemia. Cancer Res 37: 535
78. Ranney HM, Gellhorn A (1957) The effect of massive prednisone and prednisolone therapy on acute leukemia and malignant lymphomas. Am J Med 22: 405
79. Riehm H, Gadner H, Henze G, Langermann HJ, Odenwald E (1980) The Berlin childhood acute lymphoblastic leukemia therapy study, 1970–1976. Am J Pediatr Hematol Oncol 2: 299
80. Rivera G, Bowman P, Ochs J, Abromowitch M, Pui CH (1982) Cyclic combination chemotherapy for recurrent childhood lymphocytic leukemia (ALL) after elective cessation of therapy. Proc Am Soc Clin Oncol 1: 126 (abstract C-489)
81. Rivera G, Dahl GV, Bowman WP, Avery TL, Wood A, Aur RJ (1980) VM-26 and cytosine arabinoside combination chemotherapy for initial induction failures in childhood lymphocytic leukemia. Cancer 46: 1727
82. Rodriguez V, Hart JS, Freireich EJ et al. (1973) POMP combination chemotherapy of adult acute leukemia. Cancer 32: 69
83. Rodriguez V, McCredie KB, Keating MJ et al. (1978) Isophosphamide therapy for hematologic malignancies in patients refractory to prior treatment. Cancer Treat Rep 62: 493
84. Royston I, Minowada J, LeBien T et al. (1983) Phenotypes of adult acute lymphoblastic leukemia (ALL) defined by monoclonal antibodies (MoAbs). Proc Am Soc Clin Oncol 2: 177 (abstract C-690)
85. Ruggero D, Baccarani M, Gobbi M, Tura S (1979) Adult acute lymphoblastic leukaemia: study of 32 patients and analysis of prognostic factors. Scand J Haematol 22: 154
86. Sackmann-Muriel F, Svarch E, Eppinger-Helft M et al. (1978) Evaluation of intensification and maintenance programs in the treatment of acute lymphoblastic leukemia. Cancer 42: 1730
87. Sallan SE, Camitta BM, Cassady JR, Nathan DG, Frei E (1978) Intermittent combination chemotherapy with adriamycin for childhood acute lymphoblastic leukemia. Clinical results. Blood 51: 425
88. Scavino HF, George JN, Sears DA (1976) Remission induction in adult acute lymphocytic leukemia. Cancer 38: 672
89. Shanbron E, Miller S (1962) Critical evaluation of massive steroid therapy of acute leukemia. N engl J Med 266: 1354

90. Simone JV, Verzosa MS, Rudy JA (1975) Initial features and prognosis in 363 children with acute lymphocytic leukemia. Cancer 36:2099
91. Smyth AC, Wiernik PH (1976) Combination chemotherapy of adult acute lymphocytic leukemia. Clin Pharmacol Ther 19:240
92. Sullivan MP, Moon TE, Trueworthy R, Vietti TJ, Humphrey GB, Komp D (1977) Combination intrathecal therapy for central nervous system leukemia: two versus three drugs. Blood 50:471
93. Tan CT, Phoa J, Plyman M (1961) Hematological remissions in acute leukemia with cyclophosphamide. Blood 18:808 (abstract)
94. Thiel E, Rodt H, Huhn D et al. (1980) Multimarker classification of acute lymphoblastic leukemia: evidence for further T subgroups and evaluation of their clinical significance. Blood 56:759
95. Thöne I, Kabisch H, Müller J, Winkler K, Landbeck G (1982) Immunologische Klassifizierung der akuten lymphoblastischen Leukämien (ALL) des Kindesalters. Monatsschr Kinderheilkd 131:883
96. de Vries EGE, Mulder NH, Houwen B, Haaxma-Reiche H (1982) Combination chemotherapy for acute lymphocytic leukaemia in 25 adults. Blut 44:151
97. Whitecar JP, Bodey GP, Freireich EJ, McCredie KB, Hart JS (1972) Cyclophosphamide (NSC-26271), vincristine (NSC-67574), cytosine arabinoside (NSC-63878), and prednisone (NSC-10023) (COAP) combination chemotherapy for acute leukemia in adults. Cancer Chemother Rep 56:543
98. Willemze R, Hillen H, Hartgrink-Groeneveld CA et al. (1975) Treatment of acute lymphoblastic leukemia in adolescents and adults: a retrospective study of 41 patients (1970–1973). Blood 46:823
99. Willemze R, Drenthe-Schonk AM, van Rossum J, Haanen C (1980) Treatment of acute lymphoblastic leukaemia in adolescents and adults. Comparison of two schedules for CNS leukaemia prophylaxis. Scand J Haematol 24:421
100. Willemze R, Zwaan FE, Colpin GGD, Keuning JJ (1982) High dose cytosine arabinoside in the management of refractory acute leukaemia. Scand J Haematol 29:141
101. Wilson HE, Bodey GP, Moon TG (1977) Adriamycin therapy in previously treated adult acute leukemia. Cancer Treat Rep 61:905
102. Winton EF, Vogler WR, Rose KL (1980) Phase II study of acridinyl anisidide (m-AMSA) (NSC-249992) in refractory adult acute leukemia. Proc AACR/ASCO 21:437 (abstract)
103. Wolk RW, Masse SR, Conklin R, Freireich EJ (1974) The incidence of central nervous system leukemia in adults with acute leukemia. Cancer 33:864
104. Woodruff RK, Lister TA, Paxton AM, Whitehouse JMA, Malpas JS (1978) Combination cheotherapy for haematological relapse in adult acute lymphoblastic leukaemia (ALL). Am J Hematol 4:173
105. Yap BS, McCredie KB, Benjamin RS, Bodey GP, Freireich EJ (1978) Refractory acute leukaemia in adults treated with sequential colaspase and high-dose methotrexate. Br Med J 2:791
106. Young C, Currie V, Cvitknovic E et al. (1978) Early Phase II evaluation of vindesine in patients with advanced cancer. In: Siegenthaler W, Luthy R (eds) Current chemotherapy. Proceedings of the tenth international congress of chemotherapy II. American Society of Microbiology Washington, p 1330
107. Zintl F, Herman J, Katenkamp D, Malke H, Plenert W (1983) Results of LSA_2-L_2 therapy in children with high-risk acute lymphoblastic leukemia and non-Hodgkin's lymphoma. In: Neth R, Gallo RC, Greaves M, Moore R, Winkler K (eds) Modern trends in human leukemia 5. Springer, Berlin Heidelberg New York, p 36 (Hämatologie und Bluttransfusion, vol 28)

Acute Myelogenous Leukemia: Current Status of Therapy in Children

J. Ritter, U. Creutzig, H.-J. Riehm, and G. Schellong

Universitäts-Kinderklinik, Robert-Koch-Strasse 31, 4400 Münster, FRG

Introduction

In contrast to the major advances in the treatment of childhood acute lymphoblastic leukemia (ALL), the progress achieved in the therapy of children with acute myelogenous leukemia (AML) has not been satisfactory. Until recently, no differences in therapeutic response and prognosis were found between children and adults with AML. While the majority of patients obtain a complete remission, remission duration has remained disappointingly short, ranging from 8 to 15 months [2, 10, 12, 19, 20, 25, 36, 39, 42, 44, 49]. Recent data from a study in the United States [55] and a multicenter trial in the Federal Republic of Germany [14, 15], however, suggest that a significant increase in the proportion of long-term survivors and possible cures in childhood AML have been achieved with prolonged, aggressive chemotherapy. In addition, bone marrow transplantation in first remission may provde a new approach for improvement of treatment results for AML, both in children and in young adults [23, 41, 52].

Incidence, Age, and Sex Distribution

AML is a rare disease in children, accounting for only 15%–20% of all childhood acute leukemias [35, 46, 58]. AML occurs at a frequency of approximately 10 per million children less than 15 years of age per year [58]. The incidence of childhood AML is evenly distributed over all age groups, with a median at 9.5 years [13, 15, 35, 55]. In contrast, the incidence of childhood ALL decreases continuously with age after a maximum occurrence rate between 3 and 7 years [35, 45, 46]. The frequency of childhood AML is evenly distributed among sexes, in contrast to the slight predominance of male patients in ALL (Table 1) [15, 35, 45, 46].

Classification

The morphologic classification of childhood AML is usually based on the criteria defined by the French-American-British (FAB) committee [5]. The distribution of AML subtypes is similar in children and adults, except that acute monoblastic leukemia (AMOL; FAB M5) is more frequent in children less than 2 years of age [11, 15, 22, 38, 55, 56].
In addition to morphology, AML is classified by cytochemical techniques, especially the myeloperoxydase reaction and staining for nonspecific esterase [5]. Other approaches have been applied for the classification of morphologically and cytochemically undifferentiated

Recent Results in Cancer Research. Vol. 93

Table 1. Age and sex distribution of childhood ALL and AML Data from the BFM study-group

Age (years)	Acute lymphoblastic leukemia (%) (n = 1,086)	Acute myelogenous leukemia (%) (n = 151)
0– 3	23.5	19
3– 7	37	18
7–10	15	15
10–13	13.5	23
Over 13	11	25
Male : female	58 : 42	54 : 46

acute leukemias, such as immunologic techniques (Chap. 5), biochemical assays (TdT activity) [32], determinations of serum and urine lysozyme [57] and cationic leukocyte antigen [53] levels, and flow cytometry of cellular DNA and RNA [1]. Some acute leukemias remain unclassifiable, and cases with two distinct blastic populations have even been described [13a, 37a].

Chemotherapy

Cytostatic therapy in childhood AML is based on the same drugs found to be active against AML in adults. A review of published pediatric trials reveals remission rates between 59% and 79% for nine different induction regimens, most of which consist in the combination of a pyrimidine analog with an anthracycline, with or without the addition of a purine analog. Most protocols for childhood AML also include vincristine, prednisone, and cyclophosphamide (Table 2). The major cause of failure of induction therapy remains death from severe bleeding or uncontrollable infectious complications, whereas primary resistance of leukemic blasts to aggressive induction regimens is rather infrequent [2, 15, 44, 55].

For the treatment of children in complete remission, continuous or intermittent maintenance therapy with alternating combinations of cytotoxic drugs is administered (Table 2). More aggressive consolidation or intensification cycles have been included in more recent studies [15, 55].

Different modalities of CNS prophylaxis have been applied in studies published by Haghbin [25] and Dahl et al. [18], and in the German Berlin–Frankfurt–Münster (BFM) trial [14, 15, 47]. In patients treated according to the Children's Cancer Study Group (CCSG) protocol, CNS relapse prevention is not carried out until a patient has completed 6 months in continuous bone marrow and CNS remission [2].

In spite of high remission rates obtained by intensive induction therapy, the duration of complete remission is short in most pediatric trials (Table 3). The majority of relapses occur in the bone marrow, although a considerable proportion of extramedullary relapses has been reported in all series, especially with involvement of the CNS [21, 33, 37, 40, 44].

Encouraging results have recently been reported by Weinstein and co-authors [55], who apply aggressive induction therapy with vincristine, cytosine arabinoside, prednisone, and adriamycin (VAPA) followed by early and late intensification with alternating drug combinations. Their study aimed at maximum reduction and possible eradication of the

Table 2. Study design of nine regimens for treatment of childhood acute myelogenous leukemia

References	Institution	Remission induction[a]	CNS prophylaxis	Consolidation	Intensification	Maintenance
Haghbin et al. [25]	MSKCC, New York	ADR, TG, ARA-C (ATA) × 3	MTX IT	ATA × 2	∅	L2 Protocol [24]
Chard et al. [12]	Children's Cancer Study Group	PRED, ARA-C, TG, CTX, VCR (PATCO) × 4	∅	∅	∅	TG, ARA-C, CTX, VCR
Madanat et al. [36]	M. D. Anderson, Houston	CTX, VCR, ARA-C, PRED (COAP)	∅	COAP × 4	∅	COAP
Baehner et al. [2]	Children's Cancer Study Group	DNR, AZA, ARA-C PRED, VCR (D-ZAPO) × 4	After 6 months in CCR, MTX IT	∅	∅	TG, AZA, ARA-C, VCR
Pluess et al. [44]	Dept. of Pediatrics, Zürich	ARA-C, DNR or ADR × 1–2	∅	∅	∅	ARA-C, TG, ± VCR, ± ADR
Dahl et al. [19]	St. Jude's, Memphis	DNR, VCR, AZA, ARA-C × 2–5	MTX IT	∅	PRED, VCR, MTX, 6-MP (POMP)	ADR, CTX, VCR, ARA-C 6-MP
Weinstein et al. [55]	Sidney Farber, Boston	VCR, PRED, ADR, ARA-C (VAPA) × 2	∅	Intensive sequential maintenance I ADR + ARA-C × 4 II ADR + AZA × 4 II POMP × 4 V ARA-C × 4		
Scheer et al. [47]	Dept. of Pediatrics, Münster	VCR, PRED, ADR, TG, ARA-C, CTX (8 weeks) × 1	Cranial irradiation: 18 Gy MTX IT	Prolonged and intensified remission induction		ADR, ARA-C, TG
Creutzig et al. [15]	German BFM Study Group					

[a] *ADR*, adriamycin; *TG*, thioguanine; *ARA-C*, cytosine-arabinoside; *MTX*, metrothexate; *CTX*, cyclophosphamide; *VCR*, vincristine; *PRED*, prednisone; *AZA*, azacytidine; *DNR*, daunorubicin

Table 3. Results of nine recent chemotherapy studies in childhood acute myelogenous leukaemia

Reference	No. of patients (recruitment-period)	% CR	No. of relapses (CNS involved)	Median duration of CCR (months) (life-table method)	CCR % of patients in CR (life-table method)	Survival % of all patients treated (life-table method)
Haghbin et al. [25]	21 (1971–1976)	76%	8 (1)	15	50% (after 6 years)	38% (after 6 years)
Chard et al. [12]	163 (1972–1974)	59%	69 (12)	11.5	28.5 (after 4 years)	19% (after 4 years)
Madanat et al. [36]	43 (1968–1976)	51%	15 (?)	8	32% (after 4 years)	19% (after 4 years)
Baehner et al. [2]	163 (1974–1977)	72%	72 (9)	12	30% (after 3 years)	20% (after 3 years)
Pluess et al. [44]	38 (1971–1977)	79%	21 (7)	10	22% (after 8 years)	16% (after 8 years)
Dahl et al. [19]	95 (1976–1980)	72%	48 (6)	10	29% (after 5 years)	16% (after 5 years)
Weinstein et al. [55]; + 1983 update [37]	61 (1976–1980)	72%	19 (8)	Not yet reached	52% (after 6 years)	44% (after 6 years)
Scheer et al. [47]; + 1983 update [15]	23 (1974–1978)	74%	10 (1)	46.5	37% (after 8 years)	39% (after 8 years)
Creutzig et al. [15]	151 (1979–1982)	79%	40 (6)	Not yet reached	56% (after $3^3/_4$ years)	43% (after $3^3/_4$ years)

For therapy outlines see Table 2

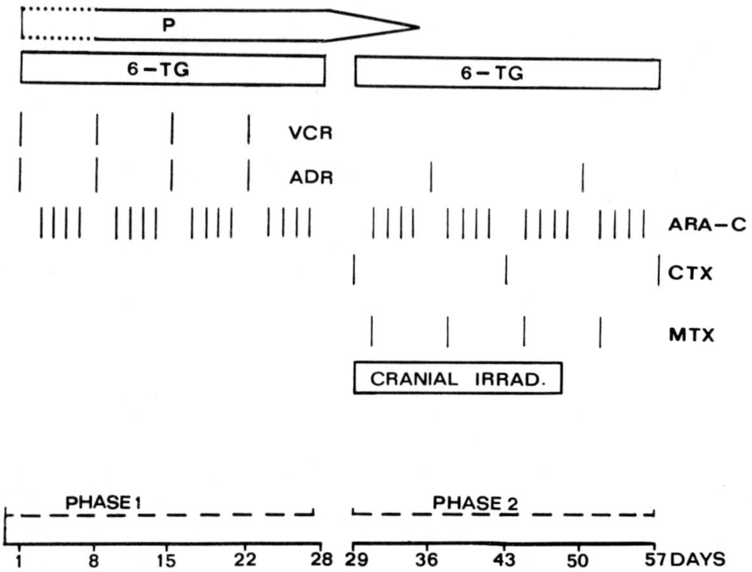

Fig. 1. Induction regimen of the German Cooperative Childhood AML Study BFM-78. *P*, prednisone 60 mg/m^2 PO (withheld initially for some days in the event of bleeding or coagulation problems); *6-TG*, thioguanine 60 mg/m^2 PO; *VCR*, vincristine 1.5 mg/m^2 IV (maximum single dose 2.0 mg); *ARA-C*, cytosine arabinoside 75 mg/m^2 IV; *CTX*, cyclophosphamide 500 mg/m^2 IV; *MTX*, methotrexate 12.5 mg/m^2 IV (maximum single dose 15 mg); cranial irradiation: age 0–12 months: 12 Gy; 13–24 months: Gy; over 24 months: 18 Gy

leukemic cell burden, and prevention of the emergence of drug-resistant cell clones. In all, 61 children with AML entered this study, the results being updated in 1982 [37]. Though the remission rate of 74% is similar to that obtained in most other pediatric trials, the duration of complete continuous remission (CCR) exceeds all previously published data considerably: the probability of remaining in first complete remission after 6 years is 52% (Table 3). These results emphasize the probability of cure for a significant proportion of children with AML as a consequence of intensive remission induction and intensive postremission multidrug treatment.

Promising results with a remission rate of 74% and a median duration of CCR of 46.5 months were obtained in a German BFM pilot study in Münster by prolonged intensive induction therapy [15, 47] derived from the BFM protocol for childhood ALL [45]. On the basis of these results a nationwide multicenter cooperative trial was initiated by the BFM study group in 1978 using an almost identical protocol.

Induction chemotherapy consisted of vincristine, prednisone, adriamycin, cytosine arabinoside, and 6-thioguanine for the first 4 weeks. After a treatment-free interval of 1–2 weeks a combination of cyclophosphamide, cytosine arabinoside, 6-thioguanine, and adriamycin was administered for a further 4 weeks, together with CNS prophylaxis consisting of four intrathecal methotrexate injections and cranial irradiation (Fig. 1). For remission maintenance daily 6-thioguanine was given, together with monthly cycles of cytosine arabinoside SC for 4 days. In the first year patients also received one dose of adriamycin every 8 weeks. In children in CCR maintenance therapy was stopped after 2 years. The results of the life-table analysis of this cooperative study from 30 participating

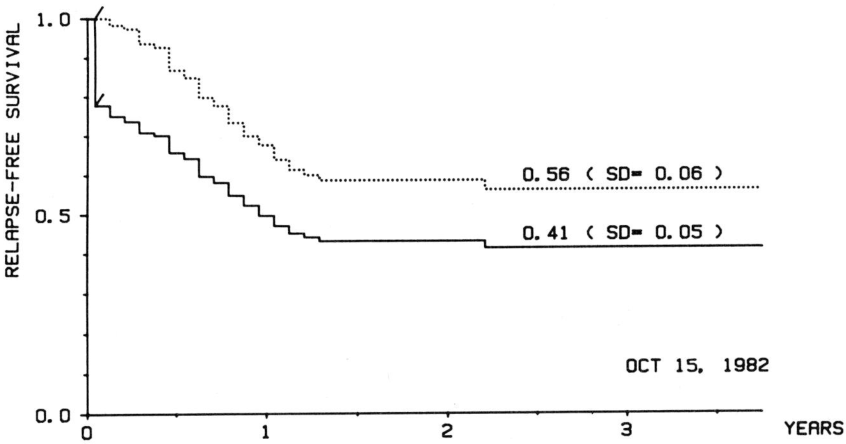

Fig. 2. Probability of relapse-free survival in the German Cooperative Childhood AML Study BFM-78. ———, all patients (*n* = 151; 71 in CCR); ·····, remission group (*n* = 119; 71 in CCR); *tick* indicates last patient entering the study

centers in Germany are given in Fig. 2. A total of 151 patients entered the study between December 1978 and October 1982. Of all these, 79% (*n* = 119) achieved complete remission. The median duration of CR has not yet been reached after a median observation time of 23 months (October 1982). Life-table analysis reveals a probability of 56% ± 6% for remaining in CR at 45 months for patients having achieved a complete remission, and of 41% ± 5% for all patients who entered the trial.

In Table 4 the data from the BFM study and the VAPA trial are compared. While the remission and relapse rates are similar in both studies, there are considerable differences with respect to the sites of relapses. In the BFM trial the vast majority of relapses occurred in the bone marrow and there was a low incidence of CNS relapses [14, 15]. In contrast, the CNS was the primary site of relapse in 8/18 pediatric patients in the VAPA study [37]. This difference is likely to be the consequence of the CNS prophylaxis applied in the BFM protocol; in the VAPA trial no specific treatment at prevention of CNS relapse was included. On the basis of these results intrathecal chemotherapy with cytosine arabinoside was added to the modified VAPA regimen currently in use (H. J. Weinstein, personal communication, 1982).

CNS Therapy

Recent improvements in the therapy of childhood AML and the increasing numbers of long-term survivors emphasize the need for effective prevention of CNS relapse. As in experience with childhood ALL two decades ago, an increase in remission duration in children with AML is complicated by a concurrent rise in the frequency of CNS relapses [21, 33, 37, 40, 44]. The design and intensity of prophylactic CNS treatment, however, remains controversial as in childhood ALL. Intrathecal methotrexate [14, 15, 25] and cytosine arabinoside [33], with or without simultaneous cranial or cranial and spinal irradiation [15, 18], are currently under investigation. Dahl et al. [18] reported a significant reduction in meningeal relapses following combined cranial and spinal irradiation. The

Table 4. Treatment results of the VAPA study and the German cooperative BFM study in childhood acute myelogenous leukemia

	VAPA [55] Updated in 1982 [37]	BFM [15]
No. of patients	61	151
Age (median)	0–17 years (9.5 years)	0–17 years (9.9 years)
Early deaths	No. not available	17
Complete remission (%)	45 (74%)	119 (79%)
Death in CR	0	6
Withdrawal/ lost to follow-up	5	2
Relapses	18	40
Bone marrow	9	29
CNS involved	8	6
Testes	0	3
Other sites	1	2
CCR	22	71
Survival	27	77
Follow-up (median)	18–72 months (38 months)	1–45 months (23 months)
Life-table analysis		
CCR (% of patients with CR)	52% (after 6 years)	56% (after 3¾ years)
Survival (% of all patients treated)	44% (after 6 years)	43% (after 3¾ years)

overall survival was not improved, however, which is probably due to a delay in systemic chemotherapy because of radiation-induced bone marrow suppression. In spite of the low incidence of CNS relapses in the BFM 78 study [14, 15], which clearly indicates that CNS disease can be prevented in most children by prophylactic CNS treatment early in remission, in respect of disease-free survival no advantage was observed over the VAPA study, which had a relatively high frequency of CNS relapses, but more intensive maintenance therapy [37, 55].

Prognostic Factors

In childhood ALL analyses of the prognostic significance of pretreatment characteristics have provided a means of identifying patients at high and low risk for relapse and of stratifying patients to different therapeutic regimens [27, 28, 48]. In childhood AML, however, no generally accepted parameters of clinical relevance for initial response to chemotherapy of remission duration have yet been defined. Hence no rationale exists for a risk-adapted therapeutic strategy. Similarly, in adult AML evaluations of the significance of prognostic factors have revealed contradictory results of have not yet proven useful for pretreatment assignment that patients to different therapeutic approaches [6, 7, 9, 16, 26, 34, 38]. As for childhood ALL, the discrepancies between the reported prognostic factors for adult AML might be the result of different treatment protocols and differences in age and AML subtype distribution.

Multivariate analysis of the data from two AML studies of the CCSG indicated that age between 3 and 10 years and a short time to eradication of the leukemic cell infiltrate in the bone marrow were the only parameters associated with a prolonged remission duration [3]. Data from the VAPA study suggest a short remission duration for patients with acute monoblastic leukemia (AMOL) [37, 55]. Since six out of the nine children with AMOL in this study were under the age of 2 years, the independent prognostic significance of morphology from age requires further confirmation. In contrast, multivariate analysis of data from the German cooperative BFM study reveals no increased risk for relapse in children with AMOL [14, 15]. However, patients with AMOL are at a higher risk for early death due to intracranial hemorrhage in this study [14, 15].

Supportive Care

Intensive multidrug induction therapy for acute leukemia, aiming at eradication of the leukemic cell population, is almost inevitably followed by severe bone marrow hypoplasia. Aggressive treatment has to be complemented, therefore, by, supportive care, which is an essential element of successful antileukemic therapy. The principles of supportive care are similar for children with AML and ALL. However, platelet transfusions have to be administered to almost all children receiving AML therapy, either prophylactically, to prevent bleeding complications if the platelet count drops below 15,000–20,000/μl, or therapeutically, to treat hemorrhagic manifestations. Granulocyte transfusions are given only to children with severe granulocytopenia and proven Gram-negative septicemia in life-threating situations. Systemic antimycotic drugs should be given if systemic fungal infection is suspected. In patients presenting with disseminated intravascular coagulation (DIC) or hyperfibrinolysis, transfusion of fresh-frozen plasma and platelets, possibly in combination with low-dose heparin treatment, is recommended.

Bone Marrow Transplantation

The currently available results of BMT in AML in first remission suggest a low relapse rate of approximately 15%–20% and a 50%–70% chance of long-term disease-free survival [23, 51, 52, 59]. The overall survival after BMT is considerably lower, however, because of the severe side-effects of this approach, incuding graft-versus-host disease and infectious complications. Randomized studies on the significance of BMT versus chemotherapy for maintaining remission in childhood AML have recently been initiated and firm conclusions are not yet available. One study is under way to compare two intensive postinduction regimens with bone marrow transplantation. A preliminary analysis reveals no significant differences among the three treatment arms (D. R. Miller, personal communication, 1982). Similar results have been obtained by the study at UCLA (Chap. 9). Therefore, the question as to whether a child with AML who has an HLA-identical sibling should receive a transplant in first remission or be treated by intensive postinduction chemotherapy is still open at present [43].

Conclusions

The results of aggressive therapy, such as high-dose sequential postinduction chemotherapy or prolonged intensified induction treatment, followed by intensive maintenance therapy or by allogeneic BMT in first remission strongly suggest that a substantial number of pediatric patients with AML can be cured of their disease. Although the recent results of therapy in childhood AML are encouraging, it must be borne in mind that the achievement of high complete remission rates and of an increasing number of long-term disease-free survivors still remains a difficult task for the therapist, requiring a high degree of clinical experience and extensive facilities for supportive care. Despite these efforts, a considerable proportion of children die before or during remission induction, mostly of hemorrhage or infectious complications.

The major cause of ultimate failure in antileukemic treatment, however, is the recurrence of leukemia. Hence the goal for further improvements in AML therapy remains the eradication of the leukemic cell clone. One way to achieve this goal may be the definition of risk factors and the adaptation of therapy in the individual patient, althouth no prognostic factors have yet been identified in childhood AML. Preliminary results indicate that the monitoring of treatment-induced cell kinetic effects [8] and the quantitative evaluation of therapy-induced cell kill [29] may give some indication of therapeutic response and possible remission duration. It remains to be seen whether early detection of leukemic relapse by close surveillance of the remission status by highly sophisticated techniques [4, 30, 31] will result in an increase in the cure rate of childhood leukemia.

More effective use of such current therapeutic modalities as early and late intensification by nonresistant drug combinations and the introduction of new effective drugs may further increase the rate of long-term survivors in childhood AML.

References

1. Andreeff M, Darzynkiewiez Z, Sharpless TK, Clarkson BD, Melamend MR (1980) Discrimination of human leukemia subtypes by flow cytometric analysis of cellular DNA and rNA. Blood 55: 282–292
2. Beahner RL, Bernstein ID, Sather H, Higgins G, McCreadie S, Chard RL, Hammond D (1979) Improved remission induction rate with D-ZAPO but unimproved remission duration with additionof immunotherapy to chemotherapy in previously untreated children with ANLL. Med Pediatro Oncol 7: 127–139
3. Baehner RL, Kennedy A, Sather H, Chard RL, Hammond D (1981) Characteristics of children with acute nonlymphocytic leukemia in long-term continuous remission: a report for Childrens Cancer Study Group. Med Pediatr Oncol 9: 393–403
4. Baker MA, Falk JA, Carter WH, Taub RN, and the Toronto Leukemic Study Group (1979) Early diagnosis of relapse in acute myeloblastic leukemia. N Engl J MEd 301: 1353–1357
5. Bennett JM, Catovsky D, Danial MT, Flandrin G, Galton DAG, Gralnick HR, Sultan C (1976) Proposals for the classification of the acute leukaemias. Br J Maematol 33: 451–548
6. Brandmann J, Bukowski R, Greenstein R, Hewlet J, Hoffmann G (1979) Prognostic factors affecting remission, remission duration and survival in acute adult nonlymphocytic leukemia. Cancer 44: 1062–1065
7. Bloomfield CD (1980) Treatment of adult acute nonlymphocytic leukemia. Ann Intern Med 93: 133–134
8. Büchner T, Hiddemann W, Wörmann B, Gödhe W, Schumann J (1980) Flow cytometry and cell kinetic during treatment of human leukemia. Kinetic manipulations of leukemic cells by ARA-C in correlation to therapeutic response. In: Laerum O, Lindmo T, Thorud E (eds) Flow cytometry IV. Univeritetsforlaget, Bergen
9. Büchner T, Urbanitz D, Emmerich B, Fischer JT, Fülle HH, Heinecke A, Hossfeld DK, Koeppens KM, Labedzki L, Löffler H, Nowrousian MR, Pfreundschuh M, Pralle H, Rühl H, Wendt FC, for the AML cooperative group (1982) Multicentre study on intensified remission induction therapy for acute myeloid leukemia. Leuk Res 6: 827–831

10. Burgert EO, Nieri RL, Mills SD, Linman JW (1983) Nonlymphocytic leukemia in childhood. Mayo Clin Proc 48: 255–259
11. Burns CP, Armitage J, Frey A, Dick F, Jordan J, Woolson R (1981) Analysis of the presenting features of adult acute leukemia: The FAB classification. Cancer 47: 2460–2469
12. Chard RL Jr, Finklestein JZ, Sonley MJ, Nesbit M, McCreadie S, Weiner J, Sather H, Hammond GD (1978) Increased survival in childhood acute nonlymphocytic leukemia after treatment with prednisone, cytosine-arabinoside, 6-thioguanine, cyclophosphamide and oncivin (PATCO) combination chemotherapy. Med Pediatr Oncol 4: 263–273
13. Choi SI, Simone JV (1976) Acute nonlymphocytic leukemia in 171 children. Med Pediatr Oncol 2: 119–146
13a. Creutzig U, Eschenbach C, Ritter J, Schellong G (1981) Akute Leukämie bei einem 13jährigen Jungen mit gleichzeitigem Auftreten von Lymphoblasten und Monoblasten. Klin Pädiatr 193: 162–164
14. Creutzig U, Schellong G, Ritter J, Sutor AH, Riehm H, Langermann HJ, Niethammer D, Löffler H (1983) Ergebnisse und Risikoanalysen bei 130 Patienten der kooperativen Studie BFM-78 zur Behandlung der akuten myeloischen Leukämie im Kindesalter. Verh Dtsch Krebsges 4: 207–215
15. Creutzig U, Ritter J, Langermann HJ, Riehm H, Henze G, Niethammer D, Jürgens H, Stollmann B, Lasson U, Kabisch H, Wahlen W, Löffler H, Schellong G (1983) Akute myeloische Leukämie bei Kindern: Ergebnisse der kooperativen Therapiestunde BFM-78 nach 3¾ Jahren. Klin Pädiatr 196: 152–160
16. Crowther D, Beard M, Bateman C, Sawell R (1975) Factors influencing prognosis in adults with acute myelogenous leukaemia. Br J Cancer 32: 456–461
17. Cutler S, Ederer F (1958) Maximum utilization of life-table-method in analyzing survival. J Chron Dis 4: 699–731
18. Dahl GV, Simone JV, Hustu HO, Mason C (1978) Preventive central nervous system irradiation in children with acute nonlymphocytic leukemia. Cancer 42: 2187–2192
19. Dahl GV, Kalwinsky DK, Murphy S, Look AT, Amadori S, Kumar M, Novak R, George SL, Mason C, Mauer AM, Simone JV (1982) Cytokinetically based induction chemotherapy and splenectomy for childhood acute nonlymphocytic leukemia. Blood 60: 856–863
20. Evans DIK, Jones PHM, Morley CJ (1975) Treatment of acute myeloid leukemia of childhood with cytosine arabinoside, daunorubicin, prednisone, and mercaptopurine or thioguanine. Cancer 36: 1547–1551
21. Fleming I, Simone J, Jackson R, Johnson W, Walters T, Mason C (1974) Splenectomy and chemotherapy in acute myelocytic leukemia in childhood. Cancer 33: 427–434
22. Foon K, Naiem F, Yale C, Gale R (1979) Acute myelocytic leukemia: Morphologic classification and response to therapy. Leuk Res 3: 171–173
23. Gale RP, Kay HEM, Rimm AA, Bortin MM (1982) Bone marrow transplantation for acute leukaemia in first remission. Lancet 2: 1006–1009
24. Haghbin M, Tan CC, Clarkson BD, Mike V, Burchenal JH, Murphy ML (1974) Intensive chemotherapy in children with ALL (L –2 protocol). Cancer 33: 1491–1498
25. Haghbin M, Murphy ML, Tan C (1977) Treatment of acute nonlymphoblastic leukemia in children with a multiple-drug protocol. Cancer 40: 1417–1421
26. Hart J, George S, Frei E, Bodey G, Nickerson R, Freireich E (1977) Prognostic significance of pretreatment proliferative activity in adult acute leukemia. Cancer 39: 1603–1617
27. Henze G, Langermann HJ, Ritter J, Schellong G, Riehm H (1981) Treatment strategy for different risk groups in childhood acute lymphoblastic leukemia: a report from the BFM study group. In: Neth R, Gallo RC, Graf T, Mannweiler K, Winkler K (eds) Modern trends in human leukemia 4. Springer, Berlin Heidelberg New York, Haematology and Blood Transfusion, vol 26, pp 87–93
28. Henze G, Langermann HJ, Fengler R, Brandeis M, Evers KG, Gadner H, Hinderfeld L, Jobke A, Kornhuber B, Lampert F, Lasson U, Ludwig R, Müller-Weihrich S, Neidhardt M, Nessler G, Niethammer D, Rister M, Ritter J, Schaaff A, Schellong G, Stollmann B, Treuner J, Wahlen W,

Weinel W, Wehinger H, Riehm H (1982) Therapiestudie BFM 79/81 zur Behandlung der akuten lymphoblastischen Leukämie bei Kindern und Jugendlichen: intensivierte Reinduktionstherapie für Patientengruppen mit unterschiedlichem Rezidivrisiko. Klin Pädiatr 194: 195–203

29. Hiddemann W, Clarkson B, Büchner T, Melamed M, Adreeff M (1982) Bone marrow cell count per cubic millimeter bone marrow. A new parameter for quantitating therapy induced cytoreduction in acute leukemia. Blood 59: 216–225
30. Hiddemann W, Wörmann B, Ritter J, Henze G, Langermann HJ, Kaufmann U, Schellong G, Riehm H, Büchner T (1982) Diagnostik von Aneuploidien bei akuten Leukämien mittels Impulszytophotometrie (ICP): Häufigkeit und klinische Relevanz. Verh Dtsch Ges Inn Med 88: 934–936
31. Hittlemann WN, Broussard LC, Dosik G, Mc Credie KB (1980) Predicting relapse of human leukemia by means of premature chromosome condensation. N Engl J Med 303: 475–484
32. Janossy G, Hoffbrand A, Greaves M, Ganeshaguru K, Pair C, Bradstock K, Prentice H, Kay H (1980) Terminal transferase enzyme assay and immunological membrane markers in the diagnosis of leukaemia in a multiparameter analysis of 300 cases. Br J Haematol 44: 221–234
33. Kay HEM (1976) Development of CNS leukaemia in acute myeloid leukaemia in childhood. Arch Dis Child 51: 73–74
34. Keating MJ, Smith TL, Gehan EA, McCredie KB, Bodey GP, Spitzer G, Hersh E, Guttermann J, Freireich EJ (1980) Factors related to length of complete remission in adult acute leukemia. Cancer 45: 2017–2029
35. Kobrinsky NL, Robison LL, Nesbit ME (1980) Acute nonlymphocytic leukemia. Pediatr Clin North Am 27: 345–360
36. Madanat F, Sullivan MP (1978) Improved survival in young children with acute granulocytic leukemia (AGL) treated with combination therapy using cyclophosphamide, oncovin, cytosine arabinoside and prednisone mini-COAP. Proc Am Soc Clin Oncol 19: 417
37. Mayer RJ, Weinstein HJ, Coral FS, Rosenthal DS, Frei E (1982) The role of intensive post-induction chemotherapy in the management of patients with acute myelogenous leukemia. Cancer Treat Rep 66: 1455–1462

37a. Mertelsmann R, Koziner B, Ralph P, Filippa D, McKenzie S, Arlin ZA, Gee TS, Moore MAS, Clarkson BD (1978) Evidence for distinct lymphocytic and monocytic populations in a patient with terminal transferase-positive acute leukemia. Blood 51: 1051–1056

38. Mertelsmann R, Thaler H, To L, Gee T, McKenzie S, Schauer P, Friedman A, Arlin Z, Cirrincione C, Clarkson B (1980) Morphological classification, response to therapy and survival in 263 adult patients with acute non-lymphoblastic leukemia. Blood 56: 773–781
39. Moreno H, Castleberry RP, McCann WP (1977) Cytosine arabinoside and 6-thioguanine in the treatment of childhood acute myeloblastic leukemia. Cancer 40: 998–1004
40. Necheles TF (1979) Acute myeloblastic leukemia. In: Necheles TF (ed) The acute leukemias. Thieme, Stuttgart
41. O'Leary M, Ramsay N, Nesbit M et al. (1979) Early bone marrow transplantation in acute leukemia in children and young adults. Blood [Suppl 1] 54: 201a (abstract)
42. Pizzo PA, Henderson ES, Leventhal GB (1976) Acute myelogenous leukemia in children: A preliminary report of combination chemotherapy. J Pediatr 88: 125–130
43. Preisler HD (1982) Therapy for patients with AML who enter remission. Bone marrow transplantation or chemotherapy? Cancer Treat Rep 66: 1467–1473
44. Plüss HJ, Hitzig H (1980) Die akuten myeloischen Leukämien im Kindesalter. Schweiz Med Wochenschr 110: 1459–1462
45. Riehm H, Gadner H, Henze G, Langermann HJ, Odenwald E (1980) The Berlin childhood lymphoblastic leukemia therapy study, 1970–1976. Am J Pediatr Hematol Oncol 2: 299–306
46. Robison L, Sather H, Coccia P, Nesbit M, Hammond D (1980) Assessment of the interrelationship of prognostic factors in childhood acute lymphoblastic leukemia. Am J Pediatr Haematol Oncol 2: 5–13
47. Scheer U, Schellong G, Riehm H (1979) Verbesserte Prognose der akuten myeloischen Leukämien bei Kidern nach intensivierter Anfangstherapie. Klin Pädiatr 191: 210–216

48. Simone S (1976) Annotation: factors that influence haematological remission duration in acute lymphocytic leukaemia. Br J Haematol 32: 465–472
49. Sonley MJ, Nesbit M, Thatcher LG, Karon M, Hammond D (1971) Cytosine arabinoside, cyclophosphamide and vincristine in children with acute myelogenous leukemia. Proc Am Assoc Cancer Res 12: 87
50. Sutor AH (1979) Zur Blutungsproblematik bei akuten myeloischen Leukämien. Klin Pädiatr 191: 217–220
51. Thomas ED, Buckner CD, Banaji M, Clift RA, Fefer R, Flournoy N, Goodell B, Hickman R, Lerner K, Neiman P, Sale G, Sanders J, Singer J, Stevens M, Storb R, Weiden PL (1982) One hundred patients with acute nonlymphoblastic leukemia who achieve a first remission. Cancer Treat Rep 66: 1463–1466
52. Thomas ED, Clift RA, Buckner CD (1982) Marrow transplantation for patients with acute nonlymphoblastic leukemia who achieve a first remission. Cancer Treat Rep 66: 1463–1466
53. Tischendorf F, Haas H, Tischendorf M (1978) Prognostic significance of leucocyte antigens in human leukemia. In: Rosalki S (ed) New pathway on laboratory medicine. Huber, Bern
54. Weiden PL, Fluornoy N, Thomas ED, Prentice R, Fefer R, Buckner CD, Storb R (1979) Antileukemic effect of graft-versus-host disease in human recipients of allogeneic-marrow grafts. N Engl J Med 300: 1068–1073
55. Weinstein HJ, Mayer RJ, Rosenthal DS, Camitta BM, Coral FS, Nathan DG, Frei E III (1980) Treatment of acute myelogenous leukemia in children and adults. N Engl J Med 303: 473–478
56. Whittacker J, Withey J, Powell D, Parry T, Kurshid M (1979) Leukaemia classification. A study of the accuracy of diagnosis in 456 patients. Br J Haematol 41: 177–181
57. Wiernik PH, Serpick AA (1969) Clinical significance of serum and urine muramidase in leukemia and other hematologic malignancies. Am J Med 46: 330–343
58. Young JL, Miller RW (1975) Incidence of malignant tumors in U.S. children. J Pediatr 86: 254–258
59. Zwaan FE (1980) Bone marrow transplantation for acute leukaemia in remission – European results. Blut 41: 208–213

Acute Myelogenous Leukemia: Current Status of Therapy in Adults

K. A. Foon and R. P. Gale

Monoclonal Antibody-Hybridoma Section, Biological Therapeutics Branch, Biological Response Modifiers Program, Division of Cancer Treatment, National Cancer Institute, Frederick Cancer Research Facility, Building 560, Frederick, MD 21701, USA

Introduction

Acute myelogenous leukemia (AML) is a neoplastic disease characterized by the proliferation of malignant myeloblasts and other immature myeloid cells. Infiltration of the bone marrow by these leukemia cells results in the impairment of normal hematopoiesis, with resultant anemia, granulocytopenia, and thrombocytopenia. If untreated the disease is rapidly fatal, with a median survival of less than 2 months. Death frequently results from infection, hemorrhage or both [1].

The therapeutic goal in AML is to eradicate the leukemia cells and to restore normal hematopoiesis. This goal is best accomplished by the administration of high doses of antileukemic drugs. This treatment may be followed by the cyclic readministration of chemotherapy with or without immunotherapy or central nervous system (CNS) prophylactic therapy to prevent leukemic relapse. An alternative approach is a bone marrow transplantation from an HLA-identical sibling donor while the patient is in remission.

Classification

Because of the common origin of several hematopoietic cell lines, abnormalities of proliferation or differentiation of monocytes, red cell precursors, and megakaryocytes are frequently present in patients with AML. The variability in the morphologic features of AML has led to the development of several systems of classification. A recent widely accepted scheme is that of the joint French-American-British (FAB) committee [2, 3] (Table 1). The FAB classification is based on the predominant cell type involved. Three forms of AML with granulocytic differentiation are identified: M1, which shows some evidence of granulocytic differentiation apparent either in 3% or more myeloperoxidase-positive blasts or in blasts with a few azurophilic granules, Auer rods, or both; M2, which shows maturation to or beyond the promyelocyte stage; and M3, which is characterized by hypergranular promyelocytes with abundant Auer rods (abnormal primary granules). Variant forms of M3 with minimal granulation and bilobed or multilobed nuclei have been described [4, 5]. Up to one-half of the cases of M3 have a specific chromosome abnormality, i.e., a t(15q+; 17q−) translocation. Electron microscopy may be required to identify some variants of M3. Myelomonocytic leukemia, or M4, shows both granulocytic and monocytic differentiation in varying proportions, with at least 20% promonocytes and monocytes in the bone marrow and/or peripheral blood. M5, or monocytic leukemia, shows fewer than 20% granulocytic components. Two subtypes of

Recent Results in Cancer Research. Vol. 93

Table 1. French-American-British classification of acute myelogenous leukemia

Designation	Predominant cell type(s)
M1 (undifferentiated myelocytic)	Myeloblasts
M2 (myelocytic)	Myeloblasts, promyelocytes, myelocytes
M3 (promyelocytic)	Hypergranular promyelocytes
M4 (myelomonocytic)	Promyelocytes, myelocytes, promonocytes, monocytes
M5a (monoblastic)	Monoblasts
M5b (differentiated monocytic)	Monoblasts, promonocytes, monocytes
M6 (erythroleukemia)	Erythroblasts

M5 are distinguished: M5a, poorly differentiated or monoblastic, with > 80% immature cells, and M5b, in which promonocytes and monocytes predominate with < 20% monoblasts. Erythroleukemia (M6) shows prominent involvement of erythroid precursors.

Drugs Evaluated in Acute Myelogenous Leukemia

Pyrimidine Analogs

The introduction of cytarabine represented the first major advance in the therapy of AML. Cytarabine is a pyrimidine analog that acts through its incorporation into DNA [6]. Because cytarabine has a brief half-life and is active against proliferating cells during the S-phase, its antileukemic effect is dose and schedule dependent [7]. Complete response rates of approximately 25% are achieved with a 5- to 7-day course of 100–200 mg/m^2 per day by continuous IV infusion or by IV injection twice daily [8–12] (Table 2). Very high doses (3 g/m^2 every 12 h for 4–6 days) may produce up to 50% remissions in patients with leukemia resistant to conventional doses [13, 14].
5-Azacytidine is a pyrimidine nucleotide analog resembling cytidine in chemical structure. Complete response rates of 15%–30% have been reported in relapsed AML patients treated with 5-azacytidine [15–19]. Optimal results have been obtained with doses of 150–300 mg/m^2 per day. 5-Azacytidine is inactivated by a different deaminase than is cytarabine; leukemia cells resistant to the latter may be sensitive to 5-azacytidine. Other pyrimidine analogs, including cyclocytidine [20], 3-deazauridine [21], and pyrazofurin [22], and 2,2-anhydro-1-β-D-arabinofuranosyl-5-fluorocytosine [23] have demonstrated limited activity in patients with relapsed AML.

Anthracyclines

The introduction of daunorubicin was a second major advance in the treatment of AML [24]. Daunorubicin is an anthracycline antibiotic related to doxorubicin. It is thought to inhibit DNA replication by intercalation of base pairs [25, 8]. Daunorubicin is probably the most effective single drug against AML; complete remission rates of 35%–50% have been reported with doses of 45–60 mg/m^2 per day for 3 days [26–28]. Anthracyclines can also be given by infusion rather than by bolus injection. Data in animals suggest decreased

Table 2. Active single agents for acute myelogenous leukemia

Drug class	Complete remissions (%)[a]	References
Pyrimidine analogs:		
Cytarabine	25	[8–12]
5-Azacytidine	15–30	[16, 17]
Anthracyclines:		
Daunorubicin	35–50	[23, 28, 32]
Zorubicin (rubidazone)	30–60	[32–34]
Carubicine (carminomycin)	10–30	[27, 28, 32]
Aclacinomycin	20–30	[32, 35, 36]
Purine analogs:		
6-Mercaptopurine	10–14	[40, 41]
Acridine derivatives:		
AMSA	20–30	[43, 44]
Epipodophyllotoxins:		
VP-16-216	5–15	[46–50]

[a] Approximate rates

cardiotoxocity without loss of antitumor efficacy. Comparable data in man are lacking and in most studies bolus injections are used. Daunorubicin-DNA complex was reported to have similar clinical results to free daunorubicin with fewer "minor" cardiac complications [29].

Doxorubicin is the 14-hydroxyl derivative of daunorubicin. There are limited studies of doxorubicin as a single agent in untreated patients with AML. Doxorubicin used in combination chemotherapy appears to give results comparable to those obtained with daunorubicin [30, 31]; however, doxorubicin has considerably more gastrointestinal toxicity. Because of this, most investigators consider daunorubicin the drug of choice in AML. Patients who are resistant to daunorubicin are very unlikely to respond to doxorubicin, with a crossover response ratio of < 10% in several small studies.

Several new anthracycline antibiotics related to daunorubicin have recently been evaluated in patients with AML [32]. Zorubicin (rubidazone), a daunorubicin analog, produced remission in 30%–60% of previously untreated patients, but is relatively ineffective in patients resistant to other anthracyclines [33, 34]. Carubicine (carminomycin) and aclacinomycin also have been reported to produce remissions in 10%–40% of patients with AML [32, 35–38]. None of these agents appears to be superior to daunorubicin for this disease.

Purine Analogs

Purine analogs have been used extensively to treat AML. The most widely studied drugs are 6-mercaptopurine and 6-thioguanine. Both drugs require activation to the ribonucleotide form for their antileukemic effect [39]. Thioguanine is more commonly used than mercaptopurine because the dose does not have to be modified in patients receiving xanthine oxidase inhibitors such as allopurinol. Purine analogs at a dose of 200–300 mg/m^2 per day PO in divided doses produce complete remission in 10%–15% of patients with

AML [40, 41]. The dose of mercaptopurine should be reduced to one-third or one-fourth when it is given concomitantly with allopurinol. Very low doses of 6-thioguanine have been reported to cause differentiation of leukemia cells in vitro, and some investigators have suggested that its mechanism of activity in AML may involve this effect rather than cytotoxicity. It is important to note that absorption of orally administered 6-thioguanine may be erratic and that controlled trials in which the drugs were given IV have not been reported. Another purine analog, β-2′-deoxythioguanosine, has been reported to have limited activity in patients with acute leukemia resistant to other purine analogs [42].

Acridine and Anthraquinone Derivatives

A new effective agent for AML is 4′-(9-acridinylamino)methanesulfon-*m*-anisidide (AMSA). Complete remission rates of 20%–30% have been reported for patients with resistant AML [43, 44]. It is not cross-resistant with cytarabine or anthracyclines. Other agents undergoing phase 1 and 2 studies include mitoxantrone (dehydroxyanthracenedione dihydrochloride) [45] and bisantrone (anthracinedione).

Epipodophyllotoxins

Two epipodophyllotoxins, VP-16-213 (Etoposide) and VM-26 (Teniposide), have been used to treat patients with resistant AML. VP-16-213 has been reported to produce remissions in 5%–15% of previously treated and untreated patients [46–50]. VP-16-213 in combination with vinblastine and 5-azacytidine or combined with cytarabine, *m*-AMSA, and 6-thioguanine produced remissions in up to 50% of patients with resistant leukemia [51, 52]. Some studies indicate that VP-16-213 may be most effective in AML with a monocytic component (M4 and M5), but these data are controversial [48, 50].

Miscellaneous

Several other drugs have been studied as single agents in patients with AML. Most of these agents have been studied in recurrent and refractory leukemia. The antitumor antibiotic neocarzinostatin (zinostatin) has shown activity against AML but failed to produce any complete remissions in 22 patients with refractory leukemia [53]. Guanazole, a triazole that blocks DNA synthesis, produced no complete remissions in patients with resistant leukemia [15]. Other agents that have not been effective in patients with resistant AML include conventional-dose methotrexate [54, 55], cyclophosphamide [56], L-asparaginase [57, 58], prednisone [59], and *cis*-diamminedichloroplatinum(II) (*cis*-platinum) [60, 61]. Certain biologicals such as human leukocyte interferon and the interferon inducer polyribinosinic-polyribocytidylic acid [poly(ICLC)] have been evaluated in limited trials [62, 63]. Poly(ICLC) was ineffective, and data regarding the action of interferon in patients with resistant AML are too limited for critical analysis.

Remission-Induction Chemotherapy

The initial objective of therapy of AML is to achieve a hematologic remission. Remission is commonly defined as the reduction of leukemia cells to undetectable levels (fewer than 5%

Table 3. Combination chemotherapy for acute myelogenous leukemia

Regimen	Complete remissions (%)	References
Cytarabine + 6-thioguanine or mercaptopurine	35–56	[12, 64–67]
Cytarabine + vincristine + prednisone + cyclophosphamide (COAP)	48	[10]
Cytarabine + daunorubicin + 6-thioguanine (5 days)	50–85	[28, 68, 70]
Cytarabine + doxorubicin or daunorubicin (7 days)	66	[30]
Cytarabine + daunorubicin + 6-thioguanine (7 days)	60–85	[69, 70]
Cytarabine + vincristine + prednisone + doxorubicin	70	[31]
Cytarabine + 6-thioguanine + doxorubicin + vincristine + prednisone	82	[72]

myeloblasts), restoration of normal bone marrow function including normalization of hemoglobin, granulocyte and platelet counts, resolution of organomegaly, and return of the patient to a normal performance status [8].

Single agents such as cytarabine and daunorubicin produce remission in less than 50% of patients with AML (Table 2). Over the past 10 years, numerous combinations of drugs have been evaluated in controlled clinical trials (Table 3). Cytarabine combined with minimally effective drugs such as thioguanine or mercaptopurine produced remission in 35%–56% of patients, a clearly synergistic interaction [64–67]. The addition of daunorubicin (or doxorubicin) resulted in complete remissions in 50%–85% of patients [30, 31, 68–73]. These results were superior to those achieved with less intensive chemotherapy.

An overview of these studies suggests that the combination of 7-day cycles of cytarabine with three doses of daunorubicin or doxorubicin is the most effective induction regimen. Daunorubicin is generally preferred over doxorubicin as there is considerably less gastrointestinal toxicity. Addition of other drugs, including thioguanine [74] and azacytidine, does not clearly improve results. A recent prospective randomized trial has demonstrated that 7-day courses of cytarabine are more effective than 5-day courses [75], but 10-day courses of cytarabine do not appear to increase the remission rate [30] and may be associated with severe gastrointestinal toxicity [76]. The suggestion that 10-day courses of cytarabine may yield greater leukemia cytoreduction and therefore prolong survival has been proposed. Prospective randomized trials are currently under way to address this question. Continuous infusion of cytarabine (100 mg/m^2 per day) and intermittent infusion every 8–12 h (200 mg/m^2 per day) probably produce comparable results. One large group study suggested improved benefit with continuous infusion but the differences were not significant [75].

The optimal dose and schedule of daunorubicin are also controversial. One to three daily doses of 30–60 mg/m^2 have been recommended. The best results have been reported at a dose of 60 mg/m^2 per day for 3 days in patients < 60 years. Patients > 60 years of age did better when treated with daunorubicin for 3 days at 30 mg/m^2 per day than with daunorubicin at 45 mg/m^2 per day or doxorubicin at 30 mg/m^2 per day [77]. Comparable results were observed whether daunorubicin was given at the beginning or the end of the induction cycle [30, 69–71].

Since anthracycline administration may be accompanied by substantial gastrointestinal and cardiac toxicity, some investigators have developed induction regimens which limit the use of daunorubicin or doxorubicin to patients who fail to respond to cytarabine and thioguanine. In one study, all patients were treated with cytarabine and 6-thioguanine for 14 days. Daunorubicin was used only in patients who failed to respond [78]. Overall, 64% of the patients achieved a remission, and 25% of those achieving a remission did not require an anthracycline. In another study, a synchronizing dose of cytarabine was followed by continuous administration of cytarabine and 6-thioguanine until marrow aplasia developed [79]; no anthracycline was given. Out of a total of 21 patients 16 achieved a complete remission. Innovative approaches such as these require further prospective evaluation. It should be remembered that, in contrast to doxorubicin, daunorubicin produces relatively little cardiotoxicity in adults at doses < 1 g/m^2 ($< 5\%$) [80].

Consolidation and Maintenance Chemotherapies

Once hematologic remission is achieved, the next therapeutic objective is to prevent the recurrence of leukemia. Relapse is most probably related to the subclinical persistence of resistant leukemia cells. The most common approach to prevention of a leukemia relapse has been the administration of chemotherapy to patients in remission. The two most frequent types of chemotherapy are: *consolidation* chemotherapy, in which one or two courses of high doses of the same drugs that were used for remission induction are given following successful remission induction, and *maintenance* chemotherapy, in which lower doses of the same or new drugs are usually given monthly over a prolonged period of time [81]. Representative data on maintenance schedules from several centers are shown in Table 4.

The role of consolidation and maintenance chemotherapy in prolonging remission in patients with AML remains controversial; there have been few controlled trials addressing this question specifically. In a study from Johns Hopkins, patients with AML received induction chemotherapy with cytarabine and daunorubicin; consolidation and maintenance were not given [82]. Median remission duration was 10 months. This is probably not significantly different than that in numerous trials in which consolidation and maintenance chemotherapy were given. At the University of California – Los Angeles (UCLA), 38 patients who entered a complete remission and received two courses of high-dose consolidation therapy without maintenance therapy were evaluated [83]. The median duration of remission was 22 months. This was not significantly different than previous studies in which monthly cycles of maintenance chemotherapy with cytarabine, daunorubicin, and thioguanine were given [69] (Table 4). Other studies, reviewed in Table 4, have shown similar results [82, 84]. There is recent evidence that when cytarabine is given SC for maintenance therapy, rather than by IV bolus, this is of significant advantage for remission duration [75]. Overall, the above studies suggest that low-dose maintenance chemotherapy, as previously conceived, is of little value. High-dose consolidation therapy, introducing new drugs such as AMSA and 5-azacytidine, is emerging as a promising new approach for the therapy of AML. The terminology (perhaps this would more accurately be referred to as *intensification* chemotherapy) remains confusion. However, this approach of intensive postremission therapy will be further discussed in the *Intensification Chemotherapy* section.

Table 4. Maintenance chemotherapy in acute myelogenous leukemia

Center	Drug								Median remission duration (weeks)	References
	Cyt-arabine	6-Mercap-topurine/ 6-thiogua-nine	Dauno-rubicin/ doxo-rubicin	Predni-sone	Vincris-tine	Carmus-tine/ lomus-tine	Metho-trexate	Other		
Cancer & Acute Leukemia Group B	+	+	–	–	–	–	–	–	20–38	[12]
Argentine Group for the Treatment of Acute Leukemia	+	+	+	+	+	+	–	Intrathecal methotrexate	24	[86]
Baltimore Cancer Research Center	±[a]	±	+	–	–	+	–	Cyclophosphamide, guanazole	25–27	[28]
British Medical Research Council	±	+	±	±	–	–	–	–	26	[65]
Western Cancer Study Group	+	+	+	–	+	+	+	L-Asparaginase, hydroxyurea	32	[67]
Sloan-Kettering Memorial Institute	+	+	+	–	+	+	+	Cyclophosphamide, hydroxyurea	40	[64]
Roswell Park Memorial Institute	+	+	+	–	–	–	–	Methylglyoxal bis(guanylhydrazone)	54	[30]
Southwest Oncology Group	+	–	–	+	+	–	–	Cyclophosphamide	65–81	[85]
UCLA[b]	+	+	+	–	–	–	–	–	56	[69]
UCLA	–	–	–	–	–	–	–	–	76	[83]
The Johns Hopkins Oncology Center	–	–	–	–	–	–	–	–	38	[82]
University of Münster	–	–	–	–	–	–	–	–	36	[84]

[a] The ± signs denote randomization; [b] University of California – Los Angeles

Intensification Chemotherapy

Intensification chemotherapy is a relatively recent concept in the treatment of AML. Patients in remission receive intensive courses of chemotherapy designed to eradicate residual leukemia cells. *Early intensification* involves high-dose chemotherapy with drugs that the patient has not previously received. It is usually given within a few months of achieving remission. Early intensification differs from consolidation therapy in that the latter is given immediately following remission and usually uses the same drugs as have been used to induce remission. *Late intensification* takes the form of high-dose chemotherapy with new drugs in patients who have been in continuous complete remission for 1 year or more. This differs from maintenance chemotherapy, which is generally low-dose therapy and is usually given on an outpatient basis.

The role of intensification chemotherapy is controversial. Data from several centers suggest that the relapse rate may be 50% or higher [87, 88]. Although this trend is discouraging, only 1 of 24 patients who remained in unmaintained remission for 4 years after late intensification therapy at M.D. Anderson Hospital has relapsed [88]. Unfortunately, a critical analysis of these data is impossible, since the patients were highly selected and there were no concurrent controls. Weinstein and co-workers used both early and late intensification with drug combinations that were not cross-resistant. They refer to this method as "intensive postinduction chemotherapy." This was designed to maximize leukemia cytoreduction and prevent the emergence of drug-resistant cell lines. Their results are very encouraging, with a projected median duration of complete remission of 32 months [89].

Immunotherapy

Patients with AML have a large burden of leukemia cells at the time of diagnosis, usually exceeding 10^{10}. Because only a small proportion of these cells are actively dividing, cell-cycle-specific drugs such as cytarabine and thioguanine have a low probability of completely eradicating leukemia. Cell-cycle-nonspecific drugs such as daunorubicin can theoretically overcome this limitation, since they kill both dividing and nondividing cells. Unfortunately, the drugs currently available have little or no therapeutic margin; thus, substantial host toxicity limits the possibility of complete eradication of the leukemia. In theory, the contribution of immunotherapy is a high therapeutic margin, i.e., the ability to kill leukemia cells and to spare normal cells. Most experimental data indicate that immunotherapy is effective against only relatively small numbers of tumor cells (usually less than 10^5). Because of this limitation most immunotherapy trials have been directed toward prolonging duration of remission rather than toward inducing remission. Nonspecific immune stimulation has been attempted with agents such as bacillus Calmette-Guérin (BCG), methanol-extraction residue of tubercle bacillus (MER), *Corynebacterium parvum,* and levamisole. Specific immunization with leukemia cells, cell-free extracts and cultured cell lines also has been evaluated. In most trials patients have been assigned randomly to receive chemotherapy alone, immunotherapy alone, or both.

There has been a substantial number of clinical trials of immunotherapy in patients with AML [reviewed in 90–92]. Initial reports were, in most instances, encouraging and indicated a substantial benefit of immunotherapy in prolonging remission or increasing survival [93–95]. Unfortunately, most of these data were not reproduced when patients

Table 5. Clinical trials of immunotherapy in acute myelogenous leukemia

Type of immunotherapy (number of patients)	Median remission (weeks)		Data analysis	References
	Control	Immunotherapy		
Bacillus Calmette-Guerin (BCG)				
Southeastern Cancer Study Group (61)	11[a]	35	< 0.05	[96]
Southeastern Cancer Study Group (19)	56	29[b]	NS[c]	[97]
Southeastern Cancer Study Group (97)	26[d]	32	NS	[98]
University Hospital of Wales (45)	35	39	NS	[99]
Hospital Edward Herriot (63)	48	60	NS	[100]
M.D. Anderson Hospital (47)	52[e]	85	NS	[101]
Southwestern Oncology Group (49)	55	54	NS	[102]
Royal Liverpool Hospital (32)	19	24	NS	[103]
Italian (43)	64	65	NS	[104]
Bacillus Calmette-Guérin (BCG) + leukemia cells				
St. Bartholomew's and Royal Marsden Hospitals (50)	27	43	NS	[105]
British Medical Research Council (71)	20	35	NS	[106]
The Leukemia Group of Central Sweden (42)	23	66	NS	[107]
St. Mary's Hospital (41)	20	35	< 0.05	[108]
St. Bartholomew's Hospital (36)	32[f]	32	NS	[109]
Royal Marsden Hospital (45)	29[f]	35	NS	[110]
Children's Cancer Study Group (86)	44	40	NS	[111]
Southeastern Cancer Study Group (23)	56[f]	48	NS	[97]
University Hospital of Wales (34)	35	39	NS	[99]
Corynebacterium parvum (C. parvum)				
University of California – Los Angeles (48)	72	52[g]	NS	[69]
Argentine Group for the Treatment of Cancer (80)	32	20	NS	[86]
Methanol extraction residue of tubercle bacillus (MER)				
Israel (35)	32	68	< 0.002[h]	[112]
Mt Sinai Hospital (80)	24	44–88[i]	< 0.05	[94]
Androgen and BCG				
Italian (63)	64	42–54	NS	[105]
Viral oncolysates of leukemia cells				
Swiss Group for Clinical Cancer Research (44)	26	26	NS	[113]

[a] Remission duration is indicated from the onset of remission
[b] These patients had splenectomies
[c] Not significant
[d] Controls received either no therapy (24 weeks) or chemotherapy (28 weeks)
[e] Uncontrolled trial; controls were historical
[f] Controls received BCG without leukemia cells
[g] Immunotherapy group received *C. parvum* and leukemia cells
[h] Not evaluable because only two-thirds of patients were in complete remission
[i] Immunotherapy consisted of MER alone (28 weeks) or MER + neuraminidase-treated leukemia cells (44 weeks)

were followed for longer periods or when carefully controlled prospective trials with large numbers of patients were performed. Results of 21 trials of immunotherapy in 1,222 patients are summarized in Table 5. For each trial the most recent published data are indicated rather than the initial report. Nine trials have evaluated BCG immunotherapy; in only one instance was a significant prolongation in remission reported [96–105]. In three studies survival was prolonged in patients receiving BCG [99, 101, 103]; no beneficial effect was found in the remaining five studies. Nine studies evaluated BCG combined with immunization with leukemia cells [97, 99, 105–111]. Variables included allogeneic versus autologous cells, irradiated versus unirradiated cells, IV versus ID or SC BCG, and BCG and cells injected at identical or disparate sites. Only one small study of 41 patients revealed a beneficial effect of immunotherapy on remission duration [108]. The difference was due primarily to shorter than average remission in the control group rather than prolongation of remission in the immunotherapy group. Four studies reported increased survival in the immunotherapy cohort [99, 105, 107, 108], but this was not confirmed in the remaining studies. Two studies evaluated *Corynebacterium parvum* with [69] and without leukemia cells [86]. Both studies failed to show any benefit in remission duration or survival. Two studies evaluated MER. One trial of MER- and neuraminidase-treated leukemia cells was reported to show a benefit [94], and another from Israel demonstrated a benefit but was difficult to interpret because partial responders were included [112]. Finally, trials of viral oncolysates of leukemia cells and the androgen stanazol with or without BCG failed to indicate any beneficial effect [105, 113].

In summary, there is little convincing data to indicate that immunotherapy is of any benefit in the treatment of AML. Only 4 of 21 evaluable trials reported increased remission. Of those four trials, one could not be evaluated critically and the other three showed a beneficial effect that appeared to be due to a decrease in remission duration among controls, rather than an improved remission duration from immunotherapy. Eight studies were followed by reports of increased survival in patients receiving immunotherapy. This effect, even if it were substantiated, is of little impact since it resulted primarily from an increase in postrelapse survival rather than longer remission. It seems clear at this time that immunotherapy, as currently conceived, is ineffective in the treatment of AML. It is time for a careful laboratory-based re-evaluation of this approach prior to the initiation of the next phase of clinical trials.

Central Nervous System Therapy

Involvement of the CNS with leukemia is usually the result of meningeal involvement. Autopsy studies indicate a 5%–20% prevalence of CNS involvement, and a 10% incidence of clinically overt disease is not uncommon [114–117]. In one large group study, 7%–10% of patients with AML who were asymptomatic had leukemia cells in the cerebral spinal fluid at the time of diagnosis. Treatment of meningeal leukemia usually involves cranial or craniospinal irradiation and intrathecal chemotherapy with methotrexate or cytarabine. Optimal therapy remains controversial. Our own policy has been to use cranial irradiation [24 Gy) given in 12 fractions over 3 weeks. Cytarabine is also given intrathecally at a dose of 30–50 mg/m^2 at 3- to 5-day intervals until leukemia cells have cleared from the spinal fluid. Some investigators have used doses up to 100 mg, which has resulted in neurotoxicity [118].

The role of *CNS prophylaxis* in AML is also controversial. Although prophylactic cranial irradiation and intrathecal chemotherapy are probably effective in preventing meningeal leukemia, this approach does not appear to prolong systemic remissions. Because of this and the relatively low incidence of meningeal leukemia, CNS prophylaxis cannot be *routinely* recommended in patients with AML. Recently, Weinstein and co-workers reported a high incidence of CNS disease in children with AML, suggesting that the concept of CNS prophylaxis in children with AML may require re-examination [31]. This might be related to a high number of patients with myelomonocytic and monocytic leukemia in this study. It should be noted that their experience is unusual; CNS relapse was a cause of treatment failure in $< 5\%$ of children in another large study [111].

Resistant and Recurrent Leukemia

Patients who fail to achieve a remission following intensive induction chemotherapy that includes cytarabine and daunorubicin or doxorubicin have a poor prognosis. Patients who relapse after a remission also have a guarded prognosis, but are more likely to respond than those who never achieved a remission. Second remissions are generally of limited duration and median survival following relapse is usually less than 6 months, with only 10% of patients surviving at 1 year.

Several investigational drugs have been evaluated in patients who relapse or who fail to achieve a remission with intensive courses of cytarabine and daunorubicin. The results of some of these trials are discussed above. Drugs of special interest include 5-azacytidine, AMSA, and high-dose cytarabine. 5-Azacytidine at a dose of 150–300 mg/m^2 per day for 5 days is capable of producing remissions in 15%–30% of patients with resistant leukemia [16–18]. AMSA at a dose of 100–150 mg/m^2 per day for 5–10 days has been reported to have a complete response rate of 20%–30% in patients with AML resistant to cytarabine and anthracyclines [43, 44]. The combination of AMSA with 5-azacytidine or with cytarabine, VP-16-213, and thioguanine has produced $> 50\%$ remissions [52, 119, 120]. High-dose therapy with cytarabine 3 g/m^2 every 12 h for 6 days, with or without asparaginase rescue or in combination with AMSA, has been reported to produce remission in 50% of patients with resistant AML [14, 121, 122].

Intensive therapy with combinations of second-line drugs has occasionally been reported to produce remissions in patients refractory to first-line drugs. In one recent report, five of ten patients who were refractory to first-line drugs entered complete remission following combination chemotherapy with vincristine, BCNU, cyclophosphamide, methylglyoxal bis(guanylhydrazone), and high-dose methotrexate with citrovorum rescue [123]. The median remission duration was 7 months.

Peterson and Bloomfield were able to achieve a second remission in a high percentage of patients who had relapsed following a first remission [124]. Of 35 patients, 20 (i.e., 57%) achieved a second remission with high doses of cytarabine and thioguanine or of cytarabine in combination with daunorubicin (or doxorubicin), thioguanine, vincristine, and prednisone. The patients most likely to respond were those who received, during reinduction, at least one drug to which they had not been exposed previously.

The above data suggest that remissions can now be achieved in 30%–50% of patients with refractory or recurrent leukemia. None of the combinations discussed above can be specifically recommended at this time; however, it seems likely that high-dose cytarabine with or without *m*-AMSA, 5-azacytidine, and/or daunorubicin may emerge as the preferred approach.

Bone Marrow Transplantation

Bone marrow transplantation (BMT) is a potentially useful therapy in selected patients with AML. Two approaches have been studied: allogeneic transplantation from an HLA-identical sibling, and autologous transplantation of the patient's bone marrow cryopreserved during remission (see also pp 269 and 290).

Allogeneic BMT

The basic principles of allogeneic BMT in leukemia patients have been reviewed recently [125, 126]. Briefly, patients receive high-dose chemotherapy and total-body irradiation, followed by "rescue" with donor bone marrow cells. Engraftment occurs over a period of 3–4 weeks, and hematologic values usually return to normal in 2 or 3 months. Two centers have reported 15%–20% 2-year disease-free survival in selected patients with resistant AML treated by BMT [126, 127]. Survival rates may be as high as 30% when an identical-twin donor is available [128].

The high incidence of relapse following transplantation in patients with resistant leukemia has led to recent trials of transplantation in remission. The concept behind this approach is that the antileukemic effect of marrow transplantation might be greater when transplantation is performed before the development of resistant disease. Over 200 transplants in patients with AML in first remission have been reported [129–138] (Table 6). In most studies, high doses of cyclophosphamide (120 mg/kg) followed by total-body irradiation (7.5–10 Gy) have been used to prepare patients for transplantation.

Although these data are preliminary, most studies indicate 1- to 2-year relapse rates of only 20% (range, 0%–45%). Actuarial survival at 1–2 years is 55% (range, 40%–70%). Several prospective studies comparing BMT in first remission with chemotherapy without transplantation are in progress. At UCLA 22 patients received transplants during remission, while 27 were treated with two courses of consolidation therapy without maintenance chemotherapy. Only 17% of the patients who received transplants had relapsed at 2 years, while 47% of the other patients had relapsed at 2 years. Actuarial survival at 2 years in the two groups is comparable – 50% for the transplantation cohort versus 44% for the chemotherapy cohort. Although the survival data are similar, the reasons for treatment failure differ between the two groups. Most patients in the transplant cohort died of graft-versus-host disease (GVHD) or interstitial pneumonia; leukemic relapse was rare, occurring in only two of 22 patients. In contrast, all deaths in the chemotherapy group were related to leukemic relapse. Similar data have recently been obtained in an ongoing trial conducted by the Children's Cancer Study Group in children with AML. Their data, while preliminary, indicate comparable survival results at 2 years for patients treated with either BMT or chemotherapy. Most studies suggest that this interval is the greatest risk period for leukemic relapse following BMT. Thus if the chemotherapy cohort continues to experience relapses it will result in a superior result of BMT over conventional chemotherapy. Unfortunately, these data are not yet available. Furthermore, there may be a substantial bias in the selection of patients for BMT. Because of these considerations it will be essential to await results of prospective randomized trials before concluding that BMT is superior to chemotherapy.

The mechanism by which BMT effects eradication of leukemia is controversial. Although most investigators believe that chemotherapy and radiation are the most important antileukemic agents, this recently has been brought into question by the observation of a

Table 6. Allogeneic bone marrow transplantation during first remission for acute myelogenous leukemia

Center[a]	No. of patients	Actuarial relapse (%)	Actuarial survival at 1–2 years (%)	References
Seattle	72	10	55	[129]
UCLA	22	20	50	[130]
Royal Marsden	29[b]	30	70	[131]
EBMT	18	30	60	[132]
Minnesota	17	30	60	[133]
Leiden	15	30	40	[134]
SKMI	14[b]	45	55	[135]
Basel	13	15	90	[136]
Henri Mondor	11	0	70	[137]
City of Hope	20	15	60	[138]
Johns Hopkins	13	0	55	Unpublished[c]
Total	244	20 ± 16[d]	63 ± 17[d]	

[a] *UCLA*, University of California – Los Angeles; *EBMT*, European Cooperative Group for Bone Marrow Transplantation; *SKMI*, Sloan-Kettering Memorial Institute
[b] Includes two patients with identical twins as donors
[c] G. Santos, personal communication
[d] Mean ± SEM

high relapse rate in patients with AML in first remission who receive transplants from identical twins. The relapse rate in these patients (approximately 50%) is much higher than that observed in patients receiving transplants from HLA-identical siblings (less than 20%). An antileukemic effect of GVHD is well documented in animals [for review see reference 139] and in patients with acute [140, 141] or chronic GVHD [142] who receive transplants during relapse. Therefore, although GVHD is one of the leading causes of morbidity and death in transplant patients, it also may have an important antileukemic effect. This has led some investigators to try to induce GVHD intentionally in transplant recipients. Data from the trials are preliminary but suggest some benefit.

Bone marrow transplantation during remission, even if potentially useful, is limited by the age of the patient and the availability of an HLA-identical sibling donor. Most investigators agree that optimal candidates for BMT are those < 30 years and usually < 20 years of age. Thus BMT, even if superior to chemotherapy, will be applicable to only a small fraction of patients with AML, those < 30 years with an HLA-identical sibling. This is probably < 15% of all patients with AML. This figure may increase if it becomes possible to perform transplants from partially HLA-matched related donors [143] or from HLA-identical unrelated individuals [144].

Autologous Bone Marrow Transplantation

Autologous BMT is an area of considerable recent interest [145, 146]. Typically, bone marrow is cryopreserved while the patient is in remission. When relapse occurs, the patient receives high-dose chemotherapy or irradiation followed by "rescue" with the cryopreserved autologous bone marrow. This approach is attractive since it can be applied to patients who lack HLA-identical donors and avoids the immunologic problems of graft rejection and GVHD. One major reservation regarding this approach is the high probability that the cryopreserved remission bone marrow contains residual leukemia cells. It is possible that this problem can be overcome by removal of leukemia cells by physical, immune, or pharmacologic techniques. One approach for patients with acute lymphoblastic leukemia has been to treat the bone marrow in vitro with antileukemia antiserum (anti-common acute lymphoblastic leukemia serum) or monoclonal antibodies prior to reinfusion into the patient. Such experiments have been reported from three centers, and recovery of all hematopoietic cell lines has been demonstrated [147–149]. Similar experiments using AML heteroantisera or monoclonal antibodies are possible provided that they are not cytotoxic to hematopoietic stem cells.

Special Problems

Acute Promyelocytic Leukemia

Acute promyelocytic leukemia (M3) accounts for 10%–15% of cases of AML. Patients with promyelocytic leukemia often show evidence of bleeding, the severity of which is greater than would be expected from the degree of thrombocytopenia. This excessive bleeding is due to disseminated intravascular coagulation (DIC), which is thought to be related to the release of procoagulants from azurophilic granules within the leukemic promyelocyte [150, 151]. The risk of DIC may be greatest at the time drug treatment is initiated, since this correlates with the period of maximum cytoreduction and granular release.

Most investigators suggest that patients with promyelocytic leukemia should receive heparin to prevent or control DIC. Heparin usually is given prophylactically at a dose of 10–20 U/kg/h during induction chemotherapy. As there are no controlled data to support this approach, some investigators prefer fresh-frozen plasma to heparin. Remission rates in patients with promyelocytic leukemia are comparable to those achieved in other subgroups. Some data indicate that these patients may have long remissions [152–154]. Unfortunately, some large group studies have not confirmed this impression.

AML During Pregnancy

The development of AML during pregnancy is a major therapeutic problem. There is considerable concern regarding the use of cytotoxic drugs, because of their potential teratogenic effect. If treatment is withheld, however, the patient and child are likely to die from complications of the disease. The risk of fetal abnormalities is greatest during the first trimester. Fortunately, fetal malformations have rarely been reported following treatment of a pregnant patient [155, 156]. When leukemia is diagnosed during the second or third trimester of pregnancy, most data suggest that the mother and fetus tolerate high-dose chemotherapy without unacceptable complications [156, 157]. Although congenital abnormalities are uncommon, long-term follow-up to these children is required. An alternative approach is to use leukophoresis to control the leukemia until after delivery [158].

Therapy-Linked AML

An increasing incidence of therapy-linked AML has been reported in patients who have received chemotherapy, radiation therapy, or immunosuppressive drugs for neoplastic and nonneoplastic diseases. This topic has recently been reviewed [159]. The incidence is highest in patients who receive both cytotoxic drugs and radiation. The most common neoplasms associated with the subsequent development of AML include multiple myeloma, Hodgkin's disease, non-Hodgkin's lymphoma, and breast and ovarian carcinoma. Nonneoplastic conditions associated with AML include rheumatoid arthritis, nephrotic syndrome and other autoimmune diseases, and renal transplantation. In these conditions patients are usually treated with cytotoxic or immunosuppressive drugs. Patients with therapy-linked AML respond less well to induction chemotherapy than other patients with AML. Remission rates of 10%–40% have been reported in most series [160–164]. Remissions may also be briefer, ranging from 5 to 12 months in several study groups.

Preleukemia

The terms "preleukemia" and "smoldering leukemia" have been applied to a spectrum of abnormalities of bone marrow function characterized by normal to increased marrow cellularity and defective hematopoiesis [165]. Three dysmyelopoietic syndromes were recognized in the FAB classification: acquired idiopathic sideroblastic anemia (AISA); refractory anemia with an excess of blasts (RAEB); and chronic myelomonocytic leukemia (CMML) [3]. The myelodysplastic syndromes tend to occur in older patients, usually > 50 years. Malaise, weakness, infection, and bleeding, which are attributable to anemia, decreased white cell count, and thrombocytopenia, are common. The bone marrow is hypercellular, with 5%–30% myeloblasts (see pp 69–101).

The relation between the dysmyelopoietic syndromes and the development of acute leukemia is controversial. Many of these patients, particularly those with RAEB and CMML, have been classed in the group of preleukemia or smoldering leukemia in the literature. Several recent studies have indicated, however, that only 20%–30% of these patients will develop AML. A similar proportion die of infection or bleeding without ever developing overt leukemia. A small number of patients, usually < 10%, may recover. Most patients, however, continue to display evidence of abnormal hematopoiesis without developing overt leukemia. Patients with these dysmyelopoietic syndromes should generally not receive cytotoxic chemotherapy until they develop clear-cut leukemia. It is also important to distinguish patients with these dysmyelopoietic syndromes with prominent erythroid involvement from patients with erythroleukemia, which is a subgroup of AML (M6) and is treated with intensive chemotherapy.

Future Directions

Over the past 10 years there have been substantial major advances in the treatment of AML. Intensive induction chemotherapy using 7-day courses of cytarabine and daunorubicin with or without thioguanine will produce remission in 60%–85% of patients. Most patients can be expected to remain in remission for 9–16 months, and 20–40% of patients in some series remain in continuous remission for 2 years or more [31, 69]. Many of the latter patients remain in remission for 5 years or longer and some may be cured [166]. These data indicate substantial recent progress in the treatment of this disease, which was almost uniformly fatal 10 years ago.

The fact that most patients relapse within 1 year reflects a lack of progress in developing effective maintenance chemotherapy and/or immunotherapy regimens. Future progress awaits the development of sensitive methods for detecting residual leukemia [167, 168], more effective use of current therapeutic modalities, and the introduction of new effective drugs. Intensification chemotherapy for maximum leukemic cytoreduction may replace conventional consolidation and maintenance therapies. Further understanding of normal and leukemia cell growth may offer innovative approaches, including inhibition of leukemia cell growth with granulocytic chalones or manipulations that promote the maturation of leukemia cells [169, 170]. Chemicals such as phorbol esters [171, 172], dimethylsulfoxide [173, 174], *cis*-retinoic acid [175], and alkyl-lysophospholipids [176] can induce AML cell lines to differentiate into morphologically and functionally mature macrophages and granulocytes. Investigational clinical approaches, such as bone marrow transplantation in first remission, also deserve further consideration.

References

1. Tivey H (1955) The natural history of untreated acute leukemia. Ann NY Acad Sci 60:322–358
2. Bennett JM, Catavsky C, Daniel MT et al. (1976) Proposal for the classification of acute leukaemias. Br J Haematol 33:451–458
3. Gralnick HR, Galton DAG, Catovsky D et al. (1977) Classification of acute leukemia. Ann Intern Med 87:740–753
4. Gralnick HR (1980) A variant form of hypergranular promyelocytic leukemia (M3). Ann Intern Med 92:261
5. Golomb HM, Rowley JD, Vardiman JW, Testa JR, Butler A (1980) "Microgranular" acute promyelocytic leukemia: a distinct clinial, ultrastructural and cytogenic entity. Blood 55:253–259
6. Major PP, Minden MD, Beardsley GP, Kufe DW (1981) Lethality of human myeloblasts correlates with the incorporation of ara-C into DNA. Proc Natl Acad Sci USA 78(5):3235–3239
7. Skipper HE, Schable JM Jr, Wilcox WS (1967) Experimental evaluation of potential anticancer agents. XXI. Scheduling of arabinosylcytosine to take advantage of its S-phase specificity against leukemia cells. Cancer Chemother Rep 51:125–141
8. Ellison RR, Holland JF, Weil M et al. (1968) Arabinosyl cytosine: a useful agent in the treatment of acute leukemia in adults. Blood 32:507–523
9. Wang JJ, Selawry OS, Viettr TJ et al. (1970) Prolonged infusion of arabinosyl cytosine in childhood leukemia. Cancer 25:1–6
10. Bodey GP, Coltman CA, Freireich EJ et al. (1974) Chemotherapy of acute leukemia; comparison of cytarabine alone and in combination with vincristine, prednisone, and cyclophosphamide. Arch Intern Med 133:260–266
11. Southwest Oncology Group (1974) Cytarabine for acute leukemia in adults: effects of schedule on therapeutic response. Arch Intern Med 133:251–259
12. Carey RW, Ribas-Mundo M, Ellison RR et al. (1975) Comparative study of cytosine arabinoside therapy alone and combined with thioguanine mercaptopurine, or daunorubicin in acute myelocytic leukemia. Cancer 36:1560–1566
13. Early AP, Preisler HD, Slocum H, Rustum YM, Dorn P (1981) High dose cytosine arabinoside (HD-ARAC) for acute leukemia. Blood [Suppl 1] 58:138a

14. Herzig RH, Herzig GP, Lazarus HM, Wolff SN, Phillips GL (1981) Successful treatment of patients (PTS) with refractory acute nonlymphocytic leukemia (ANLL) using high-dose cytosine arabinoside (HDAra-C) with and without anthracycline. Blood [Suppl 1] 58: 141a
15. Levi JA, Wirnik PH (1976) A comparative clinical trial of 5-azacytidine and guanazole in previously treated adults with acute nonlymphocytic leukemia. Cancer 38: 36–41
16. Vogler WR, Miller DS, Keller JW (1976) 5-Azacytidine (NSC 102816): A new drug for the treatment of myeloblastic leukemia. Blood 48: 331–337
17. Von Hoff DD, Slavik M, Muggia FM (1976) 5-Azacytidine: a new anticancer drug with effectiveness in acute myelogenous leukemia. Ann Intern Med 85: 237–245
18. Omura GA (1977) Combination therapy with 5-azacytidine plus beta-2′-deoxythioguanosine in adult acute leukemia. Cancer Treat Rep 61: 915–917
19. Van Echo DA, Lichenfeld KM, Wiernik PH (1977) Vinblastine, 5-azacytidine and VP-16-213 therapy for previously treated patients with acute nonlymphocytic leukemia. Cancer Treat Rep 61: 1599–1602
20. Burgess MA, Bodey GP, Minnow RA et al. (1977) Phase I–II evaluation of cyclocytidine. Cancer Treat Rep 61: 437–43
21. Yap P-S, McCredie KB, Keating MJ et al. (1981) Phase I–II study of 3-deazauridine (NSC 126849) in adults with acute leukemia. Cancer Treat Rep 65: 521–524
22. Vogler WR, Trulock PD (1978) Phase I study of pyrazofurin in refractory acute myelogenous leukemia. Cancer Treat Rep 62: 1569–1571
23. Mertelsmann R, Drapkin RL, Gee TS et al. (1981) Treatment of acute myelogenous leukemia in adults: response to 2,2-anhydro-a-β-D-arabinofuranosyl-5-fluorocytosine and thioguanine on the L-12 protocol. Cancer 48: 2136–2142
24. Bornstein RS, Theologides A, Kennedy BJ (1969) Daunorubicin in acute myelogenous leukemia in adults. JAMA 207: 1301–1306
25. Waring M (1970) Variation in the supercoils in closed circular DNA by binding of antibiotics and drugs: evidence for molecular models involving intercalation. J Mol Biol 54: 247–279
26. Weil M, Jacquillat CL, Gemon-Auclerc MF et al. (1976) Acute granulocytic leukemia: treatment of the disease. Arch Intern Med 136: 1389–1395
27. Weil M, Glidewell OJ, Jacquillat C et al. (1973) Daunorubicin in the therapy of acute granulocyte leukemia. Cancer Res 33: 921–928
28. Wiernik PH, Schimpf SC, Schiffer CA et al. (1976) Randomized clinical comparison of daunorubicin (NSC-63878), 6-thioguanine (NSC-752), and pyrimethamine (NSC-3061) for the treatment of acute nonlymphocytic leukemia. Cancer Treat Rep 60: 41–53
29. Paul C, Bjorkholm M, Christenson I et al. (1981) Comparison of daunorubicin and daunorubicin-DNA complex in the treatment of acute nonlymphoblastic leukemia. Cancer Chemother Pharmacol 6: 65–73
30. Preisler HD, Rustum Y, Henderson ES et al. (1979) Treatment of acute nonlymphocytic leukemia: Use of anthracycline-cytosine arabinoside induction therapy and comparison of two maintenance regimens. Blood 53: 455–464
31. Weinstein HJ, Mayer RJ, Rosenthal DS et al. (1980) Treatment of acute myelogenous leukemia in children and adults. N Engl J Med 303: 473–478
32. Viung CC, Ozols CF, Myers CE (1981) The anthracycline antineoplastic drugs. N Engl J Med 305: 139–153
33. Benjamin RS, Keating MJ, McCredie KB et al. (1977) A phase 1 and 2 trial of rubidazone in patients with acute leukemia. Cancer Res 37: 4623–4628
34. Jacquillat C, Weil M, Gemon-Auderc MF et al. (1976) Clinical study of rubidazone (22-050 R.P.): a new daunorubicin-derived compound, in 170 patients with acute leukemia and other malignancies. Cancer 37: 653–659
35. Crooke ST (1977) A review of carminomycin – a new anthracycline developed in the USSR. J Med 8: 295–316
36. Fainshtein FE, Kovaleva LG, Vakhrusheva MV et al. (1977) Carminomycin in the treatment of adult patients with acute leukemia. Antibiotiki 22: 756–758

37. Warrell RP Jr, Arlin Z, Gee T et al. (1981) Phase I–II evaluation of aclacinomycin in acute leukemia. Am Assoc Cancer Res 22: 191
38. Yamada K, Nakamura T, Tsuruno T et al. (1980) A phase II study of aclacinomycin in acute leukemia in adults. Cancer Treat Rev 7: 177–182
39. Hitchings GH, Elion GB (1954) The chemistry and biochemistry of purine analogs. Ann NY Acad Sci 60: 195–199
40. Frei E III, Freireich EJ, Gehan G et al. (1961) Studies of sequential and combination antimetabolite therapy in acute leukemia: 6-mercaptopurine and methotrexate. Blood 18: 431, 454
41. Burchenal JH, Murphy ML, Ellison RR et al. (1953) Clinical evaluation of a new antimetabolite, 6-mercaptopurine, in the treatment of leukemia and allied diseases. Blood 8: 965–999
42. Omura GA, Vogler WR, Smalley RV et al. (1977) Phase II study of β-2′-deoxytheoguanosine in adult acute leukemia. Cancer Treat Rep 61: 1379–1381
43. Legha SS, Keating MJ, Zander A et al. (1980) 4′-(acridinylamino) methanesulfon-m-anisidide (AMSA): a new drug effective in the treatment of adult acute leukemia. Ann Intern Med 93: 17–21
44. Van Echo DA, Markus SD, Schimpff SC, Wiernik PH (1980) A phase II trial of 4′-(9-acridinylamino) methanesulfon-m-anisidide (AMSA) in adult relapsed acute leukemia. Proc AM Assoc Can Res 21: 477
45. Paciucci PA, Ohnuma T, Ambinder EP et al. (1981) Effects of mitoxantrone (dehydroxyanthracenedine dehydrochloride) in patients with refractory acute leukemia. Blood [Suppl 1] 58: 148a
46. Smith IC, Gerken MC, Clink HM et al. (1976) VP-16-213 in acute myelogenous leukaemia. Postgrad Med J 52: 66–70
47. Radice PA, Bunn PA Jr, Ihde DC (1979) Therapeutic trials with VP-16-213 and VM-26: active agents in small cell lung cancer, non-Hodgkins lymphomas, and other malignancies. Cancer Treat Rep 63: 1231–1239
48. Mathé G, Schwarzenberg L, Pouillart P et al. (1974) Two epidophyllotoxin derivatives, VM 26 and VP 16-213, in the treatment of leukemias, hematosorcomas and lymphomas. Cancer 34: 985–992
49. Van Echo DA, Wiernik PH, Aisner J (1980) High-dose VP 16-213 (NSC141540) for the treatment of patients with previously treated acute leukemia. Cancer Clin Trials 3: 325–328
50. European Organization for Research on the Treatment of Cancer, Clinical Screening Group (1973) Epipodophyllotoxin VP 16213 in treatment of acute leukaemias, haematosarcomas, and solid tumors. Br Med J 3: 199–202
51. Van Echo PA, Lichtenfeld KM, Wiernik PH (1977) Vinblastine (NSC-49848), 5-azacytidine (NSC 102816) and VP 16-213 (NSC 141540) in previously treated patients with acute nonlymphocytic leukemia. Cancer Treat Rep 61: 1599–1602
52. Hurd DD, Peterson BA, Bloomfield CD (1981) 4′-(9-acridinylamino) methanesulfon-m-anisidide (AMSA), VP 16-213 (VP), cytosine arabinoside (ARA-C), and G-thioguanine (GTG) in the treatment of relapsed and refractory acute nonlymphocytic leukemia (ANLL). Blood [Suppl 1] 58: 142a
53. Griffin TW, Lister TA, Rybak ME et al. (1979) Treatment of acute nonlymphocytic leukemia with neocarzinostatin. Cancer Treat Rep 63: 1853–1856
54. Frei E III, Freireich EH, Gehan G et al. (1961) Studies of sequential and combination antimetabolist therapy in acute leukemia: 6-mercaptopurine and methotrexate. Blood 18: 431–454
55. Vogler WR, Huguley CM Jr, Rundles RW (1967) Comparison of methotrexate with 6-mercaptopurine-prednisone in treatment of acute leukemia in adults. Cancer 20: 1221–1226
56. Hoogstraten B (1962) Cyclophosphamide (cytoxan) in acute leukemia. Cancer Chemother Rep 16: 167–171

57. Clarkson B, Krakoff J, Burchenal J et al. (1970) Clinical results of treatment with E. Coli L-asparaginase in adults with leukemia, lymphoma and solid tumors. Cancer 25: 279–305
58. Capizzi RL, Bertino JR, Handschumacher RE (1980) L-Asparaginase. Annu Rev Med 21: 433–444
59. Medical Research Council (1966) Treatment of acute leukemia in adults: comparison of steroid and mercaptopurine therapy, alone and in conjunction. Br Med J 1: 1383–1389
60. De Conti RC, Toftness BR, Lange RC et al. (1973) Clinical and pharmacological studies with *cis*-diamminedichloroplatinum(II). Cancer Res 33: 1310–1315
61. Rozenweig M, von Hoff DD, Slavik M et al. (1977) *Cis*-diamminedichloroplatinum(II): a new anticancer drug. Ann Intern Med 86: 803–812
62. Hill NO, Pardue A, Khan A et al. (1981) Phase I human leukocyte interferon trials in cancer leukemia. J Clin Hematol Oncol 11: 23–25
63. Levine AS, Sivulich M, Wiernik PH, Levy HB (1979) Initial clinical trials in cancer patients of polyriboinosinic – polyribocytidylic acid stabilized with poly-1-lysine, in carboxymethylcellulose [poly(ICLC)], a highly effective interferon inducer. Cancer Res 39: 1645–1650
64. Clarkson BD, Dowling MD, Gee TS et al. (1975) Treatment of acute leukaemia in adults. Cancer 36: 775–795
65. Medical Research Council (1974) Treatment of acute myeloid leukemia with daunorubicin, cytosine arabinoside, mercyptopurine, L-asparaginase, prednisone and thioguanine: results of treatment with five multipledrug schedules. Br J Haematol 27: 373–389
66. Wallace HJ, Holland JF, Glidewell OJ et al. (1975) Therapy of acute myelocytic leukemia. In: Madelli F, Amadori S, Mariani G (eds) Acute leukemia group B studies, therapy of acute leukemia. Minerva Medica, Turin, pp 255–269
67. Lewis JP, Linman HW, Marshall GJ et al. (1977) Randomized clinical trial of cytosine arabinoside and 6-thioguanine in remission induction and consolidation of adult nonlymphocytic acute leukemia. Cancer 39: 1387–1396
68. Holland JF, Glidewell O, Ellison RR et al. (1976) Acute myelocytic leukemia. Arch Intern Med 136: 1377–1381
69. Gale RP, Foon KA, Cline MJ, Zighelboim J (1981) Intensive chemotherapy for acute myelogenous leukemia. Ann Intern Med 94: 753–757
70. Glucksberg H, Buckner DE, Fefer A et al. (1975) Combination chemotherapy for acute nonlymphoblastic leukemia in adults. Cancer Chemother Rep 59: 1131–1137
71. Rees JKH, Sandler RM, Challener J, Hayhoe FGJ (1977) Treatment of acute myeloid leukemia with a triple cytotoxic regimen: DAT. Br J Cancer 36: 770–776
72. Peterson BA, Bloomfield CD, Bosi GJ, Gibbs G, Malloy M (1980) Intensive fivedrug combination chemotherapy for adult acute-non-lymphocytic leukemia. Cancer 46: 663–668
73. Foon KA, Gale RP (1982) Controversies in the therapy of acute myelogenous leukemia. Am J Med 72: 963–979
74. Finnish Leukemia Group (1979) The effect of thioguanine in a combination of daunorubicine [sic], cytyrabine and prednisone in the treatment of acute leukemia in adults. Scand J Hematol 23: 124–128
75. Rai KR, Holland JR, Glidewell OJ et al. (1981) Treatment of acute myelocytic leukemia: A study by Cancer and Leukemia Group B. Blood 58: 1203–1212
76. Slavin RE, Dias MA, Saral R (1978) Cytosine arabinoside induced gastrointestinal toxic alterations in sequential chemotherapeutic protocols. A clinical-pathologic study of 33 patients. Cancer 42: 1747–1759
77. Yates J, Gledeucll O, Wiernik P et al. (1982) Cytosine arabinoside with daunorubicin or adriamycin for therapy of acute myelocytic leukemia: A CALGB study. Blood 60: 454–462
78. Shaikh BS, Doghtery JB, Hamilton RW et al. (1980) Selective use of daunorubicin for remission-induction chemotherapy in acute non-lymphoblastic leukemia. Cancer 46: 1731–1734
79. Saponara EJ, Rothenberg SP, Villamena D (1979) Cytarabine and thioguanine for acute nonlymphocytic leukemia. Another look. Arch Intern Med 139: 1277–1280

80. Von Hoff DD, Rozencweig M, Layard M, Slavik M, Muggia FM (1977) Daunomycin induced cardiotoxicity in children and adults. A review of 110 cases. Am J Med 62: 200–208
81. Mauer AM (1975) Cell kinetics and practical consequences for therapy of acute leukemia. N Engl J Med 293: 389–393
82. Vaughan WP, Karls JE, Burke PJ (1980) Long chemotherapy-free remissions after single-cycle times-sequential chemotherapy for acute myelocytic leukemia. Cancer 45: 859–865
83. Zighelboim J, Foon K, Yale C, Gale RP (1982) Treatment of acute myelogenous leukemia with intensive induction and consolidation chemotherapy. Proc Am Soc Clin Oncol (to be published)
84. Urbanitz D, Hiddemann W, Van de Loo J, Buchner TH (1981) Intensive and rapid remission induction in acute non-lymphocytic leukemia (ANLL) followed by consolidation without maintenance therapy. Proc Am Assoc Cancer Res 22: 271
85. Coltman CA, Bodey GP, Hewlett JJ (1978) Chemotherapy of acute leukemia. A comparison of vincristine, cytarabine, and prednisone alone and in combination with cyclophosphamide or daunorubicin. Arch Intern Med 138: 1342–1348
86. Eppinger-Helft M, Pavlovsky S, Hidalgo G et al. (1980) Chemoimmunotherapy with Corynebacterium parvum in acute myelocytic leukemia. Cancer 45: 280–284
87. Glucksberg H, Cheever M, Fefer A, Forewell V, Thomas ED (1981) Intensification therapy in acute nonlymphocytic leukemia (ANL) in adults. Proc AACR/ASCO 22: 232
88. Bodey GP, Freireich EJ, McCredie KG et al. (1978) Prolonged remissions in adults with acute leukemia following late intensification chemotherapy and immunotherapy. Cancer 47: 1937–1945
89. Mayer RJ, Weinstein JH, Coral FS, Rosenthal DS, Frei E (1982) The role of intensive post-induction chemotherapy in the management of patients with acute myelogenous leukemia. Cancer Treat Rep 66: 1455–1462
90. Terry WD, Windhorst D (1978) Immunotherapy of cancer. Present status of trials in man. Raven, New York
91. Vogler WR (1980) Results of randomized trials of immunotherapy for acute leukemia. Cancer Immunol Immunother 9: 15–21
92. Foon KA, Smalley RV, Gale RP (to be published) The role of immunotherapy in acute myelogenous leukemia
93. Gutterman JU, Hersh EM, Rodriquez B et al. (1974) Chemoimmunotherapy of adult acute leukaemia: prolongation of remission in myeloblastic leukaemia with BCG. Lancet 2: 1405–1409
94. Holland JF, Bekesi JG (1978) Comparison of chemotherapy with chemotherapy plus VCN-treated cells in acute myelocytic leukemia. In: Terry WD, Windhorst D (eds) Immunotherapy of cancer: present status of trials in man. Raven, New York, pp 353–374
95. Powles RL, Crowther D, Bateman CJT (1973) Immunotherapy for acute myelogenous leukemia. Br J Cancer 28: 365–376
96. Vogler W, Bartolucci AA, Omura GA et al. (1978) A randomized clinical trial of remission induction, consolidation and chemo-immunotherapy maintenance in adult acute myeloblastic leukemia. Cancer Immunol Immunother 3: 163–170
97. Vogler WR, Gordon DS, Smalley RV et al. (1981) Serial immunologic assessment during a randomized trial of chemoimmunotherapy in acute myelogenous leukemia. A southeastern cancer study group clinical trial. Cancer Immunol Immunother 11: 97–107
98. Omura GA, Vogler WR, Lefante J et al. (to be published) Treatment of acute myelogenous leukemia: Influence of three induction regimens and maintenance with chemotherapy or BCG immunotherapy. Cancer
99. Whittaker JA, Bailey-Wood R, Hutchins S (1980) Active immunotherapy for treatment of acute myelogenous leukemia: report of two controlled trials. Br J Hematol 45: 389–400
100. Vuvan H, Fiere D, Doillon M et al. (1978) B.C.G. therapy in acute nonlymphoid leukaemias. Scand J Haematol 21: 40–46

101. Murphy S, Hersh E (1978) Immunotherapy of leukemia and lymphoma. Semin Haematol 15: 181–203
102. Hewlett JS, Belcerzak S, Gutterman J et al. (1977) Remission induction in adult acute leukemia by 10-day continuous intravenous infusion of Ara-C plus oncovin and prednisone. Maintenance with and without immunotherapy. In: Terry WD, Windhurst D (eds) Immunotherapy of cancer: present status of trials in man. Raven, New York, pp 387–391
103. Summerfield GP, Gibbs TJ, Bellingham AJ (1979) Immunotherapy using BCG during remission induction and as the sole form of maintenance in acute myeloid leukemia. Br J Cancer 40: 736–742
104. Mandelli F, Amadori S, Dini E et al. (1981) Randomized clinical trial of immunotherapy and androgenotherapy for remission maintenance in acute non-lymphocytic leukemia. Leuk Res 5: 447–452
105. Powles RL, Russell J, Lister TA (1977) Immunotherapy for acute myelogenous leukaemia: a controlled clinical study 2-1/1 years after entry of the last patient. Br J Cancer 35: 265–272
106. Medical Research Council (1978) Immunotherapy of acute myeloid leukaemia. Br J Cancer 37: 1–11
107. Lindemalm CH, S-N, Killander A, Bjorkholm M et al. (1978) Adjuvant immunotherapy in acute nonlymphocytic leukemia. Cancer Immunol Immunother 4: 179–183
108. Zuhrie SR, Harris R, Freeman CB, et al. (1980) Immunotherapy alone vs no maintenance treatment in acute myelogenous leukemia. Br J Cancer 41: 372–377
109. Lister TA, Whitehouse JMA, Oliver RTD et al. (1980) Chemotherapy and immunotherapy for acute myelogenous leukemia. Cancer 46: 2142–2148
110. Powles RL, Selby PJ, Jones DR et al. (1977) Maintenance of remission in acute myelogenous leukemia by a mixture of BCG and irradiated leukemia cells. Lancet 2: 1107–1109
111. Baehner RL, Bernstein ID, Sather H et al. (1979) Improved remission induction rate with D-ZAPO but unimproved remission duration with addition of immunotherapy to chemotherapy in previously untreated children with ANLL Med Pediatr Oncol 7: 127–139
112. Izak G, Stupp Y, Manny N et al. (1977) The immune response in acute myelogenous leukemia. Effect of methanol extraction residue fraction of tubercle bacilli (MER) on T and B cell functions and their relation to the course of the disease. Isr J Med Sci 13: 667–693
113. Sauter C, Cavalli F, Lindenmann J et al. (1978) Viral oncolysis: its application in maintenance treatment of acute myelogenous leukemia. In: Terry WD, Windhorst D (eds) Immunotherapy of cancer: present status of trials in man. Raven, New York, pp 355–363
114. Dawson DM, Rosenthal DS, Moloney WC (1979) Neurological complications of acute leukemia in adults: changing rate. Ann Intern Med 79: 541–544
115. Law IP, Blom J (1977) Adult acute leukemia: frequency of central nervous system involvement in long term survivors. Cancer 40: 1304–1306
116. Steward DJ, Keating MJ, McCredie KB et al. (1981) Natural history of central nervous system acute leukemia in adults. Cancer 47: 184–196
117. Peterson BA, Bloomfield CD (1977) Asymptomatic central nervous system (CNS) leukemia in adults with acute non-lymphocytic leukemia (ANLL) in extended remission. Proc AACR/ASCO 18: 341
118. Wolff L, Zighelboim J, Gale RP (1979) Paraplegia following intrathecal cytosine arabinoside. Cancer 43: 83–85
119. Arlin ZA, Gee TS, Kempin SJ et al. (1981) Treatment of adult nonlymphoblastic leukemia (ANLL) with AMSA in combination with cytosine arabinoside (ARA-C) and 6-thioguanine (6TG) AAT. Proc Assoc Cancer Res 22: 172
120. Kahn SB, Conroy JR, Bulova S, Biodsky J (1981) Acridinyl anisidide (AMSA) (NSC 249992) and 5-azacytidine (AZA) (NSC 102816) therapy of acute leukemia. Blood [Suppl 1] 58: 143a
121. Rudnick SA, Cadman ED, Capizzi RL et al. (1979) High dose cytosine arabinoside (HDARAC) in refractory acute leukemia. Cancer 44: 1189–1193

122. Hines JD, Oken MM, Mazza J, Keller A, Glick J (1981) High dose cytosine arabinoside (ARA-C) and M-AMSA in refractory acute non-lymphocytic leukemia. Blood [Suppl 1] 58: 142a
123. Herman TS, Durie BGM, Hutter J (1981) Treatment of refractory acute myelogenous leukemia (AML) with vincristine, high dose methotrexate, 1,3-bis-(2-choroethyl)-1-nitrosurea (BCNU), cyclophosphamide and methylglyoxal bis(guanylhydrazone) (MGBG). Proc AACR/ASCO 22: 476
124. Peterson BA, Bloomfield CD (1981) Re-induction of complete remissions in adults with acute non-lymphocytic leukemia. Leuk Res 5: 81–88
125. Gale RP (1978) Approach to leukemic relapse following bone marrow transplantation. Transplant Proc 10: 167–172
126. Thomas ED, Buckner CD, Banaji M et al. (1977) One hundred patients with acute leukemia treated with chemotherapy, total body irradiation, and allogeneic marrow transplantation. Blood 49: 511–533
127. UCLA Bone-Marrow Transplantation Team (1977) Bone-marrow transplantation in acute leukaemia. Lancet 2: 1197–1200
128. Fefer A, Einstein AB, Thomas ED et al. (1974) Bone-marrow transplantation for hematologic neoplasia in 16 patients with identical twins. N Engl J Med 290: 1389–1393
129. Thomas ED, Buckner CD, Clift RA et al. (1981) Marrow transplantation for patients with leukemia. Exp Hematol [Suppl 9] 9: 121
130. Gale RP (1981) Bone marrow transplantation for leukemia in remission. Exp Hematol [Suppl 9] 9: 125
131. Morgenstern GR (1980) Allogeneic bone marrow transplantation for acute leukaemia. Experience in 55 patients. Blut 41: 213–215
132. Zwaan FE (1980) Bone marrow transplantation for acute leukaemia in remission – European results. Blut 41: 208–213
133. Kersey J, Ramsey N, Kim T et al. (1981) Bone marrow transplantation (BMT) in first remission in young patients with acute non-lymphocytic leukemia (ANLL). Proc AACR/ASCO 22: 143
134. Zwaan FE, Jansen J, Noordijk EM (1980) Bone marrow transplantation in acute myeloid leukaemia (AML) during first remission: the Leiden experience. Blut 41: 216–220
135. Dinsmore R, Shane B, Kapoor N et al. (1981) A randomized trial of bone marrow transplantation (BMT) versus chemotherapy (CT) maintenance for acute myelogenous leukemia in first remission: preliminary results. Exp Hematol [Suppl 9] 9: 125
136. Speck B, Gratwohl A, Nissen C et al. (1981) Further experience with cylosporin –A in allogeneic bone marrow transplantation. Exp Hematol [Suppl 9] 9: 124
137. Mannoni P, Vernant JP, Rodet M et al. (1980) Marrow transplantation for acute nonlymphoblastic leukemia in first remission. Blut 41: 220–225
138. Blume KG, Forman SJ, Spruce WE et al. (1981) Bone marrow transplantion (BMT) for acute leukemia. Exp Hematol [Suppl 9] 9: 124
139. Okunewick JP, Meredith RF (1980) Graft-versus-leukemia in man and animal models. CRC, Boca Raton
140. Weiden PL, Flournoy N, Thomas ED et al. (1979) Antileukemic effect of graft-versus-host disease in human recipients of allogeneic-marrow grafts. N Engl J Med 300: 1068–1073
141. McIntyre R, Gale RP (1981) Relationship between graft-versus-leukemia and graft-versus-host in man – UCLA experience. In: Okunewick JP, Meredith RF (eds) Graft-versus-leukemia in man and animal models. CRC, Boca Raton, pp 1–9
142. Weiden PL, Sullivan KM, Flournoy N, Storb R, Thomas ED and the Seattle Marrow Transplant Team (1981) Antileukemic effect of chronic graft-versushost disease. Contribution to improved survival after allogeneic marrow transplantation. N Engl J Med 304: 1529–1533
143. Hansen JA, Clift RA, Thomas ED, Buckner CD, Mickelson EM, Storb R (1979) Histocompatibility and marrow transplantation. Transplant Proc 11: 1924–1929

144. Hansen JA, Clift RA, Thomas ED, Buckner CD, Storb R, Giblett ER (1980) Transplantation of marrow from an unrelated donor to a patient with acute leukemia. N Engl J Med 303: 565–567
145. Graze PR, Gale RP (1978) Autotransplantation for leukemia and solid tumors. Transplant Proc 10: 177–184
146. Dicke KA, McCredie KB, Spitzer G et al. (1978) Autologous bone marrow transplantation in patients with adult acute leukemia in relapse. Transplantation 26: 169–173
147. Wells JR, Billing R, Herzog P et al. (1979) Autotransplantation after in vitro immunotherapy of lymphoblastic leukemia. Exp Hematol [Suppl] 7: 164–169
148. Netzel B, Rodt H, Haas RJ et al. (1980) Immunological conditioning of bone marrow for autotransplantation in childhood acute lymphoblastic leukemia. Lancet 1: 1330–1332
149. Ritz J, Sallan SE, Bast RC et al. (1982) Autologous bone marrow transplantation in CALLA positive acute lymphoblastic leukemia after in vitro treatment with J5 monoclonal antibody and complement. Lancet 2: 60–63
150. Groopman J, Ellman L (1979) Acute promyelocytic leukemia. Am J Hematol 7: 395–408
151. Gralnick HR, Abrell E (1973) Studies of the procoagulant and fibrinolytic activity of promyelocytes in acute promyelocytic leukemia. Br J Haematol 24: 89–99
152. Daly PA, Shiffer CA, Wiernik PH (1980) Acute promyelocytic leukemia: Clincal management of 15 patients. Am J Hematol 8: 347–359
153. Bernard J, Weil M, Boiron M, Jacquillarc, Flandrin G, Geman M-F (1973) Acute promyelocytic leukemia: Results of treatment by daunorubicin. Blood 41: 489–496
154. Collins AJ, Bloomfiled CD, Paterson BA, McKenna RW, Edison JR (1978) Acute progranulocytic leukemia. Management of the coagulopathy diromg daunorubicin-prednisone induction. Arch Intern Med 138: 1677–1680
155. Lilleyman JS, Hill AS, Anderton KJ (1977) Consequences of acute myelogenous leukemia in early pregnancy. Cancer 40: 1300–1303
156. Pizzuyo J, Aviles A, Noviega L, Niz J, Morales M, Ramero F (1979) Treatment of acute leukemia during pregnancy: presentation of nine cases. Cancer Treat Rep 63: 369–371
157. Daney KC, Kraemer KG, Shepard TH (1979) Combination chemotherapy for acute myelocytic leukemia during pregnancy: three case reports. Cancer Treat Rep 63: 369–371
158. Meyer RJ, Guttner J, Truog P, Ambinder EP, Holland JH (1978) Therapeutic leukopheresis of acute myelo-monocytic leukemia in pregnancy. Med Pediatr Oncol 4: 77–81
159. Rosner F, Grunwald HW (1980) Cytotoxic drugs and leukaemogenesis. Clin Haematol 9: 663–681
160. Anonymous (1977) Therapy-linked leukaemia. Lancet 1: 519–520 (editorial)
161. Chabner BA (1977) Second neoplasm: a complication of cancer chemotherapy. N Engl J Med 197: 213–215
162. Reimer RR, Hoover R, Graumeni JF Jr et al. (1977) Acute leukemia after alkylating agent therapy of ovarian cancer. N Engl J Med 297: 177–181
163. Cadman ED, Capizzo RL, Bertino JR (1977) Acute non-lymphocytic leukemia: A delayed complication of Hodgkin's disease therapy. Analysis of 109 cases. Cancer 40: 1280–1296
164. Vaughan WD, Karp JE, Burke PJ (1981) Effective chemotherapy of acute myelocytic leukemia (AML) occurring after alkylating agent therapy (AAT) or radiation therapy (RT) for prior malignancy. Proc AACR/ASCO 22: 483
165. Koeffler HP, Golde DW (1980) Human preleukemia. Ann Intern Med 93: 347–353
166. Bloomfield CD (1980) Treatment of acute nonlymphocytic leukemia – 1980. Ann Intern Med 93: 133–135
167. Baker MA, Falk JA, Carter WH, Taub RN and the Toronto Leukemic Study Group (1979) Early diagnosis of relapse in acute myeloblastic leukemia. N Engl J Med 301: 1353–1357
168. Hittleman WN, Broussard LC, Dosik G, McCredie KB (1980) Predicting relapse of human leukemia by means of premature chromosome condensation. N Engl J Med 303: 475–484
169. Sachs L (1978) Control of normal cell differentiation and the phenotypic reversion of malignancy in myeloid leukaemia. Nature 274: 535–539

170. Koeffler HP, Golde DW (1978) Acute myelogenous leukemia: a human cell line responsive to colony-stimulating activity. Science 200: 1153–1154
171. Loten J, Sachs L (1979) Regulation of normal differentiation in mouse and human myeloid leukemia cells by phorbol esters and the mechanism of tumor promoter. Proc Natl Acad Sci USA 76: 5158
172. Rovera G, Santole D, Damsky C (1979) Human promyelocytic leukemia cells in culture differentiate into macrophage-like cells when treated with phorbol diester. Proc Natl Acad Sci USA 76: 2779
173. Collins SJ, Ruscetti RW, Gallagher RE, Gallo RC (1978) Terminal differentiation of human promyelocytic leukemia cells induced by dimethylsulfoxide and other polar compounds. Proc Natl Acad Sci USA 75: 2458–2462
174. Collins SJ, Ruscetti FW, Gallagher RE, Gallo RC (1979) Normal functional characteristics of cultured human promyelocytic leukemia cells (HL-60) after induction of differentiation by dimethylsulfoxide. J Exp Med 149: 969–974
175. Breitman TR, Collins SJ, Keene BR (1981) Terminal differentiation of human promyelocytic leukemic cells in primary culture in response to retinoic acid. Blood 57: 1000–1004
176. Honma Y, Kasukabe T, Hozumi M, Tsushima S, Nomura H (1981) Induction of differentiation of cultured human and mouse myeloid leukemia cells by alkyl-lysophospholipids. Cancer Res 41: 3211–3216

Management of CLL and Allied Disorders with Reference to Their Immunology and Proliferation Kinetics

H. Theml and H. W. L. Ziegler-Heitbrock*

St. Vincentius-Krankenhäuser, Zentrum für Innere Medizin, Abteilung II, Hämatologie/Onkologie, Südenstrasse, 7500 Karlsruhe 1, FRG

Introduction

Leukemic lymphomas, diagnosed as chronic lymphocytic leukemia or as diffuse well differentiated lymphoma, form a heterogeneous group [7, 45]. With the progress that has been achieved in recent years in the definition of phenotype and function of leukemic lymphocytes, a more clearcut distinction of the similar but separate entities of B-type chronic lymphocytic leukemia (B-CLL), prolymphocytic leukemia (PLL), immunocytoma (IC), and T-CLL has become possible. In this paper we will refer mainly to the Kiel Classification of Non-Hodgkin Lymphomas [45] because of its clear distinction of subtypes, though other classifications are also beginning to sort out such entities as IC.

New aspects of immunology and proliferation kinetics of the above conditions and the bearing of these findings on therapy will be discussed in the present review. Information on several aspects of IC, PLL, and T-CLL are limited because of their low frequency and the fact that they have only recently been defined. Our current view, based in part on a pathophysiological concept proposed in this paper, is that cytostatic therapy in B-CLL, which is still not proven to be advantageous, should be adapted to stage of disease and should take into consideration the often profound immunodeficiency and the proliferation kinetics in a given patient. In contrast, T-CLL, PLL, and IC, which are associated with a poor prognosis, might be approached more aggressively as soon as the diagnosis has been made.

Immunology

Chronic Lymphocytic Leukemia

Immunological Characterization of Leukemic Cells in CLL

Much of the progress in our understanding of the lymphoproliferative disease of CLL has come from the immunological analysis of phenotype and function of both leukemic and nonleukemic cells. The leukemic cells usually belong to the B cell lineage, since they express surface Ig.

B-CLL cells are small lymphocytes with predominantly IgM, IgD, and one light chain expressed on the cell surface. B-CLL cells are Ia positive but they are weak stimulators in

* The authors thank S. Förster for excellent secretarial work. The work of H. W. L. Ziegler-Heitbrock is supported by a grant from the VW-Stiftung

Recent Results in Cancer Research. Vol. 93

mixed lymphocyte reaction. Differentiation induction of the CLL cells to more mature cells results in strong Ia-positivity and good stimulation capacity [56]. Further, B-CLL cells are positive for Fc receptors, complement receptors, mouse red blood cell receptors, and T65, as defined, for instance, by the monoclonal antibody (MAB) T101 [5, 47, 65]. B-CLL cells do not bind MAB FMC7 [11] or MAB RFA4 [20]. With these markers the normal counterpart to CLL cells can be pinpointed at the stage of the immature B cell [34]. This type of cell is found at low frequency in tonsils and lymph nodes but not in the peripheral blood [13, 20]. The phenotype of CLL, however, is not fixed ("frozen"), since in vitro treatment with pokeweed mitogen or phorbolesters can induce differentiation to more mature antibody-secreting cells [64, 80]. These secreted products are monoclonal and are identical with the surface Ig of the CLL cells.

In some cases a degree of in vivo differentiation of the leukemic cells can occur, resulting in plasmacytoid feature with higher amounts of cellular Ig and with antibody secretion and Ig spike in serum. Such cases, however, may have to be reclassified as immunocytoma, as discussed below.

Immunological Characterization of Nonleukemic Cells in CLL

The nonleukemic cells in the peripheral blood of CLL patients, though very dilute, can also be increased in absolute numbers [12, 84]. Among these cells the predominant T cells show an imbalance of functional subsets due to an increase of cells with the phenotype of suppressor cells, i.e., cells carrying the receptor for the Fc portion of IgG (T γ cells) and reacting with monoclonal antibodies such as OKT8 [37, 59] (Fig. 1). While in some studies this imbalance was found to result in the suppression of B cell functions [36] others failed to

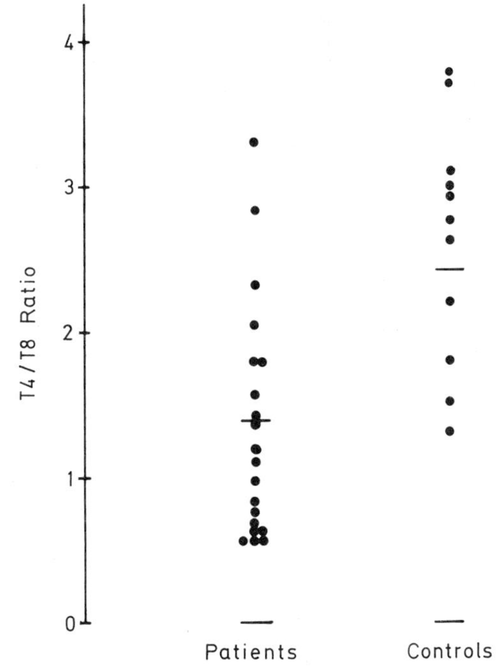

Fig. 1. Ratios of T4/T8 in CLL and controls. T4 (helper) and T8 (suppressor) T cells were determined in peripheral blood lymphocytes after removal of CLL B cells with antibody and complement according to Ziegler et al. [84]. The difference between groups is highly significant ($P < 0.001$, Student's *t*-test). H. W. L. Ziegler-Heitbrock et al., unpublished results)

confirm this, perhaps because less severely affected patients were studied [31]. Compelling evidence supporting an in vivo role of the increased OKT8$^+$ suppressor cells comes from a recent study where high ratios for OKT8$^+$ suppressor to OKT4$^+$ helper cells in CLL patients were found to correlate with low serum Ig values [59]. Specific antibody response after vaccination with bacteriophage ØX174 and with diphtheria and mumps vaccines were demonstrated to be defective [14].

In the field of cell-mediated immunity, it has been shown that some CLL patients exhibit a profound deficiency of natural killer cell activity [84], in addition to which they have a lower capacity for interferon production [18]. Recent results indicate that the patients who are deficient in NK cell activity lack the VEP13$^+$ lymphocyte subpopulation of NK cells (Ziegler-Heitbrock et al., unpublished data). Both natural killer cells and interferon are invoked as a defense mechanism against infections and tumors, and the deficiency of this system might be responsible in part for such clinical events as are seen frequently in CLL. In contrast, the T cell-mediated cellular immune response determined by means of skin tests was found to be impaired only to a moderate extent when tested with streptokinase, mumps, and *Candida,* for example. Sensitization to new antigens, e.g., DNFB, however, cannot be readily achieved [14]. In in vitro studies the generation of cytotoxic T cells against alloantigens has been demonstrated [35].

Granulocytes are known to be important for defense against bacterial infection, and were found to be decreased in absolute numbers in many CLL patients. A comparison of patients dying from infection (group A) with patients dying from some other disease (group B) revealed that 72% of group A patients had granulocytopenia, as against 7% in group B. Furthermore, patients in group A exhibited hypogammaglobulinemia in 70% of cases, as against 26% in group B [76]. These data suggest a role of both defense mechanisms in infection in CLL.

Pathophysiological Model of Immunodeficiency

The immunological findings described above are compatible with a model (Fig. 2) that begins with an expanding B cell clone. These slowly expanding CLL B cells give a signal for

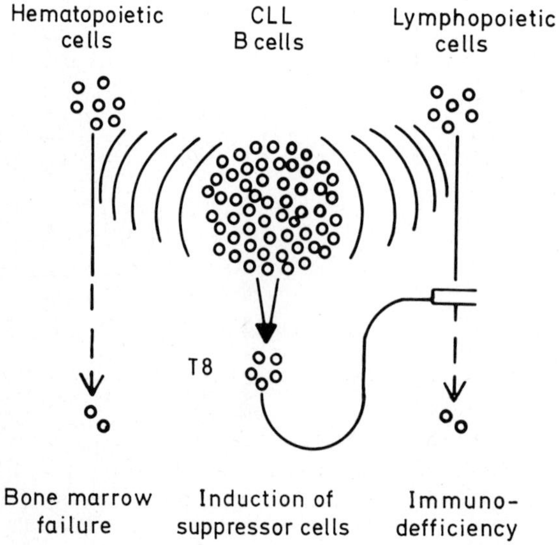

Fig. 2. Pathophysiological model for development of major clinical problems in CLL. The expanding monoclonal CLL B cells induce (>▸) T8 positive suppressor T cells, which have been shown to suppress (–[) differentiation (→) of normal B cells to plasma cells. Other branches of the immune system might be down-regulated by similar mechanisms, or both the cells of the immune system and of the hematopoietic system might be crowded out by the expanding CLL B cell clone

induction (>▸) of T8-positive, IgG Fc receptor-positive suppressor T cells, which is reminiscent of observations in in vitro studies with mitogen-stimulated or Epstein-Barr virus-transformed B cells [32]. While these suppressor cells are unable to control the malignant clone, normal B cells are effectively suppressed, resulting in an antibody deficiency syndrome. The suppressor cells increase as the disease progresses and the antibody deficiency becomes more pronounced. In addition to the functional blockade of normal B cell maturation, the overwhelming population of CLL B cells might simply crowd out the normal B cells (Fig. 2), in a similar process to that postulated as the basis of anemia, thrombocytopenia, and granulocytopenia in CLL.

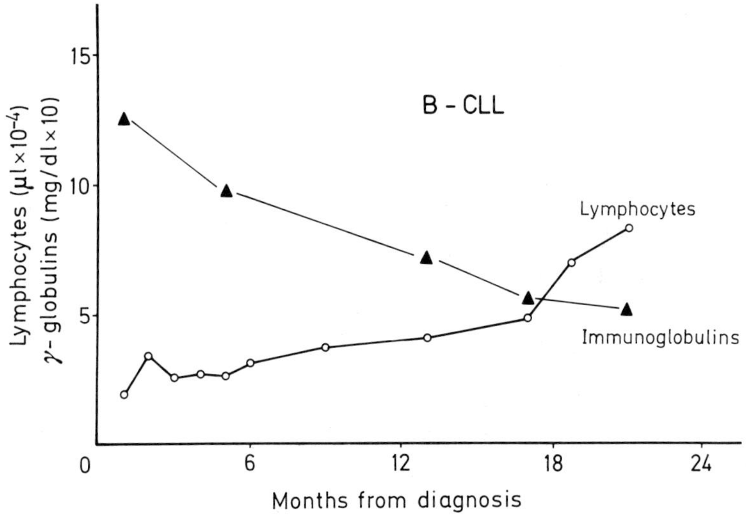

Fig. 3. Development of serum Ig and peripheral blood lymphocyte count in a patient with CLL. This case illustrates the typical development: lymphocyte counts increase while serum Ig levels decrease

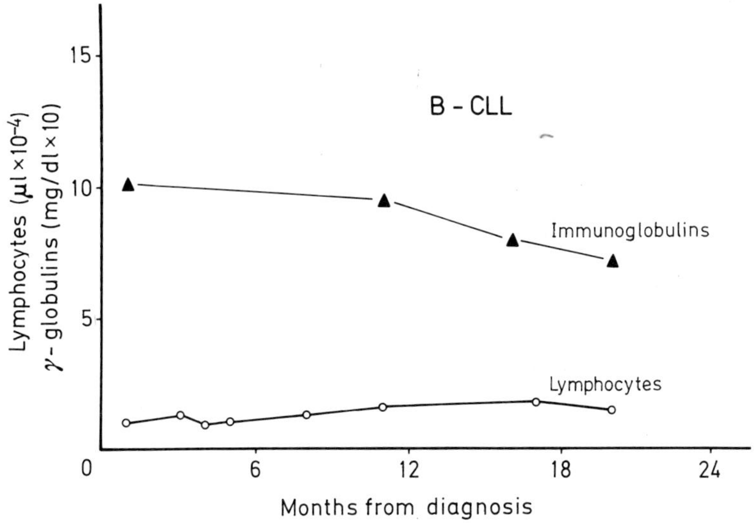

Fig. 4. Development of serum Ig and peripheral blood lymphocyte count in a patient with CLL. In this rare case, minimal expansion of the leukemic clone is observed. The continuous decline in serum Ig levels persists

In contrast to this assumption, a drastic reduction of the leukemic cell load by cytotoxic drugs leaves the antibody deficiency unaffected, but one might argue that normal B cells are damaged as well and are unable to take advantage of the free space. In favor of a role for suppressor T cells is the finding, still to be confirmed, that antibody production recovers after total-body irradiation [33], since suppressor T cells are known to be highly radiosensitive [48].

During the course of disease the Ig level continuously decreases while CLL leukemic cells increase (Fig. 3), but Ig levels also decrease in cases with minimal expansion of the leukemic cells (Fig. 4). The reason for the deficiency of the NK cell-IFN system is not yet clear.

The model outlined might serve as a guide for the design of new protocols that take into consideration the often fatal immunodeficiency in CLL.

Immunological Characterization of IC, PLL, and T CLL

The *immunocytoma* (or lymphoplasmacytoid lymphoma), in its initial description by Stein et al. [71], was characterized by a high Ig content of the lymph nodes and by the presence of plasmacytoid cells and of plasma cells in addition to CLL-like cells. The plasmacytoid IC cells contain abundant cytoplasmic Ig. This amount of cIg is readily detectable with conventional immunofluorescence techniques, in contrast to CLL, where cIg was detected only in one study [23] while another study demonstrated no cIg [44], probably reflecting different quantities of Ig and the use of assays differing in sensitivity. Intracellular Ig can be detected with the PAS reaction in the lymph node cells [45]. The Ig can be secreted, resulting in a serum Ig spike. If the Ig is IgM, the IC is of the type formerly termed Waldenström's disease. The cell surface phenotype can be similar to CLL i.e., sIg positive and T65 positive [53], but recently an MAB has been described (RF A-4) that reacts with secreting IC and with PLL, but not with CLL [20]. According to these morphological and functional characteristics IC can be placed within the B cell lineage between CLL and plasmocytoma.

As observed in CLL, polyclonal serum Ig levels decrease continuously in secreting as well as nonsecreting forms of IC [27, 74]. This decrease does not correlate with proliferation kinetics. We postulate that the pathophysiological model of Ig deficiency outlined for CLL (Fig. 1) also applies in IC.

The *PLL* of the B-type has a large lymphocyte (12 μm compared with 7 μm in CLL) with moderate amounts of cytoplasm, a prominent nucleolus, and strong expression of surface Ig. In contrast to B-CLL, these leukemic cells are reported to be negative for the monoclonal antibody-defined T cell antigen, T65, in all or most cases [13, 53], but they are reported to react with the FMC7 MAB [11] and RFA-4 MAB [20] and to be positive for mouse red blood cell receptors [44]. Few cases of PLL belong to the T cell lineage. PLL is a rare form of leukemic lymphoma and no data are available on the nonleukemic cells. Ig levels, however, have been observed to be decreased [19].

T-CLL is a rare form of leukemic lymphoma characterized by lack of production of surface or cytoplasmic Ig and by the presence of T cell markers such as SRBC receptor and T3 and T4 MAB-defined antigens [25, 30, 61, 79]. T-CLL cells can be representative of various types of normal T cell subsets. T-CLL in Japanese patients with helper phenotype and suppressor function [25, 83], with suppressor phenotype and function [57], with helper function [30], and with NK function [30] have been described. T-CLL is not usually accompanied by an antibody deficiency syndrome.

Cytokinetic Analysis

It was hypothesized very early that peripheral blood lymphocytes in CLL are long-lived, and Dameshek defined CLL as an "accumulative disease of immunologically incompetent lymphocytes" [15]. This assumption is supported by autoradiographic studies with infusions of radiolabeled thymidine, which demonstrated a that CLL B cells had a lifespan five times longer than that of normal lymphocytes [78]. In addition, however, CLL is also a proliferative disease; cytokinetic studies [17] demonstrated that ten times as many CLL cells as normal lymphocytes are produced per unit of time. This fact is somewhat obscured by the large number of nonproliferating CLL cells, which means that a small fraction of the total leukemic cell number forms the growth fraction.

The decreased cell decay and the increased fraction of proliferating cells results in exponential growth with a continuous increase of peripheral blood leukocyte counts and infiltration of all organs, especially bone marrow. The increase in the peripheral blood leukocyte count can be expressed as lymphocyte doubling time. This is simply determined by monthly measurement of leukocyte counts over 3–12 months. A graph is drawn with

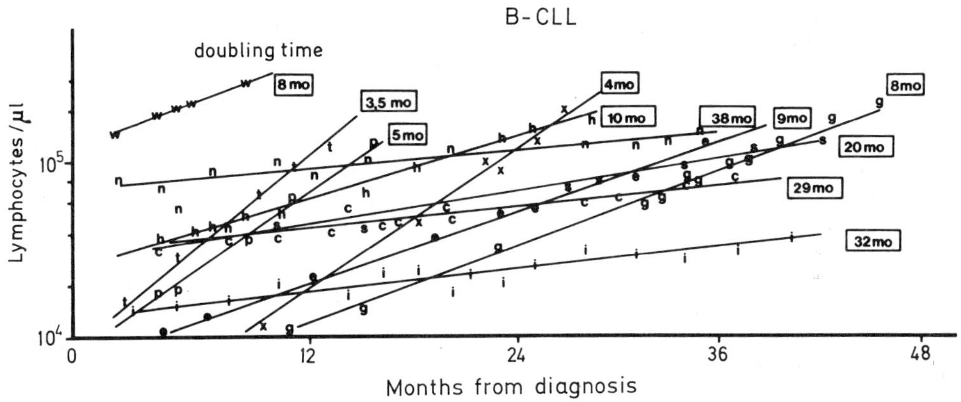

Fig. 5. Lymphocyte doubling in patients with B CLL without therapy. Time is plotted on the *x*-axis and lymphocyte count on the *y*-axis in log scale. Lymphocyte doubling times determined from these *curves* ranged from 3 to 38 months in the cases shown

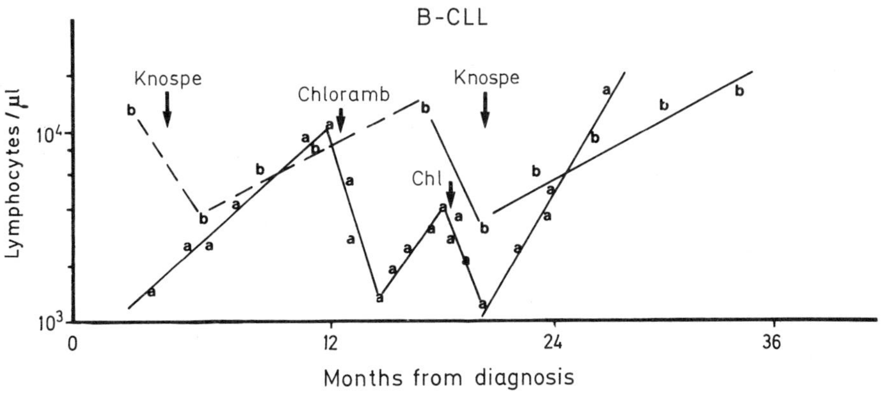

Fig. 6. Lymphocyte doubling in two patients (*a* and *b*) receiving therapy. Therapy has little or no effect on lymphocyte doubling

time in months on the x-axis and lymphocyte count on the semilogarithmic y-axis, giving a straight line, from which the time required for doubling of the lymphocyte count can be easily determined.

The doubling time is a constant, characteristic feature of any given patient; there are patients with very short doubling times and patients with very long doubling times (range 3–38, mean 15.1, months) (Fig. 5). The doubling time is usually not influenced by therapy

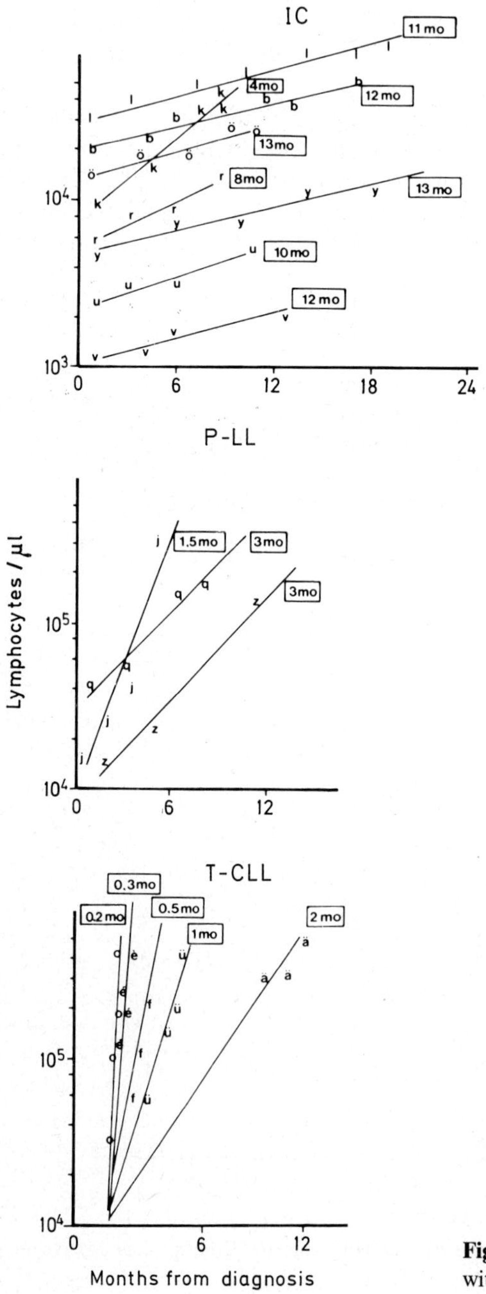

Fig. 7. Lymphocyte doubling in patients with IC, PLL, and TCLL

(Fig. 6); only in a few cases has a shortening of the doubling time been observed after cytotoxic therapy [6].

While extensive studies, including ^{3}H-thymidine labeling, have been performed in CLL, cytokinetic data for *IC, PLL* and *T-CLL* are restricted to determination of doubling times. For all types a constant expansion of leukemic cells can be observed with a medium doubling time of 10.3, 3.0, and 0.8 months for IC, PLL, and T-CLL, respectively (Fig. 7). In IC, as opposed to the other types, the lymphoma cells have a lower tendency to spread to blood and bone marrow and the tumor cells tend to expand within lymph nodes.

Prognosis and Staging

Survival times in *CLL* range from 1 to 20 years. With the complications induced by chemotherapy and with the inability to achieve what can be considered a complete remission, it is essential to have prognostic indicators to select patients at high risk. Table 1 summarizes prognostic indicators for CLL as assessed upon intial diagnosis. Most of these indicators reflect the leukemic load. A staging system according to Rai et al. [60] combines some of these indicators, which are lymphocytosis (stage 0), lymph node enlargement (stage I), spleno- and hepatomegaly (stage II), anemia (stage III), and thrombocytopenia (stage IV). Table 2 demonstrates that these stages correlate with survival, as initially described [60] and confirmed [4, 24].

A more concise staging system proposed by Binet et al. [3] (Table 3) also appears to give a good correlation with survival.

Table 1. Factor indicating poor prognosis in CLL and ICC

Factor	References
CLL	
Age over 70 years	[24, 26, 85]
Male sex	[2, 3, 85]
Large lymphoma and large spleen	[24, 72]
Enlarged liver	[2]
Leukocytosis > 50,000	[2, 85]
Anemia and thrombocytopenia	[24, 60]
Extensive bone marrow infiltration	[31, 85]
Diffuse type of bone marrow infiltration	[2, 22]
Diffuse type of lymph node infiltration	[74]
Low specific cell density	[29, 55]
Rapid lymphocyte doubling	[6, 75]
High proliferation index in blood cells and in lymph node cells	[29, 69, 70]
IC	
Stage IV, Ann Arbor pathological staging	[74]
B symptoms	[27]
Anemia and thrombocytopenia	[74]
Polymorphism in histology	[27]
Low specific cell density	[55]
High proliferation index	[69]

Table 2. Stages in B-CLL according to Rai et al. [60]

Stage	Characterized by	Mean survival from diagnosis (months)
0	Peripheral blood lymphocyte count higher than 15,000/mm^3, bone marrow infiltration greater than 40%	> 150
I	0 + enlarged lymph nodes	101
II	0 or I + enlarged liver and/or spleen	71
III	0 or I or II + anemia (Hb less than 11 g/dl)	19
IV	0 or I or II or III + thrombocytopenia (less than 100,000/mm^3)	19
All stages		71

Table 3. Stages in B-CLL according to Binet et al. [3]

Stage	Characterized by
A	Up to two areas enlarged[a] No anemia No thrombocytopenia
B	Three or more areas enlarged[a] No anemia No thrombocytopenia
C	Anemia (less than 10 g/dl) and/or Thrombocytopenia (less than 100,000/μl), with any number of enlarged areas

[a] Each of the cervical, axillary and inguinal lymph node areas (uni- or bilateral), the liver, and the pleen counts as one area

The stage of a CLL patient at diagnosis does not indicate how long it has taken for the disease to reach this stage; that is to say, the speed of disease progression is not covered. An easy estimate can be obtained by straightforward determination of lymphocyte doubling time, as described above. In a retrospective study a highly significant correlation was found between doubling time and survival time [76] (Fig. 8). Furthermore, rapid cell doubling is accompanied by rapid progression to higher clinical stages [6]. Thus for more adequate allocation of patients to risk groups the stage of disease and the doubling time appear to be important parameters. Since IC, PLL, and TCLL have a worse prognosis than CLL (see below) determination of the type of leukemia is also of great importance. The antibody deficiency as one outstanding indicator of the complex immunodeficiency observed in CLL at the time of diagnosis does not correlate with prognosis [24], in contrast to earlier reports [82]. This lack of correlation might be explained by the observation that the deficiency develops in almost all patients during the course of disease (Figs. 3 and 4). The importance of hypogammaglobulinemia for the fate of the patient is stressed by its three-fold higher frequency in patients dying from infection than in patients dying from other disease (see below). Since high susceptibility to infections appears to be the major

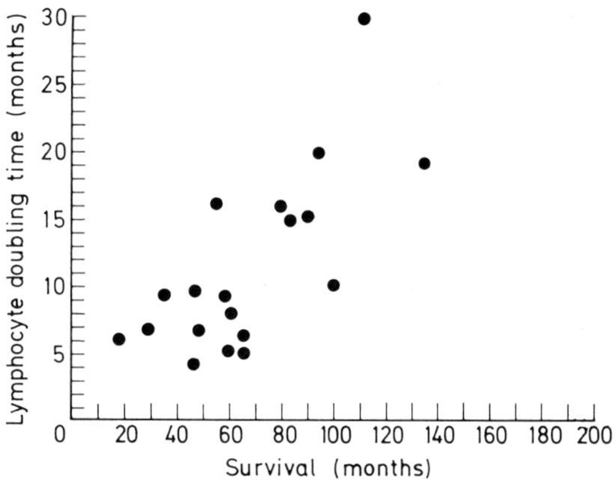

Fig. 8. Correlation of lymphocyte doubling time and survival. The Gehan test revealed a highly significant correlation with $r = 0.71$ and $P < 0.001$

cause of death in CLL, hypogammaglobulinemia and the additional deficiencies of the NK cell system, of IFN production, and of granulocytes or a combination of these appear to be crucial for the outcome of disease.

Prognosis in leukemic *IC*, which is comparable to that in CLL, was found to correlate with stages as defined by Rai [74]. In contrast to CLL, B symptoms (fever, night sweats, weight losse) are correlated with poor prognosis. Patients without generalization of lymphoma cells (5% of patients, with skin or spleen predominance) have a better prognosis. Finally, secretory and nonsecretory IC do not differ in prognosis. Compared with CLL the prognosis of IC is worse. For *PLL* and *T-CLL* no prognostic indicators other than the diagnosis itself are reported. A sequence of improving prognosis for these four entities would be the following: B-CLL – IC – PLL – T-CLL, which is similar to the sequence of increasing leukemia cell doubling in these conditions.

Clinical Course

As already indicated in a pathophysiological model (Fig. 2), the major clinical problems in *CLL* arise from bone marrow impairment resulting in anemia and thrombocytopenia, from the immunodeficiency resulting in susceptibilitiy of infections, and from the enlargement of infiltrated organs resulting in mechanical problems. The disease progresses unaffected by therapeutic maneuvers and the major cause of death in three separate studies has been infection (Table 4). In contrast, only 3%–8% of patients die of the direct consequences of bone marrow failure. Since the incidence of CLL peaks at 67 years, many patients pose additional problems of geriatric medicine and die of some disease other than CLL, e.g., cardiovascular disease.

Variants of the usual clinical course include anemia and thrombocytopenia either due to hypersplenism in splenomegalic forms or to autoantibodies. Further, two types of transformations, probably resulting from phenotypic changes of the B-CLL clone, are described, one type leading to PLL [8, 40] and the other to immunoblastic lymphoma (or DHL according to Rappaport), as first described by Richter [63].

The clinical course in *IC* in our experience is comparable to that in CLL, with a predominance of infections (10 deaths out of 23).

B-PLL and *T-CLL* are both characterized by a rapid course with short survival times and complications arising mainly from bone marrow infiltration and failure.

Table 4. Causes of death in CLL and IC

Cause of death	CLL			IC	
	Hansen [24] (n = 196)	Theml et al. unpublished (n = 100)	Trono et al. [81] (n = 50)	Theml et al. unpublished (n = 50)	Trono et al. [21] (n = 13)
Infection	63[a]	40	36	45	37
Marasmus	14	18	4	0	0
Bleeding	3	15	8	0	0
Infiltration of vital organs	0	0	4	18	7
Second malignancy	0	7	0	9	0
Independent disease	19	17	40	18	15
Unknown	1	8	8	9	28

[a] Given as percentage of total deaths

Feasibility of Obtaining Complete Remission

The intermediate aim in leukemia therapy is to achieve complete remission. For CLL this term was defined as the condition in which lymphocyte, thrombocyte, and erythrocyte counts are normal, bone marrow cytology is almost normal, and all lymphomas and all enlargement of organs have disappeared [39, 67].

This definition, however, does not include the complete elimination of the malignant clone evidenced for instance with idiotypic markers or the recovery of normal B cell function.

Recovery of B cell function, as reflected in sIg levels, has been reported to occur after total-body irradiation in 80% and 40% of cases [33, 62]. Kempin reported improvement of one Ig class only after intensive polychemotherapy in 15 of 49 patients. What is usually observed, however, is that after cytotoxic therapy sIg levels remain low or continue to decrease [21, 24, 39, 49, 66]. The impossibility of removing the malignant clone with the aggressive M2 protocol [39] is readily demonstrated by relapses occurring after 42 and 11 months with and without maintenance therapy, respectively.

The study by Kempin, who advocates such aggressive therapy, has to be interpreted with caution, since the study was not prospective or randomized, and was conducted in a selected group of patients with a historical control group. Finally, mortality due to infection was high in patients treated according to the M2 protocol, and its effect on survival was small. Kempin et al. [39] suggest that alternate protocols are needed for eradication of disease, but we must emphasize that complete remission induction with cytotoxic therapy is currently not a desirable aim.

Does Therapy Improve Survival?

For CLL, including the subtypes discussed in this chapter, it has been shown that responders to therapy with chlorambucil and steroids have a better prognosis than nonresponders (for review see [67]) with nonresponders found predominantly in advanced stages [3, 38, 41]. Controlled studies comparing matched patients treated and untreated are not available and several observations suggest a better prognosis for untreated patients [26, 28]. Further, patients who can be classified in a lower stage of disease after cytotoxic therapy than before do not acquire the better prognosis of the new stage [60, 67]. These observations are readily explained when it is taken into consideration that death in CLL results mainly from immunodeficiency and from geriatric disease, in both of which cytotoxic therapy is detrimental rather than helpful. In IC the situation is similar but less well documented, while for PLL and T-CLL the rapid progression justifies intense therapy which, however, is not convincingly efficient at present.

Rational Therapy of Leukemic Lymphomas

Chronic Lymphocytic Leukemia

The three major possibilities of treatment in CLL are cytotoxic chemotherapy, radiotherapy, and substitution.

Chemotherapy

The recommended standard strategy in treatment of CLL is to restrict cytotoxic therapy to reduction of the leukemic load in cases with bone marrow failure. Hence, only patients in stages III and IV [60] or C [3] are eligible for cytotoxic therapy. Furthermore, taking into account the aforementioned findings on doubling times, above it might be justifiable to treat any patients in earlier stages in whom a lymphocyte doubling time of less than 10 months indicates a rapid progression and incipient bone marrow failure.

The most widely used single agent is chlorambucil, which can lower lymphocyte counts to normal values in 75% of cases. The recommended dosage is 0.1–0.3 mg/kg daily for several weeks. The dosage is reduced by 50% when lymphocyte counts are reduced by 50%. Responses can be expected to be seen after 2–3 weeks and maximal effects after 8 weeks. One-third of the responders also experience an improvement of anemia and thrombocytopenia [24, 77].

Intermittent therapy with chlorambucil, according to Knospe et al. [41], appears to result in less suppression of hematopoiesis. This protocol involves dosing at 2-week therapy-free intervals, starting at 0.4 mg/kg and increasing by 0.1 mg/kg until response or bone marrow impairment is seen. Therapy is given for about 6 months with average total dosage of 8.3 (1.6–15.3) mg chlorambucil/kg and average single doses of 45 (20–83) mg. Complete remission were seen in 5 of 62 patients [41].

In cases with rapid course and nonresponsiveness to such therapy a COP regimen [1] can be tried, provided the patient is in good condition. Such therapy can induce 40% complete remissions and 28% partial remissions [46].

A much more aggressive regimen, the M2 protocol (vincristine, BCNU, cyclophosphamide, melphalan, prednisone) was used by Kempin et al. [39]. Complete remission was obtained in 17% and partial remission in 44% of patients. Three of seven patients who relapsed presented with acute myeloid leukemia; 80% of all deaths in this study were due to infection.

Radiotherapy

Radiotherapy is very effective in CLL in reducing the size of huge lymphomas and spleens with low total doses of 5–10 Gy, usually delivered as fractionated irradiation. Irradiation of the spleen with 0.2 Gy per session, besides reducing spleen size, can also effectively decrease lymphocyte numbers in peripheral blood [58] and increase hemoglobin values in one-third patients [77]. Irradiation of the mediastinal area has also been reported to give decreased lymphocyte counts and increased hemoglobin and thrombocyte levels, probably due to irradiation of lymph nodes and the blood pool in this area [62].
Extracorporeal irradiation of blood and leukopheresis can only be advocated for patients with excessive lymphocyte counts and resulting hyperviscosity syndrome. Total-body irradiation (0.05–0.1 Gy per session up to 1–2 Gy total dose) was reported to normalize all peripheral blood cell counts in one-third of patients, in addition to which many patients experienced an improvement of serum Ig values [33]. These studies need to be confirmed before such regimens can be considered for routine treatment and caution must be exercised since radiation damage of megakaryocytes can result in severe thrombocytopenia and bleeding.

Substitution

Substitution therapy in the case of bacterial infections, in addition to specific antibiotic therapy, can include the administration of Ig preparations and the infusion of granulocytes. Ig substitution is initiated in antibody-deficient patients as early as infection is apparent. In viral infections we use antiviral therapy and transfer factor with a good degree of success. Thrombocytopenia and anemia can be alleviated for a short period by substitution of the appropriate blood products. An effective adjunct to support therapy in elderly, often marasmic patients is, in our experience, substitution with adrenocorticotropic hormone (0.2 mg twice weekly), which enhances hematopoiesis in addition to improving general performance [76]. Substitution of erythrocytes and platelets is performed according to standard hematological rules but these measures should be applied even more selectively than in acute leukemia, since in CLL we are dealing with a chronic type of anemia and thrombocytopenia.

Immunocytoma

The most common type of *IC* is leukemic; some patients have normal white blood cell counts that still exhibit a monoclonal B cell population and discrete sparse bone marrow infiltration. This type of IC is similar to CLL in clinical management, in that complete removal of the malignant clone cannot be achieved. In IC patients, however, the clinical course is often more aggressive and B symptoms are more frequent, both events justifying early chemotherapy, even before hematopoiesis is impaired. Defective immune defense with a high incidence of infections in IC has also to be taken into consideration before institution of chemotherapy.
The recommended regimens include chlorambucil/prednisone or COP, as described for CLL. First results indicate that responders to therapy have a better prognosis than nonresponders [74]. Specific problems in IC are encountered (a) in secretory forms and (b) in forms with splenic dominance. Secretory IC (in most cases representing the former

entity of Waldenström's disease) can result in high serum Ig levels with hyperviscosity syndrome. Treatment consists of chemotherapy plus plasmapheresis.
To prevent recurrence of such a complication long-term maintenance therapy is recommended. In some cases of IC with splenic dominance, normalization of hematological parameters results after splenectomy, as in hairy cell leukemia. The disease can be stable for years after such treatment [14]. Large lymphomas and skin involvement respond well to radiotherapy (20 Gy) without local relapse.

Prolymphocytic Leukemia

PLL can currently be handled in a similar way to CLL, but chemotherapy, irradiation and splenectomy [10], and leukophoresis [9] bring only a transient response and the rapid course of the disease continues, so that few patients survive 1 year. Several new chemotherapeutic approaches have been tried. Catovsky et al. [10], using the CHOP regimen together with splenectomy, observed moderate responses. König et al. [42] achieved stable partial remission of 30 and 26 months in two patients with a HOP regimen (adriblastin 80 mg/m^2 day 1, vincristine 1.4 mg/m^2 day 1, prednisone 100 mg, days 1–5, with cycles repeated after a 3-week therapy-free interval until the maximum adriblastin dose of 500 mg/m^2 is reached).

T Chronic Lymphocytic Leukemia

T-CLL is characterized by rapid progression with bone marrow failure, while infections are less frequent. Chemotherapy with the COP regimen resulted in a complete remission for 20 months in one patient [54]. Usually, however, the response to chemotherapy, including the Knospe regimen, and to radiotherapy is poor. In the absence of any effective remission induction, in our experience a therapy with corticoids is able to slow the course of disease.
New therapeutic approaches are required for T-CLL. These might include the extensive use of antimetabolites or the use of monoclonal antibodies [50, 51]. Therapy that can be adapted for the lymphocyte subsets making up T-CLL might be advantageous, but at present information on these rare forms is limited.

Experimental Therapy

We have already pointed out that the improvement that can be achieved by therapy in CLL should be in balance with the side-effects of therapy. Alternate approaches to standard cytotoxic polychemotherapy are needed, approaches that take into consideration the proliferation kinetics and the defective defense mechanism in leukemic lymphoma. New therapeutic approaches that are not yet suitable for routine clinical treatment have been tried in the field of radiotherapy and immunology.
Total-body irradiation appears to be quite effective according to the first reports [33]. In addition to the reduction of leukemic B cells, a recovery of serum immunoglobulin levels has been reported. The latter effect, probably resulting from the elimination of radiosensitive suppressor T cells, could be very important, since immunodeficiency is responsible for the majority of life-threatening complications in CLL.

Interferon treatment in CLL might be expected to be effective, since in plasmacytoma the first clinical reports showed a response to treatment and in CLL interferon has been shown to increase the deficient NK cell activity. Clinical studies in malignant lymphomas including CLL, however, gave disappointing results with respect to lymphocyte counts [68]. Interferon treatment in CLL might still be useful in supporting the immune system and in improving long-term survival.

Monoclonal antibody (MAB) technology has revolutionized immunology, and early clinical trials with these highly specific reagents have been reported [51]. MAB specifically produced against the idiotype of lymphoma cells induced complete remission in one patient [52]. In a mouse model of B-CLL, antibodies against IgD in combination with cytotoxic therapy gave complete remission [43]. The use of T101 MAB against the T65 antigen for treatment of human BCLL resulted in only a transient reduction of lymphocyte counts [16]. Removal of suppressor T cells with MAB has not yet been reported but could be expected to improve immune defense. Such new approaches might give new stimulus to therapy in CLL, but we should keep in mind that the comparatively mild progression of the leukemia in many cases means that aggressive therapy with the goal of complete remission, is not justified.

References

1. Bagley CM Jr, DeVita VT Jr, Berard CW, Canellos GP (1972) Advanced lymphosarcoma: intensive cyclical combination chemotherapy with cyclophosphamide, vincristine, and prednisone. Ann Intern Med 76: 227–234
2. Bartl R, Frisch B, Burkhardt R, Hoffmann-Feser G, Demmler K, Sund M (1982) Predictive value of combined clinical staging and histologic bone marrow classification in chronic lymphocytic leukaemia. Br J Haematol 51: 361–376
3. Binet JL, Auquier A, Dighiero G, Chastang C, Piguet H, Goasguen J, Vaugier G, Potron G, Colona P, Oberling F, Thomas M, Tchernia G, Jacquillat C, Boivin P, Lesty C, Duault MT, Monconduit M, Belabbes S, Gremy F (1981) A new prognostic classification of chronic lymphocytic leukemia derived from a multivariate survival analysis. Cancer 48: 198–206
4. Boggs DR, Sofferman SA, Wintrobe MM, Cartwright GE (1966) Factors influencing the duration of survival of patients with chronic lymphocytic leucemia. Am J Med 40: 243
5. Boumsell L, Coppin H, Pham D, Raynal B, Lemerle J, Dausset J, Bernard A (1980) An antigen shared by a human T cell subset and B cell chronic lymphocytic leukemic cells. Distribution on normal and malignant lymphoid cells. J Exp Med 152: 229–234
6. Bremer K, Schmalhorst U, Grisar T, Jansen H, Mattheus-Selter J, Brittinger G (1980) Die prognostische Relevanz der verschiedenen Stadieneinteilungen und der Lymphozytenverdoppelungszeit bei der chronischen lymphatischen Leukämie. Verh Dtsch Ges Inn Med 86: 1072
7. Brittinger G, Schmalhorst U, Bartels H, Fülle HH, Gerhartz H, Gremmel G, Grisar T, Grupp HJ, Gunzer U, Huhn D, Koeppen K-M, Kubanek B, Leopold H, Löffler H, Löhr GW, Nowicki L, Rühl U, Schmidt M, Stacher A, Theml H, Lennert K (1981) Principles and present status of a prospective multicenter study of the kiel classification. Blut 43: 155
8. Brouet J-C, Preudhomme J-L, Seligman M, Bernard J (1973) Blast cells with monoclonal surface immunoglobulin in two cases of acute blast crisis supervening on chronic lymphocytic leukaemia. Br Med J IV: 23
9. Buskard NA, Catovsky D, Okos A, Goldman JJ, Galton DAG (1976) Prolymphocytic leukaemia: cell studies and treatment by leukapheresis. In: Loffler H (ed) Maligne Lymphome und monoklonale Gammopathien. Lehmann, München, pp 237–254
10. Catovsky D (1977) Hairy-cell leukaemia and prolymphocytic leukaemia. Clin Hematol 6: 245–268

11. Catovsky D, Cherchi M, Brooks D, Bradley J, Zola H (1981) Heterogeneity of B-cell leukemias demonstrated by the monoclonal antibody FMC 7. Blood 58: 406–408
12. Catovsky D, Miliani E, Okos A, Galton DAG (1974) Clinical significance of T-cells in chronic lymphocytic leukaemia. Lancet 1: 751–752
13. Caligaris-Cappio G, Gobbi M, Bofill M, Janossy G (1982) Infrequent normal B lymphocytes express features of B-chronic lymphocytic leukemia. J Exp Med 155: 623–628
14. Cone L, Uhr JW (1964) Immunological definiency disorders associated with chronic lymphocytic leukemia and multiple myeloma. J Clin Invest 43: 2241–2248
15. Dameshek W (1967) Chronic lymphocytic leukemia – an accumulative disease of immunologically incompetent lymphocytes. Blood 29: 566
16. Dillman RO, Shawler DL, Sobol RE, Collins HA, Beauregard JC, Wormsley SB, Royston I (1982) Murine monoclonal antibody therapy in two patients with chronic lymphocytic leukemia. Blood 59: 1036–1045
17. Dörmer P, Theml H, Lau B (1983) Chronic lymphocytic leukemia: a proliferative or accumulative disorder? Leuk Res 7: 1–10
18. Epstein LB, Cline MJ (1974) Chronic lymphocytic leukemia. Studies on mitogen-stimulated lymphocyte interferon as a new technique for assessing T lymphocyte effector function. Clin Exp Immunol 16: 553–563
19. Galton DAG, Goldman JM, Wiltshaw E, Catovsky T, Henry K, Goldenberg GJ (1974) Prolymphocytic leukaemia. Br J Haematol 27: 7–23
20. Gobbi M, Cligaris-Cappio F, Janossy G (1983) Normal equivalent cells of B cell malignancies: analysis with monclonal antibodies. Br J Haematol 54: 393–403
21. Gordon DS, Spira TJ (1977) Immunologic status of patients with chronic lymphocytic leukemia at presentation and in remission. Blood 50: 191 (abstract)
22. Gray JL, Jacobs A, Block M (1974) Bone-marrow and peripheral blood lymphocytosis in the prognosis of chronic lymphocytic leukemia. Cancer 33: 1169–1178
23. Han T, Ozer H, Bloom M, Sagawa K, Minowada J (1982) The presence of monoclonal cytoplasmic immunoglobulins in leukemic B cells from patients with chronic lymphocytic leukemia. Blood 59: 435–438
24. Hansen MM (1973) Chronic lymphocytic leukemia. Scand J Haematol Suppl 18
25. Hattori T, Uchiyama T, Toibana T, Takatsuki K, Uchino H (1981) Surface phenotype of Japanese adult T-cell leukemia cells characterized by monoclonal antibodies. Blood 58: 645–647
26. Heilmann E, Schreck B (1978/79) Prognose der chronischen lymphatischen Leukämie. Haematologica 12: 231–245
27. Heinz R, Stacher A, Pralle H, Theml H, Brunswicker F, Burkert M, Common H, Fülle HH, Grisar T, Grüneisen A, Herrmann F, Leopold H, Liffers R, Meusers P, Nowicki L, Nürnberger R, Rengshausen H, Rühl U, Schoengen A, Schmidt M, Wirtimüller R, Schwarze E-W, Brittinger G (1981) Lymphoplasmacytic/lymphoplasmacytoid lymphoma: a clinical entity distinct from chronic lymphocytic leukaemia? Blut 43: 183–192
28. Holmes FF, Westphal DM (1971) Survival in treated and untreated chronic lymphocytic leukemia 1942–1968. Oncology 25: 137
29. Huber C, Zier K, Michlmayr G, Rodt H, Nilsson K, Theml H, Lutz O, Braunsteiner H (1978) A comparative study of the buoyant density distribution of normal and malignant lymphocytes. Br J Hematol 40: 93
30. Huhn D, Thiel E, Rodt H, Schlimok G, Theml H, Rieber P (1983) Subtypes of T-cell chronic lymphatic leukemia. Cancer 51: 1434–1447
31. Inoshita T, Whiteside TL (1981) Imbalance of T-cell subpopulations does not result defective helper function in chronic lymphocytic leukemia. Cancer 48: 1754–1760
32. James SP, Yenokida GG, Graeff AS, Strober W (1983) Activation of suppressor T cells by autologous lymphoblastoid cells: a mechanism for feedback regulation of immunoglobulin synthesis. J Immunol 128: 1149–1154
33. Johnson RE (1970) Total body irradiation of chronic lymphocytic leukemia: incidence and duration of remission. Cancer 25: 523

34. Johnstone AP (1982) Chronic lymphocytic leukaemia and its relationship to normal B lymphopoiesis. Immunol Today 12: 343–348
35. Kabelitz D, Fink U, Reichert A, Rastetter J (1982) Alloantigen-induced suppressor and memory cells in chronic lymphocytic leukemia. Immunobiology 161: 457–463
36. Kay NE (1981) Abnormal T-cell subpopulation function in CLL: Excessive suppressor (Ty) and deficient helper (Ty) activity with respect to B-cell proliferation. Blood 57: 3
37. Kay NE, Johnson JD, Stanek R, Douglas SD (1979) T-cell subpopulations in chronic lymphocytic leukemia: abnormalities in distribution and in in vitro receptor maturation. Blood 54: 540–544
38. Keller JW, Knospe WH, Huguley CM, Moffitt S, Johnson L (1978) Treatment of chronic lymphocytic leukemia (CLL) with chlorambucil (CB) and prednisone (PRED) every two weeks. Blood 50: 256 (abstract)
39. Kempin S, Lee BJ, Thaler HT, Keziner B, Hecht S, Gee T, Arlin Z, Little C, Straus D, Reich L, Phillips E, Al-Medhiry H, Dowling M, Mayer K, Clarkson B (1982) Combination chemotherapy of advanced chronic lymphocytic leukemia: the M-2 protocol (vincristine, BCNU, cyclophosphamide, Melphalan, and prednisone). Blood 60: 1110–1121
40. Kjeldsberg CR, Marty J (1981) Prolymphocytic transformation of chronic lymphocytic leukemia. Cancer 48: 2447–2457
41. Knospe WH, Loeb V, Huguley CM (1974) Bi-weekly chlorambucil treatment of chronic lymphocytic leukemia. Cancer 33: 555–562
42. König E, Meusers P, Brittinger G (1979) Efficacy of doxorubicin in prolymphocytic leukemia. Br J Haematol 42: 487–488
43. Krolick KA, Uhr JW, Slavin S, Vitetta ES (1982) In vivo therapy of a murine B cell tumor (BCL1) using antibody-ricin a chain immunotoxins. J Exp Med 155: 1797–1809
44. Koziner B, Kempin S, Passe S, Gee T, Good RA, Clarkson BD (1980) Characterization of B-cell leukemias: a tentative immunomorphological scheme. Blood 56: 815–822
45. Lennert K (1978) Malignant lymphomas other than Hodgkin's disease. Springer, Berlin Heidelberg New York (Handbuch der speziellen pathologischen Anatomie und Histologie I, 3 B
46. Liepman M, Votaw ML (1978) The treatment of chronic lymphocytic leukemia with COP-chemotherapy. Cancer 41: 1664–1669
47. Martin PJ, Hansen JA, Siadak AW, Nowinski RC (1981) Monoclonal antibodies recognizing normal human T lymphocytes and malignant human B lymphocytes: a comparative study. J Immunol 127: 1920–1923
48. McMichael AJ, Sasazuki T (1977) A suppressor T-cell in the human mixed lymphocyte reaction. J Exp Med 146: 368–380
49. Miller DG, Karnofsky DA (1961) Immunological factors and resistance to infection in chronic lymphocytic leukemia. Am J Med 31: 748
50. Miller RA, Levy R (1981) Response of cutaneous T cell lymphoma to therapy with hybridoma monoclonal antibody. Lancet 2: 226–230
51. Miller RA, Maloney DG, McKillop J, Levy R (1981) In vivo effects of murine hybridoma monoclonal antibody in a patient with T-cell leukemia. Blood 58: 78–86
52. Miller RA, Maloney DG, Warnke R, Levy R (1982) Treatment of B-cell lymphoma with monoclonal anti-idiotype antibody. N Engl J Med 306: 517–522
53. Munker R, Thiel E, Kummer U, Rodt H, Thierfelder S (1983) Crossreaction of monoclonal anti-T-cell antibodies: implications for classifying B-cell leukemias. Blut 46: 1–6
54. Nair KG, Han T, Minowada J (1979) T-cell chronic lymphocytic leukaemia. Report of a case and review of the literature. Cancer 44: 1652–1655
55. Niederwieser D, Huber C, Lutz D, Weiser G, Theml H, Braunsteiner H (1982) Dichteverteilung menschlicher Lymphozyten. II. Dichteverteilungsmuster maligner Lymphozyten und prognostische Signifikanz bei Patienten mit Non-Hodgkin-Lymphomen. Blut 45: 385–394
56. Okamura J, LeTarte M, Stein LD, Sigal NH, Gelfand EW (1982) Modulation of chronic lymphocytic leukemia cells by phorbol ester: increase in Ia expression, IgM secretion and MLR stimulatory capacity. J Immunol 128: 2276–2280

57. Pandolfi F, Strong DM, Slease RB, Smith ML, Ortaldo JR, Herberman RB (1980) Characterization of a suppressor T-cell lymphocytic leukemia with ADCC but not NK activity. Blood 56: 653–660
58. Parmentier C, Schlienger M, Hayat M, Laugier A, Schlumberger JR, Mathe G, Tubiana M (1968) L'irradiation splenique dans le leukmies lymphocytaires chroniques decompensees. J Radiol 49: 187
59. Platsoucas CD, Galinski M, Kempin S, Reich L, Clarkson B, Good R (1982) Abnormal T-Lymphocyte subpopulations in patients with B cell chronic lymphocytic leukemia. An analysis by monoclonal antibodies. J Immunol 129: 2305–2312
60. Rai K, Sawitsky A, Cronkite EP, Chanana AD, Levy RN, Pasternack BS (1975) Clinical staging of chronic lymphocytic leukemia. Blood 46: 219–234
61. Reinherz EL, Nadler LM, Rosenthal DS, Moloney WC, Schlossman SF (1979) T-cell subset characterization of human T-CLL. Blood 53: 1066–1075
62. Richards F, Spurr C, Pajak T, Blake D, Raben M (1974) Thymic irradiation. An approach to chronic lymphocytic leukemia. Am J Med 57: 862
63. Richter MN (1928) Generalized reticular cell sarcoma of lymph nodes associated with lymphatic leukemia. Am J Pathol 4: 285–299
64. Robert K-H, Bird AG, Müller E (1979) Mitogen-induced differentiation of human CLL lymphocytes to antibody-secreting cells. Scand J Immunol 10: 447–452
65. Royston I, Omary MB, Trowbridge IS (1981) Monoclonal antibodies to a human T-cell antigen and Ia-like antigen in the characterization of lymphoid leukemia. Transplant Proc 13: 761–766
66. Rundles W (1972) Chronic lymphocytic leukemia. In: Williams WJ et al. (eds) Hematology. McGraw Hill, New York
67. Sawitsky A, Rai KR, Glidewell O, Silver RT (1977) Comparison of daily versus intermittent chlorambucil and prednisone therapy in the treatment of patients with chronic lymphocytic leukemia. Blood 50: 1049–1059
68. Siegert W, Theml H, Fink U, Emmerich B, Kaudewitz P, Huhn D, Böning L, Abb J, Joester K-E, Bartl R, Riethmüller G, Wilmanns W (1982) Treatment of non-hodgkin's lymphoma of low-grade malignancy with human fibroblast interferon. Anticancer Res 2: 193–198
69. Silvestrini R, Piazza R, Riccardi A, Rilke F (1977) Correlation of cell kinetic findings with morphology of Non-Hodgkin's malignant lymphomas. J Natl Cancer Inst 58: 499–504
70. Simonsson B, Nilsson K (1980) ^{3}H-Thymidine uptake in chronic lymphocytic leukaemia cells. Scand J Haematol 24: 169–173
71. Stein H, Kaiserling E, Lennert K, Parwaresch MR (1973) Makroglobulinbildende chronische lymphatische Leukämie ohne Markoglobulinämie. Klin Wochenschr 51: 389–396
72. Steinkamp RG, Lawrence JH, Born JL (1963) Long term experiences with the use of P^{32} in the treatment of chronic lymphocytic leukemia. J Nucl Med 4: 92
73. Theml H (1977) Die chronische lymphatische Leukaemie. In: Begemann H (ed) Handbuch der inneren Medizin II/6. Springer, Berlin Heidelberg New York
74. Theml H, Bartels H, Brittinger G, Common H, Dühmke E, Fülle HH, Gunzer U, Gyenes T, Heinz R, König E, Meusers P, Paukstat M, Pralle H, Lennert K, Feller AC, Köpcke W, Thieme C, Musshoff K, Stacher A, Herrmann F, Burger-Schüler A, Gremmel H, Gerhartz H, Koeppen K-M, Huhn D, Schoengen A, Nowicki L, Pees HW, Wannenmacher M, Schmidt M, Michlmayr G, Zettel R, Rühl U (to be published) Klinik und Prognose der Non-Hodgkin-Lymphome von niedrigem Malignitätsgrad: Ergebnisse einer multizentrischen prospektiven Studie an 1127 Fällen. Verh Dtsch Ges Inn Med 89
75. Theml H, Begemann H (1982) Therapeutische Ziele und Ansätze bei chronischer lymphatischer Leukämie im Alter. In: Stacher A (ed) Hämatologie im Alter. Urban and Schwarzenberg, Wien
76. Theml H, Begemann H, Rastetter J (1982) Erwägungen zur Therapie der chronischen Lymphadenosen auf dem Boden pathophysiologischer Daten. In: Scheurlen PG, Pees HW (eds) Therapie bösartiger Blutkrankheiten. Springer, Berlin Heidelberg New York

77. Theml H, Höft E, Helmbrecht H, Burger A, Brehm G, Kaboth W (1976) Der Stellenwert depletorischer Methoden in der Therapie von Nicht-Hodgkin-Lymphomen. In: Löffler H (ed) Maligne Lymphome und Monoklonale Gammopathien. Lehmann, München
78. Theml H, Trepel F, Schick P, Kaboth W, Begemann H (1973) Kinetics of lymphocytes in chronic lymphocytic leukemia: studies using continous ^{3}H-thymidine infusion in two patients. Blood 42: 623
79. Thiel E, Rodt H, Huhn D, Thierfelder S (1976) Decrease and altered distribution of human T-antigen on chronic lymphatic leukemia cells of T-type, suggesting a clonal origin. Blood 47: 723–736
80. Tötterman T, Nilsson K, Sundström C (1980) Phorbolester induced differentiation of chronic lymphocytic leukemia cells. Nature 288: 176–178
81. Trono D, Kapanci Y (1983) Les causes de mort en cas de lympho, myelome et maladie de Hodgkin. Schweiz Med Wochenschr 113: 701–708
82. Ultmann JE, Fish W, Osserman E, Gellhorn A (1959) The clinical implications of hypogammaglobulinemia in patients with chronic lymphocytic leukemia and lymphocytic lymphosarcoma. Ann Intern Med 51: 501
83. Yamada Y (1983) Phenotypic and functional analysis of leukemic cells from 16 patients with adult T-cell leukemia/lymphoma. Blood 61: 192–199
84. Ziegler HW, Kay NE, Zarling JM (1981) Deficiency of natural killer cell activity in patients with chronic lymphocytic leukemia. Int J Cancer 27: 321–327
85. Zippin C, Cutler SJ, Reeves WJ, Lum D (1973) Survival in chronic lymphocytic leukemia. Blood 42: 367–376

Management of Chronic Myelogenous Leukemia and Blastic Crisis

K. P. Hellriegel

II. Innere Klinik, Krankenhaus Moabit, Turmstrasse 21, 1000 Berlin 21, FRG

Definition

Chronic myelogenous leukemia (CML) is a neoplastic disease of the hematopoietic system that results from a mutation in a single pluripotential stem cell. The abnormal stem cell receives a growth advantage, while for unknown reasons the proliferation of regular hematopoiesis is inhibited. Excessive and unrestrained growth of blood progenitor cells leads to an accumulation of mature and immature cells in the peripheral blood and to clinical manifestations due to organ infiltrations by extramedullary hematopoiesis.

Pathophysiology

In comparison with other neoplasias CML has some unique features which are of importance for understanding pathophysiology as well as for selecting treatment.

1. CML proceeds in two completely different phases, a chronic one and an acute one. During the chronic phase, the disease follows a relatively benign course and is oligo- or asymptomatic. The proliferation of hematopoietic cells can be suppressed by cytotoxic drugs in most cases. Nevertheless, the disease irresistibly progresses to an accelerated phase after a variable number of months or years, eventually switching over to an acute phase in the majority of patients. After transition into the acute phase, which is characterized by a rise in the number of blasts and promyelocytes and – in most cases – by the occurrence of anemia and thrombocytopenia, treatment is largely ineffective. In this so-called blastic crisis (CML-BC) prognosis is extremely poor, and death results from inanition, organ infiltrations including extramedullary blastic tumors, infection, and hemorrhage.

2. CML is one of the few neoplasias which regularly show a chromosome abnormality, the *Philadelphia chromosome* (Ph^1). The Ph^1 is an acquired karyotypic abnormality which primarily occurs in a single stem cell and is characterized by a shortening of the long arms of chromosome 22 due to a translocation of chromosome material to the long arms of chromosome 9. This 9q+; 22q− translocation is the most frequent one, but translocations of the missing part of chromosome 22 have also been found to nearly all other chromosomes. Such patients do not show different clinical symptoms, course of disease, or prognosis. It is thus concluded that the break on chromosome 22 is of greater pathophysiological relevance than the type of translocation.

The Ph^1-positive cell clone gains a growth advantage, while the proliferation and maturation of normal hematopoiesis is limited. At diagnosis, the Ph^1 is mostly demonstrable in all dividing cells of erythro-, granulo-, and megakaryocytopoiesis. The finding that only one isoenzyme variant is demonstrable in B- und T-lymphocytes of CML patients with glucose-6-phosphatedehydrogenase heterogeneity supports the hypotheses of alteration of the pluripotential stem cell and of unicellular origin [16].

In the chronic phase, chromosome abnormalities in addition to the Ph^1 are found in about 30% of cases. The chromosome abnormalities consist of gain, loss, or structural rearrangements of particular chromosomes. The chromosome number per mitosis commonly ranges between 45 and 47 [34]. Some of these abnormalities appear to be of prognostic value, whereas the prognostic significance of others is ambiguous. A loss of the Y chromosome seems to be a rather good sign. A second Ph^1, an additional no. 8, or other translocations in addition to the 9; 22 have been observed during longer phases of the stable chronic disease. Each change of the karyotype, especially the appearance of an i (17q), however, should be regarded as a bad sign. Data from cytogenetic studies indicate that the clonal evolution may be extramedullary, preferentially in the spleen. Additional chromosome abnormalities are observed in the spleen. Additional chromosome abnormalities are observed in higher frequency in spleen than in marrow cells and may precede cytological and clinical evidence of blastic crisis.

In blastic crisis, the incidence of chromosome abnormalities in addition to the Ph^1 is about 80% [34], the number of chromosomes per mitosis commonly ranging between 47 and 52; hypodiploidy is found in only 5% of cases. The gain of certain chromosomes occurs far more often than loss. The chromosome abnormalities most often observed in the acute phase of CML are additional no. 8 (95/242), i (17q) (56/242), additional no. 17 (11/242), additional no. 19 (38/242), additional Ph^1 (73/242), and i (Ph^1) (5/242).

Chromosome losses most frequently affect no. 7 (5/242) and No. 17 (4/242). Rowley, who collected these data, stresses the point that the occurrence of additional chromosome abnormalities is not random, but follows distinct principles. In patients with only a single new chromosome abnormality, and additional no. 8, an i (17q), and an additional Ph^1 are found with approximately the same frequency; a supernumerary no. 17 or no. 19, however, only once in this series. None of the 242 patients had the combination of an i (17q) with an additional no. 19 or an additional Ph^1. Patients with myeloid-type CML-BC seem to have a hyperdiploid karyotype, whereas those with lymphoid type show a pseudodiploid or hypodiploid chromosome pattern [7, 34].

The specificity of the Ph^1 is a subject of controversy in the literature. Observations of Ph^1-negative CMLs exist, as well as descriptions of the Ph^1 in other myeloproliferative disorders or other neoplasias than CML. The percentage of Ph^1-negative CMLs in the various publications seems mainly to be influenced by the proportion of atypical cases included in the evaluation. The proportion of Ph-negative CMLs and the specifity of the Ph^1 lastly depend upon how narrowlyor broadly the term CML is defined.

Ph^1-negative CML represents an ill-defined disease with a more heterogeneous hematological and clinical picture, less effective therapeutic posibilities, and a poorer prognosis.

The clinical significance of the Ph^1 leads to a better definition of CML and to the recognition of atypical courses of CML. More precise definition of the disease and the resultant more homogeneous patient groups allow better comparability of symptoms, clinical and hematological findings, and therapeutic response and enable the elaboration of prognostic factors.

Prognostic Factors in CML

Hepatomegaly
Splenomegaly
Initial hemoglobin
Platelet count
Myelofibrosis
Karyotype
Fever

Current concepts for improving the prognosis of CML

1. Prevention of BC
2. Postponement of BC
3. Suppression of first symptoms of BC
4. More effective treatment of BC

3. CML is one of the so-called minimal deviation tumors: Although in the majority of patients all erythrocytes, white blood cells, and platelets are derived from the leukemic Ph^1-positive cell clone, these cells are able to carry out their physiological functions. In addition morphologically the blood and bone marrow cells do not differ significantly from normal erythrocytes, leukocytes, and platelets and their precursor cells.
4. In CML, a true remission, i.e. an at least temporary repopulation of the bone marrow by normal, Ph^1-negative hematopoiesis as in acute leukemias, has only rarely been achieved by the usual treatment procedures. In most patients, such treatment leads only to a suppression of the leukemic cell clone; although the clinical symptoms disappear and the blood picture becomes normal, the Ph^1 persists in the bone marrow cells.
Stem cell investigations and cytogenetic findings in intensively treated CML patients give evidence that at least in some patients, as well as the leukemic, Ph^1-positive cell clone, Ph^1-negative, apparently normal, but inactivated stem cells are present which are able to repopulate the marrow after treatment-induced bone marrow hypoplasia [9, 13, 17, 36]. The only effective measure for preventing the occurrence of CML-BC is the eradication of the Ph^1-positive cell clone. Long-lasting Ph^1 negativity of the bone marrow cells has so far been reliably obtained only by isogeneic and allogeneic bone marrow transplantation [10, 15, 20, 32, 37, 42].

Approaches to prevention of CML-BC

1. Attempt to eliminate the Ph^1 cell clone e.g., L15 protocol, MSKCC New York
2. Attempt to eliminate numerical aneuploidies e.g., Brodsky and Fuscaldo, Philadelphia
3. Bone marrow transplantation – isogeneic
   – allogeneic

Clinical and Hematological Characteristics

The partially excessive leukocytosis with shift to the left in the peripheral blood is of diagnostic significance. In the differential count, mature granulocytes predominate and progenitor cells are present in diminishing frequency. The question of the specificity of the Ph^1 has been discussed above.
Findings which are usually present but not obligatory are splenomegaly, hypercellular bone marrow, diminished index of leukocyte alkaline phosphatase, basophilia, and eosinophilia. Variable symptoms are anemia, hepatomegaly, thrombocytosis, and thrombocytopenia.

The incidence of distinct symptoms at diagnosis, course and duration of the disease, and prognostic parameters have been studied in 117 patients with Ph^1-positive CML [22, 24]. Of these patients, 81% showed more or less heavy splenomegaly, only 19% having no palpable spleen enlargement. The liver was of normal size in 32%, more or less enlarged in the others. Anemia was present in 55% of the male and 76% of the female patients. The platelet counts were more than 450×10/l in 28% of cases, less than 100×10^9/l in only 10%. Thrombocytopenia is apparently an unusual finding in CML at diagnosis.

Bone marrow biopsies were performed in 54 patients at diagnosis [24]. Of the 54, 22 patients did not show a condensation of reticulin or collagen fibers, 32 had varying degrees of fibrosis: 23 had patchy, perivasal fibrosis, seven moderate diffuse fibrosis, and two advanced fibrosis with a dense lattice of fibers. The median survival time of the 117 patients was 36 months, but the expectancy of live was highly variable from patient to patient and ranged between some months and more than 10 years [22]. Of the prognostic factors, the platelet count seems to be the most reliable. Patients with thrombocytosis at diagnosis had an unfavorable prognosis [22].

Therapy of the Chronic Phase

The conventional treatment procedures tend to prolong the chronic phase as long as possible in order to postpone the deleterious blastic crisis. These procedures lead above all to an improvement of quality of life for the patient, but are unable to actually prevent blastic crisis. The more aggressive treatment regimens are intended to prevent CML-BC and are thus aimed at cure.

Monochemotherapy

Busulfan leads to a normalization of the blood picture lasting 6–12 months, in isolated cases even up to 10 years [17], in about 90% of patients in the chronic phase. The disease responds well to busulfan until the metamorphosis occurs. Different studies have shown that no other monotherapy is superior to busulfan or can even achieve a comparably high remission rate and duration [26, 29, 35, 39]. This is even true for *6-mercaptopurine* and *thioguanine* [26, 39], which in our experience can still be administered successfully in busulfan-resistant patients. *Dibromomannitol* has not fulfilled the expectations placed in it. The treatment-free interval after normalization of the blood picture is shorter, the side-effects are the same, and after busulfan resistance it seems to be ineffective [6, 30].

Hydroxyurea turned out to be effective in busulfan resistancy and at the beginning of metamorphosis [8]. Preliminary results in a small group of patients suggest a prolongation in survival, but a proper prospective clinical trial is needed [2].

Melphalan has a profound effect on platelets, and its use can be recommended in patients with high platelet counts but relatively low leukocyte counts.

Irradiation

Irradiation was one of the first treatment procedures in CML, being introduced at the turn of the century. Both total-body irradiation and local irradiation, i.e., over the spleen or the long bones, have improved clinical condition and quality of life. Several trials have, however, demonstrated the superiority of alkylating agents [12, 21, 33].

Splenectomy

The pros and contras of splenectomy in CML have been discussed for decades. Some years ago it was reasoned that the spleen is important in the evolution of CML and that the blastic crises might be postponed by splenectomy. In the meantime, several studies have confirmed the obvious assumption that a change in motivation for splenectomy does not change the results, i.e., that splenectomy can neither prevent the occurrence of blastic crises nor significantly influence survival time [13, 27, 38, 41]. The patients only benefit from the fact that symptoms due to massive splenectomy in the terminal phase of the disease do not occur. The conception is still that splenectomy is possible in CML, but by no means generally necessary. It is indicated when the wellbeing of a patient is disturbed by displacement symptoms of a heavily enlarged spleen or by repeated spleen infarctions or when hypersplenism occurs.

Leukapheresis

Leukapheresis using a blood cell separator is indicated in patients with extremely high leukocyte counts who are jeopardized by disturbances of the microcirculation, by leukocyte thrombi, and by hyperuricemia and hyperuricosuria due to chemotherapy-induced rapid cell destruction. In this group of patients, a rapid improvement of clinical condition can frequently be achieved by reduction of the leukemic cell mass [3, 25]. The use of continuous flow centrifugation is also indicated in patients with contraindications for chemotherapy and radiation. Leukapheresis is thus the treatment of choice in *pregnant women* with CML requiring therapy.

Since leukapheresis may hardly influence the course of the disease, and since the costs in staff and in material are high, it seems unsuited for continuous treatment.

Leukapheresis is also used to collect stem cells for the purpose of *autologous stem cell transfusion* (autologous bone marrow transplantation). In the chronic phase stem cells are collected, cryopreserved, and stored. Following the occurrence of blastic crisis and the conditioning of the patients, the stem cells are thawed and retransfused in order to bring them back into the chronic phase [18, 19]. As evident as this principle is in theory, it unfortunately does not work in practice: in most patients blast cells appear rather soon after an apparently successful autograft [19], so that no significant prolongation of life is obtained.

Multiple-Drug Chemotherapy

In order to improve the prognosis and to prevent CML-BC, several groups have performed trials with irradiation and/or polychemotherapy with or without splenectomy [13, 36, 41]. In some patients, true remissions with temporary Ph^1 negativity were achieved. The proportion of patients and cells becoming Ph^1 negative strongly correlates with the intensity of treatment. The best results were obtained with the L5 protocol of MSKCC [13], where those patients with partial, temporary Ph^1 negativity had a longer median survival time than the nonresponders (> 60 vs. 34 months). Since the responders are only a minority and the survival time of the individual CML patient shows a high variability (a few months to > 10 years), the question of whether or not the responders are per se a collective with a more favorable prognosis remains unanswered.

Another approach to the prevention of CML-BC is a treatment protocol which aims to eliminate newly developing cell clones. In most patients with CML-BC, additional chromosome aberrations beyond the Ph^1 are seen. These aberrations can precede the cytological manifestation of blastic crisis by months. There is evidence that prognosis can be improved if multiple-drug chemotherapy is initiated on the detection of such aneuploidies [4], but these results need confirmation by a randomized prospective study.

Bone Marrow Transplantation

Long-lasting Ph^1 negativity of the bone marrow cells has only been demonstrated after bone marrow transplantation. The successful transplantations of four identical twins in the chronic phase [15] encouraged transplantation not only of twins, but also of HLA-identical siblings [10, 20, 32, 37, 42]. From 12 identical twins transplanted in Seattle in the chronic phase, eight were clinically well and Ph^1 negative 18–62 months after grafting. In the same group, five of nine patients transplanted in the chronic phase with an HLA-identical sibling as donor were alive and Ph^1-negative 2–27 months after grafting; the four died of interstitial pneumonia in the postgrafting period.

Transplantation in the acute phase is associated with a much higher mortality, although a few patients become Ph^1 negative, enter long-term remissions, and may be cured [14, 42].

It now appears that at least some patients with CML can be cured by (isogeneic and allogeneic) bone marrow transplantation. In possible candidates for bone marrow transplantation, the decision on exactly when to intervene remains a major problem. It is difficult to recommend this life-threatening therapy to a patient early in the disease when he has a good chance of staying in the chronic phase for years; on the other hand, the chance of cure diminishes significantly when the patient suddenly makes the transition into the acute phase. It is therefore recommended to carry out transplantation in the chronic phase or at the first appearance of unfavorable prognostic signs [10, 20, 32, 37, 42].

Therapy of the Acute Phase

CML-BC can be influenced very little by therapy. The median survival time is only about 8–12 months, independent of whether the antineoplastic chemotherapy employed is especially aggressive of relatively mild. Several prognostic parameters rather seem to influence the individual expectation of life, for example the percentage and cell type of blasts (myeloid, lymphoid, or both; occurring simultaneously or sequentially) and the extent of myelofibrosis and of extramedullary infiltrations. A factor impeding the presentation of therapeutic recommendations and the comparing of results, especially of therapy studies, is the lack of an exact definition of CML-BC. Signs and symptoms are extremely variable, the transition from the chronic phase to the phase of metamorphosis and on to CML-BC is continuous [1, 40]. Definitions of the response criteria are different, especially of the terms "partial remission" and "improvement". Not only is the case material influenced by prognostic factors, but the groups are also small and thus inhomogeneous. In spite of these reservations, the predominant cell type should be taken into consideration when the therapeutic procedure is chosen.

Prognostic factors in CML-BC

Type of blasts
Percentage of blasts
Karyotype
Platelet count
Myelofibrosis
Organomegaly

Cell types in CML-BC

Myeloid:
- myeloblasts
- promyelocytes
- proerythroblasts
- megacaryoblasts

Lymphoid:
- non-B-cell, non-T-cell properties
- T-cell properties

Mixed:
- simultaneously
- sequentially

Vincristine in combination with prednisone was shown to be effective in about one-third of patients with CML-BC, especially in those with the lymphoid type [5, 27, 28, 31]. The favorable effect of the combination was confirmed by prospective studies [4, 13, 16]. There was a strong correlation between the demonstration of terminal desoxynucleotidyl-transferase (TDT) and response rate: only those patients whose leukemic cells were TDT positive achieved a remission. The combination of vincristine and prednisone is at present regarded as the treatment of choice in the lymphoid type of CML-BC [28], although the remissions are mostly of short duration.

In the myeloid type of CML-BC, only few remissions can be achieved with multiple-drug chemotherapy regimens developed for the treatment of acute leukemia, including anthracyclines and cytosine-arabinoside. Some published data, as well as our own experience, argue in favor of the use of the combination of vindesine and prednisone [23], which is able to produce complete remissions. In comparison with more aggressive chemotherapy protocols, for example the randomized trial of the CALGB [11], the remission rates are in the same range but the survival time is somewhat shorter. In contrast to the more aggressive regimens, the rate and the intensity of side effects are lower and thus the quality of life is better. Although this regimen does not definitely improve the prognosis of the majority of patients with CML-BC, those patients who enter remission mostly profit. The survival times of three patients with complete remission were 23, 34, and 78 weeks and of four patients with partial remission 7, 9, 18, and 25 weeks [23, 24].

Conclusions

Despite all the progress in antineoplastic therapy, the survival time of most patients with CML has not been significantly changed in the past decades. For the majority of patients, the diagnosis of CML is a sentence of death. CML is still one of the most malignant diseases, and CML-BC is the neoplastic disease with the most unfavorable prognosis of all. Bone marrow transplantation has opened the chance of cure for a minority of the patients, but all other therapeutic procedures are only able to improve the quality of life, not to prolong survival or to prevent blastic crisis.

In the chronic phase of the disease, busulfan remains the treatment of choice and the standard for measuring the efficacy of other therapeutic programs, until randomized studies demonstrate the superiority of alternative therapeutic modalities. In the blastic phase, the vinca alkaloids might not be surpassed by other drugs or drug combinations.

References

1. Baikie AG (1966) Chromosomes and leukaemia. Acta Haematol (Basel) 36: 157
2. Bolin RW, Robinson WA, Sutherland J, Hamman RF (1982) Busulfan versus hydroxyurea in long-term therapy of chronic myelogenous leukemia. Cancer 50: 1683
3. Borberg H, Hellriegel KP, Müller T (1976) Die Leukapheresebehandlung chronischer myeloischer Leukämien zur Leukozytensubstitution bei akuten Leukämien. In: Stacher A, Höcker P (eds) Erkrankungen der Myelopoese. Urban & Schwarzenberg. München Berlin Wien. p 294
4. Brodsky I, Fuscaldo KE (1978) CML: Correlation of cytogenetic and clinical data and survival in patients in an experimental program (Abstr.) 17th Congr Int Soc Hemat, Paris, vol I., p 86
5. Canellos GP, DeVita VT, Whang-Peng J, Carbone PP (1971) Hematologic and cytogenetic remission of blastic transformation in chronic granulocytic leukemia. Blood 38: 671–679
6. Canellos GP, Young RC, Nieman PE, DeVita VT Jr (1975) Dibromomannitol in the treatment of chronic granulocytic leukemia: A prospective randomized comparison with busulfan. Blood 45: 197
7. Canellos GP, DeVita VT, Whang-Peng J, Chabner BA, Schein PS, Young RC (1976) Chemotherapy of the blastic phase of chronic granulocytic leukemia: Hypodiploidy and response to therapy. Blood 47: 1003–1009
8. Canellos GP (1977) The treatment of chronic granulocytic leukaemia. Clin Haematol 6: 113
9. Chervenick PA, Ellis LD, Pan SF, Lawson AL (1971) Human leukemic cells: in vitro growth of colonies containing the Philadelphia (Ph^1) chromosome. Science 174: 1134
10. Clift RA, Buckner CD. Thomas ED, Doney K, Fefer A, Neimann PE, Singer E, Sanders J, Stewart P, Sullivan KM, Deeg J, Storb R (1982) Treatment of chronic granulocytic leukaemia in chronic phase by allogeneic marrow transplantation. Lancet 2: 621–623
11. Coleman M, Silver RT, Pajak TF, Cavalli F, Rai KR, Kostinas JF, Glidewell O, Holland JF (1980) Combination chemotherapy for terminal-phase chronic granulocytic leukemia: Cancer and leukemia group B studies. Blood 55: 29–36
12. Conrad RG (1973) Survival in chronic granulocytic leukemia. Arch Intern Med 131: 684
13. Cunningham I, Gee T, Dowling M, Chaganti R, Bailey R, Hopfan S, Bowden L, Turnbull A, Knapper W, Clarkson B (1979) Results of treatment of Ph^1 + chronic myelogenous leukemia with an intensive treatment regimen (L-5 protocol). Blood 53: 375
14. Doney K, Buckner CD, Sale GE, Ramberg R, Boyd C, Thomas ED (1978) Treatment of chronic granulocytic leukemia by chemotherapy, total body irradiation and allogeneic bone marrow transplantation. Exp Hematol 6: 738
15. Fefer A, Cheever MA, Thomas ED, Boyd C, Ramberg R, Glucksberg H, Buckner CD, Storb R (1979) Disappearance of Ph^1-positive cells in four patients with chronic granulocytic leukemia after chemotherapy, irradiation and marrow transplantation from an identical twin. N Engl J Med 300: 333
16. Fialkow PJ, Denman AM, Singer J, Jacobson RJ, Lowenthal MN (1978) Human myeloproliferative disorders: Clonal origin in pluripotent stem cells. In: Clarkson B et al. (eds.) Differentiation of normal and neoplastic hematopoietic cells. Cold Spring Harbor Conferences on Cell Proliferation, vol 5. Cold Spring Harbor Laboratories, Ann Arbor, p 131

17. Finney R, McDonald GA, Bailie AG, Douglas AS (1972) Chronic granulocytic leukaemia with Ph^1-negative cells in bone marrow and a ten year remission after busulphan hypoplasia. Br J Haematol 23: 283
18. Goldman JM, Catovsky D, Galton DAG (1978) Reversal of blast-cell crisis in C.G.L. by transfusion of stored autologous buffy-coat cells. Lancet 1: 437
19. Goldman JM, Catovsky D, Goolden AWG, Johnson SA, Galton DAG (1981) Buffy coat autografts for patients with chronic granulocytic leukaemia in transformation. Blut 42: 149
20. Goldman JM, Banghan ASJ, McCarthy DM, Worsley AM, Hows JM, Gordon-Smith EC, Catovsky D, Batchelor J, Goolden AWG, Galton DAG (1982) Marrow transplantation for patients in the chronic phase of chronic granulocytic leukaemia. Lancet 2: 623–625
21. Gollerkeri MP, Shah GB (1971) Management of chronic myeloid leukemia: A five-year survey with a comparison of oral busulfan and splenic irradiation. Cancer 21: 596
22. Hellriegel KP (1977) Die Bedeutung des Philadelphia-Chromosoms für die Klinik und Differentialdiagnose der chronischen myeloischen Leukämie. In: Schumacher K, Grosser KD (eds) Aktuelle Probleme der Inneren Medizin. Schattauer, Stuttgart New York, p 65
23. Hellriegel KP (1981) Therapie der Blastenkrise der chronischen myeloischen Leukämie. Ergebnisse einer Phasen-II-Studie mit Vindesin. Folia Haematol (Leipz) 108: 699
24. Hellriegel KP (Unpublished results)
25. Höcker P (1976) Die Behandlung der chronischen myeloischen Leukämien mittels Leukapheresen. In: Stacher A, Höcker P (eds) Erkrankungen der Myelopoese. Urban & Schwarzenberg, München Berlin Wien, p 368
26. Huguley CM, Grizzle J, Rundles RW, Bell WM, Corley CC Jr, Frommeyer WB Jr, Greenberg BG, Hammack W, Herion JC, James GW III, Larsen WE, Loeb V, Leone LA, Palmer JG, Wilson SJ (1963) Comparison of 6-mercaptopurine and busulfan in chronic granulocytic leukemia. Blood 21: 89
27. Ihde DC, Canellos GP, Schwartz JH, DeVita VT (1976) Splenectomy in the chronic phase of chronic granulocytic leukemia. Ann Intern Med 84: 17
28. Janossy G, Woodruff RK, Pippard MJ, Prentice G, Hoffbrand AV, Paxton A, Lister TA, Bunch C, Greaves MF (1979) Relation of "lymphoid" phenotype and response to chemotherapy incorporating vincristine-prednisolone in the acute phase of Ph^1 positive leukemia. Cancer 43: 426–434
29. Kaung DT, Close HP, Whittington RM, Patno ME (1971) Comparison of busulfan and cyclophosphamide in the treatment of chronic myelocytic leukemia. Cancer 27: 608
30. Levin WC, Mims CH, Haut A (1974) Dibromomannitol (NSC-94100): A clinical study of previously treated patients with refractory chronic myelocytic leukemia and blastic transformation. Cancer Treat Rep 58: 223
31. Marks SM, Baltimore D, McCaffrey R (1978) Terminal transferase as a predictor of initial responsiveness to vincristine and prednisone in blastic chronic myelogenous leukemia. N Engl J Med 298: 812–814
32. McGlave PB, Arthur D, Kim TH, Ramsay N, Hurd DD, Kersey J (1982) Successful allogeneic bone marrow transplantation for patients in the accelerated phase of chronic granulocytic leukaemia. Lancet 2: 627–629
33. Report of the Medical Research Council's Working Party for Therapeutic Trials in Leukaemia (1968) Chronic granulocytic leukaemia: Comparison of radiotherapy and busulphan therapy. Br Med J 1: 201
34. Rowley JD (1979) Ph^1-positive leukaemia, including chronic myelogenous leukaemia. Clin Haematol 9: 55
35. Rundles RW, Grizzle J, Bell WN, Corley CC, Frommeyer WB Jr, Greenberg BG, Huguley CM Jr, James GW, Jones R Jr, Larsen WE, Loeb V, Leone LA, Palmer JG, Riser WH Jr, Wilson SJ (1959) Comparison of chlorambucil and myleran inchronic lymphocytic and granulocytic leukemia. Am J Med 27: 424
36. Smalley EV, Vogel J, Huguley CJ Jr, Miller D (1977) Chronic granulocytic leukemia: Cytogenetic conversion of the bone marrow with cycle-specific chemotherapy. Blood 50: 107

37. Speck B, Gratwohl A, Nissen C, Osterwalder B, Müller M, Bannert P, Müller HJ, Jeannet M (1982) Allogene Knochenmarktransplantation bei chronischer myeloischer Leukämie. Schweiz Med Wochenschr 112: 1419–1420
38. Spiers ASD, Baikie AG, Galton DAG, Richards HGH, Wiltshaw E, Goldman JM, Catovsky D, Spencer J, Peto R (1975) Chronic granulocytic leukaemia: Effect of selective splenectomy on the course of disease. Br Med J 1: 175
39. Spiers ASD, Galton DAG, Kaur J, Goldman JM (1975) Thioguanine as primary treatment for chronic granulocytic leukaemia. Lancet 1: 829
40. Spiers ASD (1977) The clinical features of chronic granulocytic leukaemia. Clin Haematol 6: 77–95
41. Tura S, Baccarani M, Zaccaria A, Santucci AM (1976) The role of splenectomy in the therapy of chronic myeloid leukemia In: Stacher A, Höcker P (eds) Erkrankungen der Myelopoese. Urban & Schwarzenberg, München Berlin Wien, p 375
42. Thomas ED (1982) Marrow transplantation for patients with leukemia. In: Baum SJ, Ledney GD, Thierfelder S (eds) Experimental hematology today. Karger, Basel München Paris London New York Sydney, p 137

*Allogeneic Bone Marrow Transplantation in Leukemia**

H.-J. Kolb

Gesellschaft für Strahlen- und Umweltforschung mbH, Institut für Hämatologie, Abteilung Immunologie, Ingolstädter Landstrasse 1, 8042 Neuherberg/Oberschleissheim, FRG

Introduction

Over the past 20–30 years there has been considerable progress in the treatment of acute leukemia. In the majority of children with acute lymphoblastic leukemia (ALL) a cure is a possibility with intensive combination chemotherapy and prophylactic treatment of sanctuary sites [64, 90, 103] such as the central nervous system. The prognosis for patients with acute nonlymphocytic leukemia (ANL) is less favorable. However, complete remissions can be achieved in a majority and long-term survival in a minority of patients with severely myelotoxic treatment regimens [45, 138, 143]. In contrast to acute leukemia, the prognosis of chronic myeloid leukemia [CML] has changed little with modern chemotherapy [105].

Since the 1950s the possibility of treating leukemia with bone marrow transplantation has stimulated investigations in laboratory animals [6] and early trials in human patients [13]. The particular options made possible by bone marrow transplantation include the administration of otherwise lethal doses of total-body irradiation [65] and/or myelosuppressive chemotherapy [95] and the antileukemic effect of a graft-versus-host reaction [6, 12, 136]. Thomas and co-workers have worked out many of the preconditions for allogeneic marrow transplantation in dogs [111]. They have pioneered marrow transplantation for the treatment of leukemia [112] and severe aplastic anemia [113], and their success has stimulated an increasing number of clinical investigators to become active in this field. Briefly, the most important principles of allogeneic marrow transplantation derived from studies in dogs are: (a) host-versus-graft and graft-versus-host reactions can be controlled if the donor is a sibling matched for antigens of the major histocompatibility complex (MHC) [39]; (b) the dose of about 10 Gy total-body irradiation is well tolerated and is sufficient for engraftment of allogeneic marrow [111]; and (c) prophylactic administration of methotrexate after grafting can prevent fatal graft-versus-host disease (GvHD) in MHC-matched transplants [108]. Thus, most transplants have been carried out with marrow of HLA-identical siblings in leukemic patients prepared with an antileukemic and immunosuppressive regimen including total-body irradiation (TBI) with about 10 Gy in the body midline. The most widely used regimen consists of cyclophosphamide (60 mg/kg body weight) given on 2 days (days 5 and 4 before transplantation) and TBI on the day before transplantation [114], and methotrexate starting the day after transplantation. For unknown reasons success has been rare in older patients. Therefore most transplant centers have excluded patients older than 40 years. The current results of allogeneic marrow

* The work described in this paper was supported by Deutsche Forschungsgemeinschaft grant SFB 37 (subproject E4/E8) and by Euratom grant no. BIO-D-089-721

transplantation for various forms and stages of leukemia are summarized below, as are the problems and future directions of allogeneic marrow transplantation in the treatment of leukemia.

Results of Marrow Transplantation from HLA-Identical Siblings

Most experience has been accumulated with bone marrow transplantation from siblings with an identical HLA genotype. The family members are typed for HLA-A, -B, and -C with lymphocytotoxic antisera; identity of HLA-D is demonstrated by mutual nonreactivity in mixed leukocyte cultures. HLA antigens of one chromosome constitute an HLA haplotype and are inherited together. Donor and recipient possess the same *HLA* genotype if they have inherited the same paternal and maternal *HLA* haplotype.

Acute Leukemia

Grafting in Leukemic Relapse

For ethical reasons patients with leukemic relapse, most of whom were refractory to conventional chemotherapy, were the candidates for the first attempts at allogeneic marrow transplantation. Antileukemic and immunosuppressive preparation consisted of high-dose cyclophosphamide (CY) [55, 96], total-body irradiation (TBI) [112], or some combination of such drugs as BCNU (biochlorethyl nitrosourea), cytosine arabinoside (Ara-C), thioguanine (6-TG) and CY (BACT) in high doses [50]. The survival was less than 4 months in most patients and only very few survived. Only one patient treated with TBI by the Seattle group has survived [112]. Early recurrence of leukemia has been a frequent cause of failure. For improvement, the combination of CY and TBI has been used by the Seattle group in a larger number of patients (Table 1). Of 100 patients who have received transplants, 13 remained in continuous remission for more than 5 years [114]. Similar results were reported by other groups. However, the probability of leukemic relapse was still 60%–70%.

Even more intensive chemotherapy including daunorubicin, 6-TG, Ara-C (SCARI [131]) or Ara-C and BCNU (CRAB [75]), (BAC-TBI [63]) was added to CY and TBI in attempts to decrease the relapse rate. In general, these regimens were quite toxic and did not improve survival. Another attempt to increase the antileukemic effect of the preparative regimen was the increase of the radiation dose with fractionation of TBI [18, 23]. So far, variations of the conditioning regimen have not improved survival to a major extent, although none of these variations has been compared with the CY-TBI regimen in a controlled study.

The combination of CY and busulfan was investigated in patients with ANL by Santos as an alternative to TBI, with success in some patients [96]. This preparatory regimen may be less effective in ALL because of the frequent involvement of sanctuary sites for chemotherapy.

In this group of patients mortality within 3 months is about 30%–60% (Table 1) and depends on the clinical condition. The most frequent causes of death were interstitial pneumonia, GvHD and leukemic relapse [114].

Table 1. Allogeneic marrow transplantation in leukemic relapse

Preparative regimen	No. of patients					Follow-up time	References
	Studied	Surviving > 3 months	Dead from		Surviving in remission (%)		
			Leukemia	Other causes			
CY[a]	9	4	8	1	0	–	[55]
BACT	6	3	1	5	0	–	[55, 76]
CY[b]	24	–	12	12	0	–	[130]
CY[b] + BU	15	–	2	11	2 (13)	10–21 months	[130]
TBI[c]	10	2	5	4	1 (10)	> 10 years	[112]
CY[d] + TBI[c]	100	49	31	56	13 (13)	6–10 years	[114]
CY[d] + TBI[c] (ALL only)	26	19	13	9	4 (15)	> 3 years	[115]
CY[d] + TBI[c]	29	–	12	12	5 (17)	2–5 years	[9, 10]
CY[d] + TBI[c]	17	6	2	14	1 (6)	> 6 years	[107]
CY[d] + TBI[c]	11	6	4	6	1 (9)	> 4 years	[98]
SCARI	33	13	3	25	5 (15)	> 5–6 years	[132]
CRAB	11	3	4	7	0	–	[75]
BAC-TBI	18	10	9	5	4 (22)	> 2.5–5 years	[63]
CY + FTBI[e] ANL	23	15	8	9	6 (26)	> 2–4 years	[18]
CY + FTBI[f] ALL	41	27	22	10	3 (7)	> 1.5–2 years	[23]

The day of transplantation is designated day 0, days before transplantation as days −1, −2, etc.
CY[a], cyclophosphamide 45 mg/kg on days −4, −3, −2, and −1; *CY*[b], cyclophosphamide 50 mg/kg on days −5, −4, −3, and −2; *TBI*[c], total-body irradiation, single dose of 9.2–10 Gy in body midline on day −1, dose rate 4.5–12 cGy/min; *CY*[d], cyclophosphamide 60 mg/kg on days −6 an −5; *BU*, busulfan, 8–20 mg/kg over 4–8 days prior to CY[b]; BACT, CY[a] + BCNU bis-chlorethyl nitrosourea) 200 mg/m^2 on day −2 + Ara-C (cytosine arabinoside) 100 mg/m^2 × 5 every 12 h on days −4, −3, −2, and −1 + 6-TG (thioguanine) 300 mg/m^2 × 5 every 12 h on days −4, −3, −2, and −1; SCARI, CY[d], + TBI[c] + daunorubicin 60 mg/m^2 on 3 days; + Ara-C 600 mg/m^2 on 5 days + 6 TG 300 mg/m^2 every 12 h on days; CRAB, BCNU 200 mg/m^2 on day −6 + CY, 50 mg/kg on days −6, −5, −4, −3 + Ara-C 100 mg/m^2 every 12 h × 7, on days −6, −5, −4, −3 + TBI as single dose of 7.5 Gy with a dose rate of 25 cGy/min on day −1; BAC + TBI, BCNU 200 mg/m^2 on days −12 and −11 + Ara-C 200 mg/m^2 per day × 5 as continuous infusion from day −11 thru −7 + CY[d] + TBI[c]; CY + FTBI[e], CY 60 mg/kg on days −10 and −9 + FTBI (fractionated total-body irradiation) with 2 Gy × 6 on days −5 thru 0 with a dose rate of 5–8 cGy/min; CY + FTBI[f], GY 60 mg/kg on 2 consecutive days + TBI with 6 × 2 Gy, 7 × 2 Gy, 7 × 2.25 Gy, 7 × 2.5 Gy, 14 Gy in 2 days or 15 Gy in 6 days

Grafting in Remission Following Relapse

A second or subsequent remission can be induced in most patients with ALL and some patients with AML who have relapsed during maintenance therapy. However, these remissions are usually short, and further relapses are inevitable with conventional chemotherapy. The results of marrow transplantation in patients with relapsed leukemia have indicated that it may be possible to cure leukemia in a minority of patients even at this advanced stage. Therefore attempts were made to improve the results by transplantation during a second or subsequent remission. During remission the chance of eliminating the malignant clone by this procedure may be better, since the tumor load is smaller and the patient is in a better clinical condition. A concurrent trial of marrow transplantation for ALL in relapse or in second to fourth remissions was reported by Thomas et al. [114].

Survival was 32% in patients receiving grafts in remission and 15% in patients receiving grafts in relapse, but recurrences of leukemia occurred with similar frequency in both groups. These results indicate that the complications of transplantation were more easily controlled in remission, but that eradication of the leukemic clone is not easier. The proportion of patients surviving in remission was no higher when fractionated TBI with 14 Gy given in 7 daily fractions of 2 Gy was used instead of a single dose of 10 Gy for preparation [24]. In children with ALL in second or subsequent remission chemoradiotherapy and marrow transplantation was compared with conventional chemotherapy. The grafted children survived significantly better than those treated conventionally [58].

Second remissions can be achieved only in a minority of patients with ANL. Consolidation of second remissions of ANL with chemoradiotherapy and allogeneic marrow transplantation was successful in about 30% of the patients, a similar proportion to that attained in ALL [19]. In ANL patients a variety of complications including GVHD, interstitial pneumonitis, infections, toxicity, and leukemic recurrences was the cause of failures, whereas recurrence of leukemia was the predominant cause of failure in patients with ALL.

Grafting in First Remission

The majority of children with ALL can be cured by conventional chemotherapy including prophylaxis against CNS leukemia. The results of chemotherapy in childhood AML are inferior, but a substantial proportion of these patients remain in remission for prolonged periods. In adults, remission rates of acute leukemia are generally lower and in the majority of cases remissions are of limited duration.

It was again first shown by the Seattle Group that allogeneic marrow transplantation in the first remission provides the best chance for eradication of leukemia. Relapse was observed in only 6 of 75 patients treated in this way [10] (Table 3) and more than 85% of surviving patients remain in remission [117, 118]. About 50% of such patients survive longer than 4 years and may be cured [118]. The probability of survival is even higher in patients aged less than 20 years, and lower in patients older than 30 years. Fractionated TBI can be expected to be less toxic than TBI given as a single dose. Survival was superior in a group of patients given fractionated TBI instead of a single dose [119].

Several transplant groups have confirmed the possibility of eradicating leukemia in first remission with similar results. Concurrent comparative trials were reported by the groups at the Royal Marsden Hospital, London, the University of California-Los Angeles, and the

Table 2. Allogeneic marrow transplantation for acute leukemia in second or subsequent remission

Groups	No. of patients					Follow-up time	References
	Studied	Surviving > 3 months	Dead from		Surviving in remission (%)		
			Leukemia	Other causes			
ALL, 2nd–4th remission							
CY^{d} + TBI^{c}	22	20	12	3	7 (32)	> 3–5 years	[115, 116]
CY^{d} + $FTBI^{f}$ (7 × 2 Gy)	12	10	4	2	4 (33)	> 21–33 months	[24]
CY^{d} + $FTBI^{g}$ (hyperfractionated)	13	–	1	3	9 (69)	> 2–25 months	[31]
CY^{d} + TBI^{c} (children)	24	24	12	3	9 (38)	> 17–55 months	[58]
CT^{h} + TBI	32	–	7	6	19 (59)	> 1–24 months	[7, 59]
ANL, 2nd remission							
CY^{d} + TBI^{c}	14	10	3	5	6 (43)	> 4–63 months	[19]
CY^{d} + $FTBI^{e}$ (6 × 2 Gy)	10	4	1	7	1 (10)		
CY^{d} + $FTBI^{g}$ (hyperfractionated)	14	–	3	4	7 (50)	> 8 months	[31]
AL							
CY + TBI	21	–	9	5	7 (33)	> 13–40 months	[9, 10]
	10	–	1	3	5 (50)	> 1–28 months	[139]
	9	7	4	1	4 (44)	> 7–21 months	[107]

Abbreviations as in Table 1

Sloan-Kettering Memorial Institute, New York. Patients less than 40 years of age with an HLA-identical sibling as marrow donor received grafts following CY and TBI as consolidation of the first remission. The control patients were treated with conventional chemotherapy and/or immunotherapy [30, 46, 80]. These studies have not yet been concluded. Essentially, the survival rate at 2 years has been similar in the transplant group and in the chemotherapy group, but the relapse rate has been lower in the transplant group [30, 46]. The Royal Marsden Hospital group observed better survival of the transplant group at more than 2 years [66, 80].

There is general agreement that allogeneic marrow transplantation is not indicated in childhood ALL during the first remission. In contrast, the role of allogeneic marrow grafting in ALL of adults is under discussion. ALL of the B cell type has the worst prognosis, acute undifferentiated leukemia and ALL of the T cell type with a high number of blasts have a rather unfavorable prognosis; but ALL with c-ALL antigen may have a more favorable prognosis even in adults [57] (see pp 182–203). Very encouraging results with allogeneic marrow grafts in first remission of ALL have been reported by Barrett and co-workers [7].

The main causes of failures of marrow transplantation in first remission are interstitial pneumonitis with or without GVHD and infections. If these problems can be solved the survival rate may rise to about 85%.

Chronic Myeloid Leukemia (CML)

The course of chronic myeloid leukemia (CML) is characterized by a chronic phase, in which the disease can be easily controlled, and a terminal transformed phase resembling acute leukemia, which in the majority of cases is resistant to current chemotherapy. The terminal phase of CML may have a sudden onset which justifies in the term "blast crisis". It can also develop more gradually, in which case an "accelerated phase" precedes terminal blast transformation (see pp 259–268).

The median survival of patients in the chronic phase treated with conventional chemotherapy is about 3 years [105]. Between 23% and 40% of patients die of their disease each year [105] and only very few patients live 10 years or more. The survival of patients in the transformed phase is usually less than 6 months and only a minority of such patients respond transiently to chemotherapy [61]. Eradication of the disease with high-dose chemotherapy, TBI, and allogeneic marrow transplantation has been tried, first in the transformed phase and more recently in the chronic phase.

Grafting in the Transformed Phase

Allogeneic marrow transplantation in the transformed phase was complicated in one series by fatal infectious complications including interstitial pneumonia [33]. In the majority of the remaining patients the leukemic population could not be eradicated [33]. Long-term survival can be achieved in less than 20% of patients [120]. In contrast, isolated patients are reported by various groups, in whom a return to the chronic phase was achieved by means of conventional chemotherapy after which the disease could be eradicated by high-dose chemotherapy, TBI, and allogeneic marrow transplantation [21, 27, 34, 67, 133]. However, only a minority of patients in the transformed phase respond to conventional chemotherapy, and marrow transplantation at an earlier stage may be indicated for the majority of patients for whom a suitable donor is available.

Table 3. Allogeneic marrow transplantation for acute nonlymphocytic leukemia in first remission

References	No. of patients			Probability (%) of		Follow-up time
	Studied	With leukemic relapse	Surviving in remission	Relapse	Survival in remission	
Thomas et al. [117, 118, 119]	75	6	38	15	54	1–6 years
Blume et al. [9, 10]	28	3	17	–	–	11–58 months
Powles et al. [80, 83, 86]	53	8	32	22	55	4–56 months
Dinsmore et al. [31]	19	2	10	–	–	Median 9 months
Kensey et al. [60]	17	2	12	23	64	14–60 months

Table 4. Allogeneic marrow transplantation for chronic myeloid leukemia

References	Studied	No. of patients			Follow-up time (months)
		With relapse[c]	Dead from other causes	Surviving in remission[c]	
Transformed phase					
Doney et al. [33]	10	1	9	0	–
Thomas et al. [120]	27	–	–	7	≥ 2–41
Accelerated phase					
McGlave et al. [67]	9[a]	1	2	6	≥ 4.5–12.5
Curtis et al. [27]	1[a]	–	–	1	> 18
Vernant et al. [133]	1[a]	–	–	1	> 16
Champlin et al. [21]	4 (1)[a]	1	1	2	> 5, > 14
Doney et al. [33, 34]	6 (1)[a]	1	4	1	15.5 (median)
Chronic phase					
Clift et al. [25]	10	–	4	6	≥ 13–36
Doney et al. [34]	1[b]	–	1	0	–
Goldmann et al. [49]	12	–	2	10	≥ 3–16
Speck et al. [106]	8	–	2	6	≥ 5–20
Champlin et al. [21]	4	–	–	4	≥ 3–20
Curtis et al. [27]	4	–	1	3	≥ 4–18
	1[b]	–	1	0	–

[a] Patients in second chronic phase after remission from blast crisis
[b] Patients aplastic after busulfan therapy
[c] Relapse, reappearance of Ph^1-positive cells; remission, disappearance of Ph^1-positive cells

Grafting in the Accelerated Phase

Many patients experience an accelerated phase before entering the terminal transformed phase. It is characterized by a change in the previously stable clinical course with fever, night sweats, progressive leukocytosis unresponsive to previous chemotherapy, and the evolution of new cytogenetic abnormalities. At this stage the prognosis is poor because of impending transformation, but intensive chemotherapy can effectively suppress newly formed clones [17]. The results of allogeneic marrow transplantation reported by different groups are variable [33, 67]. The best results were reported by the University of Minnesota group, with 7 of 9 patients surviving [67]. The main causes of failure were infections, particularly interstitial pneumonia, and leukemic relapse [33, 67]. Most probably the chances of cure with allogeneic transplantation decrease as the accelerated phase progresses. The best chances can be expected with transplants early in acceleration, when additional chromosomal alterations are found without clinical symptoms.

Grafting in the Chronic Phase

Allogeneic marrow transplantation in the chronic phase of CML was encouraged by the following observations: first, 8 of 12 patients remained in complete remission of CML with disappearance of the Ph^1 chromosome following treatment with CY, TBI, and marrow from an identical twin donor [40]; second, transplant-related complications were predictable on the basis of experience with patients who had received grafts in first remission from ANL [117].

At present, more than 80 HLA-identical transplants have been reported [21, 25, 34, 49, 106, 144]. The survival at 1 year is about 75% [144]. The causes of failure have been infections, interstitial pneumonia, and GVHD. Leukemic relapse has not been observed [144], but the observation time is short for the great majority of patients. The indication for allogeneic transplantation is primarily influenced by the motivation of the patient after considering the hazards of transplantation. Many questions regarding allogeneic transplantation in CML remain to be answered, such as the risk or benefit of splenectomy with respect to infections and GVHD and the risk of interstitial pneumonia in relation to the cumulative dose of busulfan.

Other Forms of Hematologic Malignancy

Experience with high-dose chemotherapy, TBI, and marrow transplantation in the treatment of other forms of hematologic malignancy is limited to a few patients with disseminated lymphoma, acute myelosclerosis, poor-risk multiple myeloma, and hairy cell leukemia. One of three patients with Burkitt's lymphoma and one of two patients with T cell lymphoma survived in remission for more than 1 year following allogeneic transplantation [75]. Four of eight patients with disseminated non-Hodgkin's lymphoma refractory to conventional combination chemotherapy survived in complete remission following high-dose chemotherapy, TBI, and marrow from identical-twin donors [1]. Reversal of myelosclerosis was reported in four evaluable patients with acute myelosclerosis who received marrow transplants from HLA-identical siblings [94, 104, 142]. Similarly, myelofibrosis in a patient with CML disappeared within 5 months of allogeneic transplantation [68]. A patient with progressive hairy cell leukemia has been cured by chemotherapy with dimethylmyleran and CY, TBI, and infusion of marrow and buffy coat from an identical-twin donor [22]. This indicates the sensitivity of hairy cell leukemia to chemoradiotherapy and the absence of an environmental defect. In contrast, a patient with progressive multiple myeloma could not be cured by this procedure [78]. Most probably myeloma cells are less sensitive to the cytoreductive schedule.

Results of Marrow Transplantation from Other Donors than HLA-Identical Siblings

Only 20%–30% of patients have an HLA-identical sibling, the majority of patients lacking such a genotypically HLA-identical donor. Successful transplants from partially HLA-matched family members or unrelated persons were first reported in children with severe combined immune deficiency [77]. A few transplants had been successful in leukemic patients despite reactivity between donor and patient in MLC [37, 42]. A larger series of partially HLA-matched transplants was reported by the Seattle group [26, 51]. Donors were phenotypically HLA-identical parents; in some cases both parents had the same *HLA* haplotype. In other cases donor and recipient differed in either *HLA-D* or *HLA-A* and/or *-B* of one *HLA* haplotype as a consequence of *HLA-B/D* recombination or homozygosity. Of 29 such patients, 12 survived longer than 5 months, including eight of 12 patients who received grafts in remission [51]. In a recent follow-up of the Seattle group involving 80 patients, most of whom had received grafts after relapse, a plateau of 20% survivors was reported, with the longest survivor living for 5 years after grafting [121]. The survival rate in a subgroup of patients with ANL treated by BMT in first remission was about 45%. Therefore the results are not significantly worse than those in patients who received grafts from HLA-identical siblings. The causes of death were no different from those in HLA-identical siblings, with the possible exception of graft failures occurring in a minority of patients with HLA-mismatched donors [51]. One patient was successfully treated with marrow from an HLA-compatible unrelated donor [52]. In this case the *HLA* types were rather common – *HLA-A3-B7* and *HLA-A1-B8* – with a high linkage disequilibrium.

In 35 patients marrow from family donors was used, most of them sharing one *HLA* haplotype and differing in most antigens of the second haplotype, by the Royal Marsden Hospital team [81]. They received cyclosporin A (CsA) instead of MTX for prophylaxis of GVHD. Of 23 patients under the age of 30 years, 11 survive, whereas all 12 patients older than 30 years died. Twelve patients developed an adult respiratory distress syndrome and six died. Leukemic relapse was observed in 4/34 patients, as against 15/76 patients grafted with HLA-identical marrow [71]. Marrow grafts across major histocompatibility barriers have a strong antileukemic effect in animal models [14], but a similar effect remains to be demonstrated in human patients. Marrow transplantation across HLA incompatibility barriers may be more successful in patients under the age of 20 years.

Problems

The survival of patients for many years in unmaintained remission gives reason to hope that the disease can be cured [116]. However, many patients still succumb to the disease or to complications of its treatment. Major complications of the treatment are GVHD, interstitial pneumonitis, and infections. The host-versus-graft reaction resulting in failure of engraftment or rejection of the graft has not been a frequent problem with marrow transplantation for leukemia, in contrast to aplastic anemia [114]. The more vigorous immunosuppressive preparation, including TBI, and the previous chemotherapy for remission induction could explain the better suppression of the host-versus-graft reaction. Marrow from HLA-incompatible donors may be rejected more frequently [51]. Adverse effects of chemotherapy and TBI to vital organs may be particularly serious for patients in a poor clinical condition [114]. The value of more intensive chemotherapy for preparation of the recipient is limited by such adverse effects [63, 75, 131]. Cardiac failure following transplantation is not rare in older patients or patients who have received a high cumulative dose of anthracyclines [98]. Leukoencephalopathy is a known complication of the treatment of CNS leukemia and may occur in patients given intrathecal MTX after grafting [58]. Veno-occlusive disease of the liver is characterized by jaundice, enlargement of the liver, liver failure, ascites, and histological evidence of the occlusion of central veins [100]. There is a prevalence of veno-occlusive disease in patients treated with more intensive chemotherapy, particularly including dimethylmyleran, cytosine arabinoside, and 6-thioguanine [100]. A syndrome similar to adult respiratory distress syndrome (ARDS) with negative venous pressure and edema, probably due to damaged endothelium, was observed in patients who had received marrow from HLA-mismatched family members and had been treated with CsA [81]. Possibly the damage to the capillary endothelium is mediated by an early immune reaction.

Graft-Versus-Host Disease

Graft-versus-host disease (GVHD) is caused by an immune reaction of an immunocompetent graft against an immunocompromised host. The GVH reaction is elicited by and directed against histocompatibility antigens of the host which are foreign to the donor. These antigens may be coded by loci of the major histocompatibility complex (MHC) or "minor" histocompatibility loci. Acute GVHD of a moderate to severe degree is observed in 30%–60% of patients with the same *HLA* genotype as their donors [114, 125]. Even in this histocompatible situation about 5%–10% of the patients die with GVHD [125]. The effector cells of the GVH reaction are primarily T lymphocytes [70, 88], but natural killer cells may also be involved in GVH reactions against MHC antigens of the host that are foreign to the donor [32]. Target organs of GVH reactions are cells of the lymphatic and hematopoietic system, skin, liver, and epithelia of gut, mouth, esophagus, and bronchi. The GVH reaction damages epithelial surfaces of the gastrointestinal tract, bronchi, and skin and thereby facilitates the invasion of micro-organisms and systemic infections. As a rule the course of severe GVHD is complicated by life-threatening infections. Chronic GVHD may follow the acute form or arise de novo [101, 110]. Changes of the skin resemble "lichen ruber planus" progressing to scleroderma-like alterations [101]. It is frequently associated with dryness of the eyes and mouth similar to that in Sjögren's syndrome. The liver is involved, with elevations of enzyme and bilirubin levels; the histological picture resembles that of chronic aggressive hepatitis [101]. Chronic GVHD of the gut is rare and presents as ileitis. Depletion of lymphocytes from lymphatic tissues and atrophy of the thymus are frequent and persistent immune deficiency is a regular feature of chronic GVHD [101]. Without chronic GVHD the immune functions are successfully restored by the graft within a period of about 6 months to 2 years [79, 141]. Graft-host tolerance may be sustained by specific suppressor cells [126]; many patients with chronic GVHD have nonspecific suppressor cells [88, 127]. Chronic GVHD is a major obstacle to recovery of immune functions [141] and predisposes patients to opportunistic infections [3].

Prevention of GVHD has been attempted with various agents and methods. The most widely used method is prophylactic treatment with MTX for 3 months starting on day 1 [122]. The treatment with MTX (like that with CY) [97, 122] is based on experiments in animals. Despite prophylactic treatment with MTX, clinically significant GVHD is observed in 30%–60% of patients with an HLA-identical marrow graft [122]. The addition of antithymocyte globulin (ATG) and prednisone was successful in one study [87], but less successful in another [35]. A new promising immunosuppressive agent is CsA, which decreases the severity of GVHD [82, 128] by blocking the production and the effect of interleukin-2 on T lymphocytes [56]. Correct dosage of CsA appears still to be a problem. Oral administraton may not result in adequate blood levels because of indadequate absorption early after TBI [8]. Administration of CsA PO and IV has caused renal failure in some patients [102].

Elimination of T lymphocytes from the marrow graft has been attempted by physical separation on a density gradient of bovine serum albumin [29], agglutination with lectins [89], and cytotoxic treatment in vitro with activated cyclophosphamide (4-hydroxycyclophosphamide) [62]. The separation of hematopoietic precursor cells on discontinuous density gradients has reduced the incidence of GVHD in animals, but the results in human patients have not been convincing so far. Chemoseparation of hematopoietic stem cells by in vitro treatment with 4-hydroxycyclophosphamide or methylprednisolone gave promising results in animal studies [129]; clinical experience has not yet been reported. The use of lectins for depletion of T cells from the marrow has modified GVHD in animals and preliminary results in small children are encouraging [89]; their use in older children and adults may be limited by the small number of hematopoietic stem cells available for transplantation after this procedure. Another approach to the prevention of GVHD is the in vitro treatment of the marrow with specific anti-T-cell sera [91]. These antisera are either produced in rabbits immunized with thymocytes and rendered nontoxic against hematopoietic stem cells by multiple absorptions, or monoclonal antibodies against T cells are derived from hybridomas. Absorbed polyclonal antisera prevented or modified GVHD in animals by opsonizing T lymphocytes in the marrow graft. Certain strain combinations required the addition of complement for suppression of GVHD [92].

The in vitro treatment of human marrow grafts with specific polyclonal anti-T-cell globulin without added complement has shown little toxicity, but has not prevented GVHD in all cases [93]. Controversial results have been reported for the treatment of human marrow grafts with monoclonal T cell antibodies [44, 84]. This method needs critical evaluation in controlled clinical trials. At the same time the biological function of monoclonal antibodies should be further analysed in animal models.

On the basis of studies in germ-free mice [132], gnotobiotic techniques with microbiological decontamination and nursing of the patient in sterile environments have been advocated by some groups [134]. Patients who received grafts for treatment of aplastic anemia had a better survival when decontaminated and nursed in laminar air flow units [109]. Improved survival was at least partially due to a decreased incidence of GVHD. A similar improvement of survival was not observed in leukemic patients [20].

Treatment of established GVHD has been attempted with a variety of agents, including antithymocyte globulin (ATG), prednisone, CY, azathioprin and procarbacin. Prednisone and ATG have both been used with partial success in the treatment of acute GVHD [36]. Prednisone has less serious side-effects; recommended doses range from 2 mg/kg to 20 mg/kg daily [36, 85]. Treatment may result in resolution of signs, which usually is first seen in the skin, or in transition to chronic GVHD, or no response. Severe infections frequently complicate the course of GVHD. Chronic GVHD is best treated with the combination of prednisone and azathioprin [110]. The survival of patients with chronic GVHD can be improved by this combination from 20%–76%, with only 10% failing to respond [110].

Infections

Severe, life-threatening infections may result from exogenous sources or from reactivation of endogenous infectious agents. Soon after transplantation, destruction of mucosal barriers due to GVHD and/or irradiation and granulocytopenia facilitate bacterial and fungal infections. Gram-negative bacteria such as *E. coli, Pseudomonas aeruginosa,* and *Klebsiella pneumoniae* may invade from the gastrointestinal tract, white gram-positive *Staphylococcus albus* septicemia is frequently related to indwelling venous catheters. Fungal infections such as systemic candidiasis or aspergillosis, are serious therapeutic problems. Systemic candidiasis derives from invasion of mucosa and may be prevented by oral amphotericin and nystatin or ketokonazole. Aspergillosis is usually acquired by inhaling spores and can be prevented by filtering the air. There is a wide variety of viruses that cause infections in transplant patients. Intersitital pneumonitis associated with cytomegalovirus (CMV) is the most frequent viral infection and its mortality is high [72]. It is rare in recipients of syngeneic transplants and more frequent in patients with GVHD [2]. CMV may be an endogenous virus reactivated by GVHD, or CMV infection may be facilitated by immunosuppression due to GVHD or its immunosuppressive therapy. The risk of CMV infection is increased in patients failing to develop cytotoxic T cells against CMV-infected cells [86] and also in patients receiving granulocyte transfusions [54]. Attempts at preventing CMV infection with interferon [74] or adenine arabinoside have been largely unsuccessful [73]. The present approach consists of prophylactic administration of CMV-immune globulin and avoidance of granulocyte transfusions from CMV antibody-positive donors in CMV-negative recipients. The incidence of CMV pneumonitis may be decreased by CMV-immune globulin in patients not given granulocyte transfusions [140]. Patients with a history of recurrent *Herpes simplex* infections may develop extensive lesions of the skin, stomatitis, and esophagitis, and occasionally pneumonitis and encephalitis soon after transplantation. Mucocutaneous *Herpex simplex* virus infections after marrow transplantation have been treated with some benefit with acyclovir [135]. *Varicella zoster* (VZ) virus infections occur several months after transplantation in about 40% of patients, a minority of whom develop disseminated disease [4]. The mortality is about 8%, mainly due to *varicella* pneumonia [4]. Acyclovir may also be effective in VZ infections, VZ infections are not generally more frequent in patients with chronic GVHD [4], but may be associated with the presence of nonspecific suppressor cells in chronic GVHD [5]. Other infections occurring late after transplantation are infections with gram-positive bacteria [3]. They may be severe and recurrent in patients with chronic GVHD. In some transplant centers penicillin is given prophylactically to prevent frequent pneumococcal infections. The value of pneumococcal vaccine has still to be evaluated. *Pneumocystis carinii* pneumonitis and toxoplasmosis are the most important protozoal infections in marrow transplant recipients. Interstitial pneumonitis caused by *Pneumocystis carinii* may be due to reactivation of an endogenous infection. Co-trimoxazole is the drug of choice for prevention (5 mg/kg trimethoprim daily) and for treatment (20 mg/kg trimethoprim daily). Pentamidine isothiocyanate is an alternative drug, but involves considerable toxicity. Toxoplasmosis should be suspected in patients with rapidly

progressive CNS involvement. The most likely mode of infection is by transfusions. Selection of toxoplasmosis-negative blood donors may be an effective prophylaxis.
Our increasing knowledge about infectious complications after bone marrow transplantation is providing a basis for further prophylactic measures. Most transplant centers give oral nonabsorbable antibiotics and antifungal agents and provide some form of reverse isolation, the most stringent being laminar air-flow tents. Such protective measures have been shown to reduce the rate of severe infections against those in conventionally treated leukemia patients [11]. On the other hand, most of the bacterial infections can be controlled with the administration of systemic antibiotics and possibly granulocyte transfusions. However, these therapeutic interventions carry their own risks, i.e., transfer of infectious agents by transfusions and prolongation of the bleeding time by systemic antibiotics. Finally the influence of the gut flora on development and severity of GVHD has not yet been sufficiently evaluated in human patients.

Interstitial Pneumonitis

Interstitial pneumonitis remains the main complication of allogeneic marrow transplantation for leukemia. About half of all patients develop interstitial pneumonitis and a fourth to a third die of it [73]. Interstitial pneumonitis occurs most often in the first 100 days. The pathogenesis may be an opportunistic infection, a toxic reaction to radiation and chemotherapy, an immune reaction as part of GVH reactions, or some combination of these. In open-lung biopsies infectious agents were found in 65% of cases [73]. Most frequently cytomegalovirus and less frequently *Pneumocystis carinii, Herpes simplex* virus, *Varicella zoster* virus or adenovirus were found [73]. In about a third of the cases interstitial pneumonitis was idiopathic, i.e., no infectious agent was found. It is noteworthy that only 17 of 100 recipients of syngeneic marrow developed interstitial pneumonitis [2]. CMV-asociated pneumonitis was very rate in syngeneic recipients and most cases of pneumonitis were idiopathic. The incidence of CMV-associated pneumonitis is higher in patients with GVHD. The incidence of both CMV-associated and idiopathic pneumonitis increases with the age of the patients [69]. Effective prevention of interstitial pneumonitis has only been achieved for *Pneumocystis carinii*-associated pneumonitis by means of co-trimoxazole prophylaxis. The value of CMV-immune globulin [140] and the selection of CMV-negative blood donors [140] for prevention of CMV-associated pneumonitis has still to be confirmed.
The preparative regimen may influence the risk of idiopathic as well as of CMV-associated pneumonitis [69]. Radiation-induced pneumonitis is familiar from conventional radiotherapy. Pneumonitis related to chemotherapy has been described for a variety of cytostatic drugs such as CY, busulfan, BCNU, bleomycin, and MTX. Animal experiments [28, 124] and clinical observations [15, 99] indicate that the incidence of interstitial pneumonitis may be lowered by decreasing the dose rate of TBI to less than 6 cGy/min and by fractionation. Another attempt has been limitation of the lung dose to 8 Gy by lung shielding. Without shielding the lung is irradiated with a dose up to 25% higher than the calculated body midline dose. The effect of these measures on the inactivation of leukemic cells is presently unknown. So far the only controlled study in patients has shown an improved survival of patients given fractionated irradiation [119]. Further studies are needed to evaluate the effect of different radiation modalities on the incidence of interstitial pneumonitis.

Recurrence of Leukemia

Leukemic relapse is a major cause of failure in patients who receive grafts at an advanced stage. In a few patients leukemia has recurred in the grafted cells of the donor [38, 43, 48, 74, 123], as demonstrated by cytogenetic analysis. Although these cases are of great interest for research on leukemogenesis in man, they are exceptional. Most probably the great majority of relapses result from the regrowth of residual leukemic cells of the host [53]. Allogeneic grafts may eliminate residual leukemic cells of the host by a GVH reaction [12]. The effect of the antileukemic preparation can be estimated in recipients of syngeneic transplants from an identical-twin donor. Following preparation with CY (2 × 60 mg/kg) and TBI (single dose of 9.4 Gy) the probability of leukemic relapse for patients who had received transplants for refractory leukemia was about 70% [41]. This was not influenced by additional chemotherapy prior to CY and TBI. Similar conclusions were drawn from experience with additional chemotherapy in allogeneic recipients [47]. Preliminary results of preparation with larger doses of fractionated TBI in patients with refractory acute leukemia have also not been promising [18, 19, 23, 24]. Acute and chronic GVHD reduced the relapse rate, particularly in patients who had received transplants in relapse or as treatment for ALL [136]. However, this advantage was offset by mortality from other GVHD-related causes. Better survival due to a lower probability of relapse can be expected in patients with chronic GVHD who have survived for more than 5 months [137]. Methods for the induction of chronic GVHD may be valuable in improving the antileukemic effect without impact on survival, since chronic GVHD can be treated effectively with a combination of steroids and azathioprin. Patients with refractory ALL may be the best candidates.

In animal models a strong antileukemic effect has been exerted by hematopoietic grafts from donors differing in MHC antigens [16]. In man, experience with grafts from HLA-incompatible donors is limited [51, 81]. Recurrences of leukemia have been observed, but the possibility still exists that certain HLA incompatibilities may confer an antileukemic effect.

Outlook

During the past decade allogeneic marrow transplantation has developed from a last-resort therapeutic attempt in desperate cases of leukemia into a widely accepted part of the treatment of acute and chronic leukemia with well-defined indications. Nevertheless, the present methods of ablation of the hematopoietic system with high-dose chemotherapy and TBI followed by rescue with a marrow graft from a healthy donor are as crude as the currently available intensive chemotherapy protocols. Better preparative regimens, including fractionated TBI, may increase the therapeutic ratio of elimination of leukemia to damage to the lung and other organs. Inactivation of T lymphocytes in the marrow graft with specific antisera may prevent acute GVHD, which together with careful selection of blood donors may decrease the incidence of interstitial pneumonitis. Finally, the antileukemic effect may be better with the use of marrow from HLA-incompatible donors. Further experience of manipulating the graft in vitro and the host's responses to this must be collected before more specific methods of therapeutic intervention with hematopoietic grafts can be found.

References

1. Applebaum FR, Fefer A, Cheever MA et al. (1981) Treatment of non-Hodgkins lymphoma with marrow transplantation in identical twins. Blood 58: 509–513
2. Applebaum FR, Meyers JD, Fefer A et al. (1982) Non bacterial non fungal pneumonia following marrow transplantation in 100 identical twins. Transplantation 33: 265–268
3. Atkinson K, Storb R, Prentice RL, Weiden PL, Witherspoon RP, Sullivan K, Noel D, Thomas ED (1979) Analysis of late infections in 89 longterm survivors of bone marrow transplantation. Blood 53: 720–731
4. Atkinson K, Meyers JD, Storb R et al. (1980) Varizella-Zoster virus infection after marrow transplantation for aplastic anemia or leukemia. Transplantation 29: 47–50
5. Atkinson K, Farewell V, Storb R et al. (1982) Analysis of late infections after human bone marrow transplantation: role of genetypic nonidentity between marrow donor and recipient and of nonspecific suppressor cells in patients with chronic graft-versus host disease. Blood 60: 714–720
6. Barnes DHW, Loutit JF, Neal FE (1956) Treatment of murine leukemia with X-rays and homologous bone marrow. Br Med J 52: 626
7. Barrett AJ, Kendra JR, Lucas CF, Joss DV, Joski R, Desai M, Jones KH, Philipps RH, Rogers TR, Tabura Z, Williamson S, Hobbs JR (1982) Bone marrow transplantation for acute lymphoblastic leukemia. Br J Haematol 52: 181–188
8. Barrett AJ, Kendra JR, Lucas CF et al. (1982) Cyclosporin A as prophylaxis against graft-versus-host disease in 36 patients. Br Med J 285: 162–166
9. Blume KG, Beutler E, Bross KJ, Chillar RK, Ellington OB, Fahey JL, Farbstein MJ, Forman SJ, Schmidt GM, Scott EP, Spruce WE, Turner A, Wolf J (1980) Bone marrow ablation and allogeneic marrow transplantation in acute leukemia. N Engl J Med 302: 1041
10. Blume K, Bross KJ, Hecht Th, Schmidt G, Winkler K, Winkler U (1982) Allogene Knochenmarktransplantation zur Behandlung akuter Leukämien. Karger, Basel, pp 24–29 (Beiträge zur Onkologie, vol 13)
11. Bodey GP, Bolivar R, Fainstein V (1982) Infectious complications in leukemic patients. Semin Hematol 19: 193–226
12. Boranic M, Tonkovic I (1977) Time pattern of the antileukemic effect of graft-versus-host reaction in mice. Cancer Res 31: 1140
13. Bortin MM (1970) A compendium of reported human bone marrow transplants. Transplantation 9: 571
14. Bortin MM, Rimm AA, Rose WC, Saltzstein EC (1974) Graft- versus-host-leukemia. V. Absence of antileukemic effect using allogeneic H2 identical immunocompetent cells. Transplantation 18: 280
15. Bortin MM, Kay HEM, Gale RP, Thimm AA (1982) Factors associated with interstitial pneumonitis after bone marrow transplantation for acute leukemia. Lancet 1: 437–439
16. Bortin MM, Rimm AA, Rose WC, Truitt RL, Saltzstein EC (1976) Transplantation of hematopoietic and lymphoid cells in mice. H-2 matched unrelated adult donors compared with H-2 mismatched fetal donors. Transplantation 21: 331
17. Brodsky I, Fuscaldo KE, Kahn SB, Comroy JF (1979) Myeloproliferative disorders: II CML: clonal evolution and its role in management. Leuk Res 3: 379–393
18. Buckner CD, Clift RA, Thomas ED, Sanders JE, Stewart PS, Storb R, Sullivan KM, Hackman R (1982) Allogeneic marrow transplantation for acute non-lymphoblastic leukemia in relapse using fractionated total body irradiation. Leuk Res 6: 389–394
19. Buckner CD, Clift RA, Thomas ED, Sanders JE, Hackman R, Stewart PS, Storb R, Sullivan KM (1982) Allogeneic marrow transplantation for patients with acute nonlymphoblastic leukemia in second remission. Leuk Res 6: 395–399
20. Buckner CD, Clift RA, Sanders JE et al. (1978) Protective environment for marrow transplant recipients: a prospective study. Ann Intern Med 89: 893–901
21. Champlin R, Ho W, Arenson E, Gale RP (1982) Allogeneic bone marrow transplantation for chronic myelogenous leukemia in chronic or accelerated phase. Blood 60: 1038–1041

22. Cheever MA, Fefer A, Greenberg PD et al. (1982) Treatment of hairy cell leukemia with chemoradiotherapy and identical-twin bone marrow transplantation. N Engl J Med 307: 479–481
23. Clift RA, Buckner CD, Thomas ED, Sanders JE, Stewart PS, Sullivan KM, McGuffin R, Hersman J, Sale GE, Storb R (1982) Allogeneic marrow transplantation using fractionated total body irradiation in patients with acute lymphoblastic leukemia in relapse. Leuk Res 6: 401–407
24. Clift RA, Buckner CD, Thomas ED, Sanders JE, Stewart PS, McGuffin R, Hersman J, Sullivan KM, Sale GE, Storb R (1982) Allogeneic marrow transplantation for acute lymphoblastic leukemia in remission using fractionated total body irradiation. Leuk Res 6: 409–412
25. Clift RA, Buckner CD, Thomas ED et al. (1982) Treatment of chronic granulocytic leukemia in chronic phase by allogeneic marrow transplantation. Lancet 2: 621–623
26. Clift RA, Hansen JA, Thomas ED et al. (1979) Marrow transplantation from donors other than HLA-identical siblings. Transplantation 28: 235–242
27. Curtis JE, Messner HA (1982) Bone marrow transplantation for leukemia and aplastic anemia: management of ABO in compatibility. Can Med Assoc 126: 649–655
28. Depledge MH, Barrett A (1982) Dose rate dependence of lung damage after total body irradiation in mice. Int J Radiat Biol 41: 325–334
29. Dicke KA, van Bekkum DW (1971) Allogeneic bone marrow transplantation after elimination of immunocompetent cells by means of density gradient centrifugation. Transplant Proc 3: 666–68
30. Dinsmore R, Shank B, Kapoor N et al. (1981) A randomized trial of marrow transplantation (BMT) vs. chemotherapy (CT) maintenance for acute myelogenous leukemia in first remission: preliminary results. Exp Hematol [Suppl 9] 9: 125 (abstract)
31. Dinsmore R, Kapoor N, Kirkpatrick D, Teitelbaum H, Shank B, O'Reilly RJ (1981) Bone marrow transplantation for acute leukemia in remission. Proc Am Soc Clin Oncol 22: 491
32. Dokhelar MC, Wiels J, Lipinski M et al. (1981) Natural killer cell activity in human bone marrow recipients. Transplantation 31: 61
33. Doney K, Buckner CD, Gale GE et al. (1978) Treatment of chronic granulocytic leukemia by chemotherapy, total body irradiation and allogeneic bone marrow transplantation. Exp Hematol 6: 738–747
34. Doney KC, Buckner CD, Thomas ED et al. (1981) Allogeneic bone marrow transplantation for chronic granulocytic leukemia. Exp Hematol 9: 966–971
35. Doney K, Weiden PL, Storb R, Thomas ED (1981) Failure of early administration of antithymocyte globulin to lessen graft-versus-host disease in human allogeneic marrow transplant recipients. Transplantation 31: 141–143
36. Doney KC, Weiden PL, Storb R, Thomas ED (1981) Treatment of graft-versus-host disease in human allogeneic marrow graft recipients: a randomized trial comparing antithymocyte globulin and corticosteroids. Am J Hematol 11: 1–8
37. Dupont B, O'Reilly RJ, Pollack MS, Good RA (1979) Use of genotypically different donors in bone marrow transplantation. Transplant Proc 11: 219–224
38. Elfenbein GJ, Brogaonkar DS, Bias WB et al. (1978) Cytogenetic evidence for recurrence of acute myelogenous leukemia after allogeneic bone marrow transplantation in donor hematopoietic cells. Blood 52: 627–636
39. Epstein EB, Storb R, Radge H, Thomas ED (1968) Cytotoxic typing antisera for marrow grafting in littermate dogs. Transplantation 6: 45–58
40. Fefer A, Cheever MA, Greenberg PD et al. (1982) Treatment of chronic granulocytic leukemia with chemoradiotherapy and transplantation of marrow from identical twins. N Engl J Med 306: 63–68
41. Fefer A, Cheever MA, Thomas ED et al. (1981) Bone marrow transplantation for refractory acute leukemia in 34 patients with identical twins. Blood 57: 421–430
42. Feig SA, Opelz G, Winter HS, Falk PM, Neerhout RC, Sparkes R, Gale RP (1976) Successful bone marrow transplantation against mixed lymphocyte culture barrier. Blood 48: 385

43. Fialkow PJ, Thomas ED, Bryant JI et al. (1971) Leukaemic transformation of engrafted human marrow cells in vivo. Lancet 1: 251–255
44. Filipovich AH, McGlave PB, Ramsay NKC et al. (1982) Pretreatment of donor bone marrow with monoclonal antibody OKT 3 for prevention of acute graft-versus-host disease in allogeneic histocompatible bone marrow transplantation. Lancet 1: 1266–1269
45. Gale RP, Cline MJ (1977) High remission-induction rate in acute leukemia. Lancet 1: 497
46. Gale RP for the Transplantation Biology Unit, UCLA, School of Medicine (1981) Bone marrow transplantation for leukemia in remission. Exp Hematol [Suppl 9] 9: 125 (abstract)
47. Gale RP for the UCLA Marrow Transplant Team (1978) Approaches to leukemic relapse following bone marrow transplantation. Transplant Proc 10: 167–171
48. Goh KO, Klemperer MR (1977) In vivo leukemic transformation: cytogenetic evidence of in vivo leukemic transformation of engrafted marrow cells. Am J Hematol 2: 283–290
49. Goldman JM, Baughan ASJ, McCarthy DM et al. (1982) Marrow transplantation for patients in the chronic phase of chronic granulocytic leukemia. Lancet 2: 623–625
50. Graw RG, Lohrmann HP, Bull MC, Decter J, Herzig GP, Bull JM, Leventhal BG, Yankee RA, Herzig RH, Krüger GRF, Bleyer WA, Buja ML, McGiniuss MH, Alter HJ, Whang-Peng J, Gralnick HR, Krikpatrick CH, Henderson ES (1974) Bone marrow transplantation following combination chemotherapy immunosuppression (B.A.C.T.) in patients with acute leukemia. Transplant Proc 6: 349
51. Hansen JA, Clift RA, Mickelson EM et al. (1981) Marrow transplantation from donors other than HLA identical siblings. Hum Immunol 1: 31–40
52. Hansen JA, Clift RA, Thomas ED, Buckner CD, Storb R, Giblett ER (1980) Transplantation of marrow from an unrelated donor to a patient with acute leukemia. N Engl J Med 303: 565–567
53. Harrison DT, Flournoy N, Ramberg R et al. (1978) Relapse following marrow transplantation for acute leukemia. Am J Hematol 5: 191–303
54. Hersman J, Meyers JD, Thomas ED et al. (1982) The effect of granulocyte transfusions on the incidence of cytomegalovirus infection after allogeneic marrow transplantation. Ann Intern Med 96: 149–152
55. Herzig GP, Bull MI, Decter J, Lohrmann HP, Herzig RH, Krueger G, Pomeroy T, Henderson ES, Graw RG Jr (1975) Bone marrow transplantation in leukemia and aplastic anemia. – NCI experience with four grafting regimens. Transplant Proc 7: 817–882
56. Hess AD, Tutschka PJ, Santos GW (1982) The effect of cyclosporin A on T-lymphocyte subpopulations. In: White DJG (ed) Cyclosporin A. Elsevier Biomedical, Amsterdam, pp 209–231
57. Hoelzer D, Thiel E, Löffler H et al. (to be published) Multicentre trial acute lymphatic leukemia (ALL) and acute undifferentiated leukemia (AUL) in adults. Blood (in press)
58. Johnson FL, Thomas ED, Clark BS, Chard RL, Hartmann JR, Storb R (1981) A comparison of marrow transplantation with chemotherapy for children with acute lymphoblastic leukemia in second or subsequent remissions. N Engl J Med 305: 846
59. Kendra JR, Salleem N, Ingram L, Joski R, Rogers TR, Phillips R, Barrett A, James DCO, Hugh-Jones K, Hobbs JR, Barrett AJ (to be published) Marrow transplantation for acute lymphoblastic leukemia in remission. Exp Hematol [Suppl]
60. Kersey JH, Ramsay NKC, Kim T, McGlasve P, Krivit W, Levitt S, Filipovich A, Woods W, O'Leary M, Coccia P, Nesbit ME (1982) Allogeneic bone marrow transplantation in acute non lymphocytic leukemia: a pilot study. Blood 60: 400–403
61. Koeffler HP, Golde DW (1981) Chronic myelogenous leukemia – new concepts. N Engl J Med 304: 1201–1209, 1269–1973
62. Körbling M, Hess AD, Tuschka PJ et al. (1982) 4-Hydroperoxycyclophosphamide: a model for eliminating residual human tumor cells and T-lymphocytes from the bone marrow graft. Br J Haematol 52: 89–96
63. Kolb HJ, Bender-Götze Ch, Albert ED et al. (1981) Knochenmarktransplantation bei rezidivierter, akuter Leukämie. Klin Wochenschr 59: 251–266

64. Lampert F (1977) Kombinations-Chemotherapie und Hirnschädelbestrahlung bei 530 Kindern mit akuter lymphoblastischer Leukämie. Dtsch Med Wochenschr 102: 917
65. Lorenz E, Uphoff DE, Shelton E, Ried T (1951) Modification of irradiation injury in mice and guinea pigs by bone marrow injection. J Natl Cancer Inst 12: 197–201
66. Lumley HS, Powles RL, Morgenstern GR, Clink HM (1982) Matched allogeneic sibling bone marrow transplantation for acute myeloid leukemia in first remission. Exp Hematol [Suppl 10] 10: 70–71
67. McGlave PB, Arthur DC, Kim TH et al. (1982) Successful allogeneic bone marrow transplantation for patients in the accelerated phase of chronic granulocytic leukemia. Lancet 2: 625–627
68. McGlave PB, Brunning RD, Hurd DD, Kim TH (1982) Reversal of severe bone marrow fibroisis and osteosclerosis following allogeneic bone marrow transplantation for chronic granulocytic leukemia. Br J Haematol 52: 189–194
69. Meyers JD, Flournoy N, Thomas ED (1982) Non bacterial pneumonia after allogeneic marrow transplantation – review of ten years experience. Rev Infect Dis 4: 1119
70. Miller JFAP, Marshal HE, White RG (1962) Immunological significance of the thymus. Adv Immunol 2: 111
71. Morgenstern GR, Powles RL, Leigh M (to be published) Relapse following allogeneic marrow transplantation for acute myeloid leukemia. Exp Hematol [Suppl]
72. Neimann PE, Reeves W, Ray G et al. (1977) A prospective analysis of interstitial pneumonia and opportunistic viral infection among recipients of allogeneic bone marrow grafts. J Infect Dis 136: 754
73. Neimann PE, Meyers JD, Medeiros E et al. (1980) Interstitial pneumonia following marrow transplantation for leukemia and aplastic anemia. In: Gale RP, Fox CF (eds) Biology of bone marrow transplantation. Academic, New York (ICN-UCLA symposia on molecular and cellular biology, vol 17)
74. Newburger PE, Latt SA, Pesando JM et al. (1981) Leukemia relapse in donor cells after allogeneic bone marrow transplantation. N Engl J Med 304: 712–714
75. O'Leary M, Ramsey NKC, Nesbit ME, Krivit W, Coccis PF, Kim TH, Woods WG, Kersey JH (to be published) Bone marrow transplantation for hematologic malignancy. In: O'Kunewick JP (ed) Graft-versus-host leukemia in man and animal models
76. Oliff A, Ramu NP, Poplack D (1978) Leukemic relapse $5^1/_2$ years after allogeneic bone marrow transplantation. Blood 52: 281–284
77. O'Reilly RJ, Pahwa R, Dupont B, Good RA (1978) Severe combined immunodefiency: transplantation approaches for patients lacking a HLA genotypically identical sibling. In: Gale RP, Opelz G (eds) Immunobiology of bone marrow transplantion. Grune and Stratton, New York, pp 187–199
78. Osserman EF, DiRe LB, Sherman WH et al. (1982) Identical twin marrow transplantation in multiple myeloma. Acta Haematol (Basel) 66: 815–223
79. Pahwa SG, Pahwa RN, Friedrich W et al. (1982) Abnormal humoral immune responses in periphal blood lymphocyte cultures of bone marrow transplant recipients. Proc Natl Acad Sci USA 79: 2663–2667
80. Powles RL, Watson JG, Morgenstern GR, Kay HEM (1982) Bone marrow transplantation in leukemia remission. Lancet 1: 336–337
81. Powles RL, Morgenstern GR, Kay HEM et al. (1983) Mismatched family donors for bone marrow transplantation as treatment for acute leukemia. Lancet 1: 612–615
82. Powles RL, Link HM, Spence D, Morgenstern G, Watson JG, Selby PJ, Woods M, Barrett A, Jamieson B, Sloane J, Lawler SD, Kay HEM, Lawson D, McElwain TJ, Alexander P (1980) Cyclosporin A to prevent Graft-versus-host disease in man after allogeneic bone marrow transplantation. Lancet 1: 327–330
83. Powles RL, Morgenstern G, Clink HM et al. (1980) The place of bone marrow transplantation in acute myelogenous leukemia. Lancet 1: 1047–1050

84. Prentice HG, Blacklock HH, Janossy G et al. (1982) Use of anti-T-cell monoclonal antibody OKT 3 to prevent acute graft-versus-host disease in allogeneic bone marrow transplantation for acute leukemia. Lancet 1: 700–703
85. Prentice HG, Bateman SM, Bradstock KF, Hoffbrand AV (1980) Highdose methyl prednisone therapy in established acute graft-versus-host disease. Blut 20: 175–177
86. Quinnan GV, Kirmani N, Rook AH et al. (1982) Cytotoxic T-cells in cytomegalovirus infection. HLA-restricted T lymphocyte and non-T-lymphocyte cytotoxic responses correlate with recovery from cytomegalovirus infection in bone marrow transplant recipients. N Engl J Med 307: 6–13
87. Ramsay NKC, Kersey JH, Robinson L et al. (1982) A randomized study of the prevention of acute graft-versus-host disease. N Engl J Med 306: 392–397
88. Reinherz EL, Parkman R, Rappaport J, Rosen FS, Schlossman SF (1979) Abberations of suppressor T cells in human graft-versus-host disease. N Engl J Med 300: 1061
89. Reisner Y, Kapoor N, Kirkpatrick D et al. (1981) Transplantation for acute leukemia with HLA-A and -B non identical parental marrow cells fractionated with soya bean agglutinin and sheep red blood cells. Lancet 1: 327–332
90. Riehm H, Gadner H, Welte K (1977) Die Westberliner Studie zur Behandlung der akuten lymphoblastischen Leukemie des Kindes – Erfahrungsbericht nach 6 Jahren. Klin Pädiat 189: 89
91. Rodt H, Thiefelder S, Hoffmann-Fezer G (1980) Influence of the recipient thymus on the maturation of T-lymphocytes in H-2 different radiation chimeras. In: Thierfelder S, Rodt H, Kolb HJ (eds) Immunobiology of bone marrow transplantation. Springer, Berlin Heidelberg New York, p 179
92. Rodt H, Thierfelder S, Kummer U (1982) Suppression of GVHD by monoclonal antisera. Exp Hematol [Suppl] 10: 107–109
93. Rodt H, Kobl HJ, Netzel B et al. (1981) Effect of anti T cell globulin on GVHD in leukemic patients treated with BMT. Transplant Proc 13: 257–261
94. Rozman C, Granena A, Hernandez-Prieto M et al. (1982) Bone marrow transplantation for acute myelofibrosis. Lancet 1: 618
95. Santos GW (1966) Effect of syngeneic, allogeneic and parental marrow infusions in busulfan-injected rats with a note concerning effects of busulfan on antibody production. Exp Hematol 9: 61–63
96. Santos GW, Sensenbrenner LL, Burke BJ, Colvin M, Owens AH, Bias WB, Slavin RE (1971) Marrow transplantation in man following cyclophosphamide. Transplant Proc 3: 400
97. Santos GW, Owens AH (1966) Production of graft-versus-host disease in the rat and its treatment with cytotoxic agents. Nature 210: 139
98. Schäfer UW, Schmidt CG, Ruther U, Schuning F, Becher R, Beyer JH, Hossfeld DK, Nowrousian MR, Öhl S, Wetter O, Bamberg M, Schmitt G, Bormann U, Scherer E, Harlambie E, Linzenmeier G, Grosse-Wilde H, Hierholzer E, Kuwert E, Henneberg KB, Luboldt W, Richter HJ, Leder LD, Hentschke D (1982) Knochenmarktransplantation bei Panmyelopathie und akuter Leukämie. Dtsch Med Wochenschr 107: 803–808
99. Shank B, Hopfen S, Kim JH et al. (1981) Hyperfractionated total body irradiation for bone marrow transplantation: I early results in leukemia patients. Int J Radiat Oncol Biol Phys 7: 1109–1115
100. Shulman HM, McDonald GB, Matthews D et al. (1980) An analysis of hepatic veno-occlusive disease and centro-lobular hepatic degeneration following bone marrow transplantation. Gastroenterology 79: 1178–1191
101. Shulman HM, Sullivan KM, Weiden DL et al. (1980) Chronic graft-versus-host syndrome in man. A long-term clinico-pathologic study of 20 Seattle patients. Am J Med 69: 204–217
102. Shulman H, Striker G (1981) Nephrotoxicity of cycloporin A after allogeneic marrow transplantation: glomerular thromboses and tubular injury. N Engl J Med 305: 1392
103. Simone J (1974) Acute lymphocytic leukemia in childhood. Semin Hematol 11: 25–39
104. Smith JW, Shulman HM, Thomas ED et al. (1981) Bone marrow transplantation for acute myelosclerosis. Cancer 48: 2198–2203

105. Sokal JE (1976) Evaluation of survival data for chronic myelocytic leukemia. Am J Hematol 1: 493–500
106. Speck B, Gratwohl A, Nissen C et al. (1982) Allogene Knochenmarktransplantation bei chronischer myeloischer Leukämie. Schweiz Med Wochenschr 112: 1419–1420
107. Speck B, Gratewohl A, Nissen C, Osterwalder B, Müller M, Lutley A, Signer E, Burri HP, Jeannet M (1981) Neue Entwicklung in der klinischen Knochenmarktransplantation bei Leukämie. Schweiz Med Wochenschr 111: 1975–1977
108. Storb R, Rudolph RH, Kolb HJ, Graham TC, Mickelson E, Erikson V, Lerner KG, Kolb H, Thomas ED (1973) Marrow grafts between DLA-matched canine littermates. Transplantation 15: 92–100
109. Storb R, Prentice RL, Buckner CD et al. (1983) Graft-versus-host disease and survival in patients with aplastic anemia treated by marrow grafts from HLA-identical siblings. Beneficial effect of a protective environment. N Engl J Med 308: 302–307
110. Sullivan KM, Shulman HM, Storb R et al. (1981) Chronic graft-versus-host disease in 52 patients: adverse natural course and successful treatment with combination in immunosupression. Blood 57: 267–276
111. Thomas ED, Ashley CA, Lochte HL, Jaretzki A, Sahler OD, Ferrebee JW (1959) Homografts of bone marrow in dogs after total body irradiation. Blood 14: 720–736
112. Thomas ED, Buckner CD, Rudolph RH, Fefer A, Storb R, Neiman PE, Bryant JI, Chard RL, Clift RA, Epstein RB, Fialkow PJ, Funk DD, Giblett ER, Lerner KG, Reynolds FA, Slichter S (1971) Allogeneic marrow grafting for hematologic malignancy using HLA matched donor recipient sibling pairs. Blood 38: 267–287
113. Thomas ED, Buckner CD, Storb R et al. (1972) Aplastic anemia treated by marrow transplantation. Lancet 1: 284–289
114. Thomas ED, Buckner CD, Banaij M, Clift RA, Fefer A, Flournoy N, Goodell BW, Hickman RO, Lerner KG, Neiman PE, Sale GE, Sanders JE, Singer J, Stevens M, Storb R, Weiden PL (1977) One hundred patients with acute leukemia treated by chemotherapy, total body irradiation and allogeneic marrow transplantation. Blood 49: 511–533
115. Thomas ED, Sanders JE, Flournoy N, Johnson FL, Buckner CD, Clift RA, Fefer A, Goodwell BW, Storb R, Weiden PL (1979) Marrow transplantation for patients with acute lymphoblastic leukemia in remission. Blood 54: 468
116. Thomas ED (1981) Bone marrow transplantation. In: Burchenal JH, Oettgen HF (eds) Cancer – achievements, challenges and prospects for the 1980s, vol 2. Grune and Stratton, New York, pp 625–638
117. Thomas ED, Buckner CD, Clift RA, Fefer A, Johnson FL, Neiman PE, Sale GE, Sanders JE, Singer JW, Shulman H, Storb R, Weiden PL (1979) Marrow transplantation for acute non lymphoblastic leukemia in first remission. N Engl J Med 301: 597–599
118. Thomas ED, Clift RA, Buckner CD (1982) Marrow transplantation for patients with acute non-lymphoblastic leukemia who achieve a first remission. Cancer Treat Rep 66: 1463–1466
119. Thomas ED, Clift RA, Hersman J, Sanders JE, Stewart P, Buckner CD, Fefer A, McGuffin R, Smith JW, Storb R (1982) Marrow transplantation for acute nonlymphoblastic leukemia in first remission using fractionated or single-dose irradiation. Int J Radiat Oncol Biol Phys 8: 817–821
120. Thomas ED (1982) The role of marrow transplantation in the eradication of malignant disease. Cancer 49: 1963–1969
121. Thomas ED for the Seattle Marrow Transplant Team (1982) Marrow transplantation for hematologic malignancies. Exp Hematol [Suppl 11] 10: 2 (abstract)
122. Thomas ED, Storb R, Clift RA, Fefer A, Johnson FL, Neiman PE, Lerner KG, Glucksberg H, Buchner CD (1975) Bone marrow transplantation. N Engl J Med 292: 832–843
123. Thomas ED, Bryant JI, Buckner CD et al. (1972) Leukaemic transformation of engrafted human marrow cells in vivo. Lancet 1: 1310–1330
124. Travis EL, Down JD (1981) Repair in mouse lung after split doses of x rays. Radiat Res 87: 166–174

125. Tsoi MS (1982) Immunological mechanismus of graft-versus-host disease in man. Transplantation 33: 459–464
126. Tsoi MS, Storb R, Dobbs S, Thoams ED (1981) Specific suppressor cells in graft-host tolerance of HLA-identical marrow transplantation. Nature 292: 355–357
127. Tsoi MS, Storb R, Dobbs S et al. (1979) Non-specific suppressor cells in patients with chronic graft-versus-host disease after marrow grafting. J Immunol 123: 1970–1976
128. Tutschka PJ, Beschorner W, Allison AC, Burns WH, Santos GW (1979) Use of Cyclosporin A in allogeneic bone marrow transplantation in the rat. Nature 280: 148–151
129. Tutschka PJ, Körbling M (1981) Prevention of graft-versus-host disease (GVHD) by chemo-separation of marrow cells. Transplant Proc 13: 374
130. Tutschka PJ, Santos GW, Elfenbein GJ (1980) Marrow transplantation in acute leukemia following busulfan and cyclophosphamide. In: Thierfelder S, Rodt H, Kolb HJ (eds) Immunbiology of bone marrow transplantation. Springer, Berlin Heidelberg New York, pp 375–380
131. UCLA Bone Marrow Transplantation Group (1977) Bone marrow transplantation with intensive combination chemotherapy radiation therapy (SCARI) in acute leukemia. Ann Intern Med 86: 155
132. van Bekkum DW, Roodenburg J, Heidt PJ (1974) Mitigation of secondary disease of allogeneic mouse radiation chimeras by modification of the intestinal microflora. J Natl Cancer Inst 52: 401–404
133. Vernant JP, Rodet M, Rochant H et al. (1981) Successful allogeneic bone marrow transplantation after reversion to chronic phase of blast crisis in chronic myeloid leukemia. Am J Hematol 11: 205–207
134. Vossen JM, van der Waaij D (1972) Reverse isolation in bone marrow transplantation: Ultra clean room compared with laminar flow technique. II. Microbiological and clinical results. Rev Eur Etud Clin Biol 17: 564
135. Wade JC, Newton B, McLaren C et al. (1982) Intravenous acyclovir to treat mucocutaneous herpes simplex virus infection after bone marrow transplantation. Ann Intern Med 96: 265–269
136. Weiden PL, Flournoy N, Thomas ED, Prentice R, Fefer A, Bruckner CD, Storb R (1979) Antileukemic effect of graft-versus-host disease in marrow transplantation. N Engl J Med 300: 1068
137. Weiden PL, Sullivan KM, Flournoy N et al. (1981) Antileukemic effect of chronic graft-versus-host disease. Contribution to improved survival after allogeneic marrow transplantation. N Engl J Med 304: 1529–1533
138. Weinstein HJ, Mayer RJ, Rosenthal DS et al. (1980) Treatment of acute myelogenous leukemia in children and adults. N Engl J Med 303: 473–478
139. Wilms K, Link H, Meyer P et al. (1982) Knochenmarktransplantation bei Patienten mit Leukämien. Klin Wochenschr 60: 1279–1287
140. Winston DJ, Pollard RB, Ho WG et al. (1982) Cytomegalovirus immune plasma in bone marrow transplant recipients. Ann Intern Med 97: 11–18
141. Witherspoon RP, Storb R, Ochs HD et al. (1981) Recovery of antibody production in human allogeneic marrow graft recipients: influence of time posttransplantation, the presence or absence of chronic graft-versus-host disease and antithymocyte globulin treatment. Blood 58: 360–368
142. Wolf JL, Spruce WE, Bearman RM et al. (1982) Reversal of acute ("malignant") myelosclerosis by allogeneic bone marrow transplantation. Blood 59: 191–193
143. Yates J, Glidewell O, Wiernik P et al. (1982) Cytosine arabinoside with daunorubicin or adriamycin for therapy of acute myelocytic leukemia: a CALGB study. Blood 60: 454–462
144. Zwaan FE for European Cooperative Group for Bone Marrow Transplantation (to be published) Marrow transplantation for leukemia – summary of European results. Exp Hematol [Suppl]

*Autologous Bone Marrow Transplantation in Leukemia**

B. Netzel, R. I. Haas, and S. Thierfelder

Thierschstrasse 19, 8000 München 22, FRG

Summary

In patients without HLA-identical donors autologous bone marrow transplantation should be considered as an alternative to conservative treatment of recurrent malignancies. Any patient in complete remission is suitable for an autologous bone marrow transplantation. Bone marrow is aspirated from the patient during complete remission, frozen, and stored at −196° C, and it can be used for hematopoietic reconstitution after high-dose chemotherapy and radiotherapy of the patient.

In patients with solid malignant tumors or leukemia the elimination of clonogenic tumor cells from the graft by means of physical separation techniques has not been successful. However, studies in mice and more recently in patients indicate that antibodies destroy residual leukemic cells of the bone marrow transplant without jeopardizing the capacity for regeneration.

During our first study in children with acute lymphoblastic leukemia, bone marrow was taken from 50 patients in remission and cryopreserved. Preservation time ranged from 1 to 60 months and the mean number of aspirated nucleated bone marrow cells was 4×10^8/kg body weight ($1.9-7.4 \times 10^8$/kg). After cryopreservation the stem cell viability of the standard samples was 80%−100%.

Autologous bone marrow was transplanted in five patients with common ALL (cALL). The transplant was prepared by incubation with specific antisera of high cytotoxic, selective activity against cALL cells.

Our preliminary results show that bone marrow cells aspirated in remission and prepared with antileukemic antisera stimulate repopulation of the recipient's bone marrow and effect hematopoietic regeneration.

Introduction

Treatment of leukemia by allogeneic bone marrow transplantation is limited to patients with histocompatible donors. The majority of patients lack such donors (see pp 269−289). Thus it was appropriate to ask whether remission bone marrow autografts represent an alternative to allogeneic bone marrow transplantation for protection of the patient against fatal marrow aplasia induced by maximal chemo- and radiotherapy. Clearly, autologous bone marrow transplantation circumvents problems of donor procurement and histoincompatibility. But would a patient in remission have sufficient stem cells − and if so at what

* The work described in this paper was supported by the Deutsche Forschungsgemeinschaft (SFB 37) and by Deutsche Krebshilfe, Bonn

Recent Results in Cancer Research. Vol. 93

Table 1. Indications for autologous bone marrow transplantation

Leukemias
No HLA-identical donor
Bone marrow in remission
Elimination of residual leukemic cells from the bone marrow (e.g., by antibodies)
Solid tumors
No HLA-identical donor
Bone marrow without tumor cells at diagnosis or collection

point in remission – not only to fully reconstitute his own hematopoiesis but also to achieve this after months if not years of cryopreservation? The answer is yes, as has been documented in several clinical centers by the collection, preservation, and engraftment of patients' own bone marrow [5, 7, 9, 10].

Before autologous bone marrow transplantation is accepted in principle for leukemic patients it is also necessary to clarify whether this treatment eradicates or reduces the leukemic clone sufficiently for cure or at least stable remissions to be obtained. Of course relapses must be expected, which arise from residual leukemia that has withstood chemotherapy. Neoplastic cells may have been reimplanted with the patient's hematopoietic stem cells. Selective manipulation of such leukemic cells has been attempted by physical means – differential centrifugation in albumin gradients – or and chemoseparation, i.e., in vitro treatment of the marrow with certain cyclophosphamides or steroids [13].

The immunological approach has attracted great interest. This consists in pretreatment of the marrow to be reimplanted with antibodies against the leukemic cells [18, 27]. Several experimental and clinical studies are currently investigating the potential of this "purging of the marrow from leukemic cells".

But even if the autograft is successfully purged it is still not known whether the leukemic clone has been eradicated in the patient by the conditioning treatment. Can we expect that the promising results of allogeneic bone marrow transplantation will be reproduced under the conditions of autologous bone marrow transplantation – at least for certain types of leukemia? It is true that immunological graft-versus-leukemia effects have been reported only after allogeneic bone marrow transplantation [3]. However, long-term remissions after transplantation of marrow from identical twins [8] indicate that autologous bone marrow grafting may indeed become a successful therapy in certain leukemias (Table 1).

Autologous bone marrow transplantation has also been attempted in patients with solid malignant tumors, although its therapeutic use has remained a rare event in children with solid tumors such as neuroblastomas in stages III and IV, Ewing's sarcoma, rhabdomyosarcoma, Burkitt's lymphoma, and non-Hodgkin's lymphoma. Partial and complete remissions have been achieved, with tumor-free survival of 1–19 months [2, 5, 14]. Autologous bone marrow transplantation should of course be applied only in patients without evidence of tumorous bone marrow infiltration at the time of diagnosis.

Animal Studies

Autologous bone marrow transplantation cannot be checked by genetic markers. Also, elimination of leukemic cells can only be assumed after long-term clinical follow-up.

Observations recorded in the more standardized conditions of animal experiments are therefore particularly important.

Autologous bone marrow transplantation is possible in splenectomized mice, whose stem cell-containing spleen cells have been reinfused as a cure for radiation-induced aplasia. In fact hematopoietic reconstitution following irradiation of mice with shielded spleens was a classic experiment to demonstrate the regenerative capacity of hematopoiesis [11]. Autologous bone marrow transplantation has also been performed in other species, such as dog and monkey [4, 16].

The experimental model for autologous bone marrow transplantation in leukemia is syngeneic transplantation, i.e., bone marrow grafting within an inbred strain, preferably the AKR mouse strain with its high incidence of thymic lymphoma/leukemias. Leukemias of other strains and species, mostly rats, have also been studied in this context, however. Since the onset of leukemia can unfortunately not be diagnosed early enough in a given mouse, investigators preferred to inject mice with cells of a spontaneous leukemia which had been kept alive by passage through syngeneic mice. Antileukemic treatment was applied either in vitro before, or in vivo after, the cells had been injected into the experimental animal. The use of passaged leukemias makes it possible to work under standardized conditions, but on the other hand entails the disadvantages inherent in working with "difficult" leukemias, whose kinetics have usually accelerated during the passages.

Purging of the Leukemic Marrow with Antibodies

A first study with antibodies was performed in irradiated AKR mice [27]. These received injections of AKR bone marrow mixed with a lethal number of cells from an AKR T cell leukemia. Pretreatment of the leukemic marrow with polyclonal rabbit antiserum which after absorption and fractionation reacted only with T cells resulted in long-term survival of 40%–75% of the animals. But mice dying earlier also showed no symptoms of leukemia. Interestingly, complement had to be added to the antibody treatment (Table 2). The bone marrow recipients' reticuloendothelial system was apparently not capable of eliminating enough leukemic cells by opsonization if antibody alone bound to the T cells. In vitro complement had to lyse the leukemic cells incubated with antibody. Recipients of bone marrow pretreated with anti-T did not develop T cell deficiency. As long as they had a thymus, normal immune reconstitution was observed (Table 3). This important fact indicated that purging bone marrow of normal and leukemic T cells did not prevent hematopoietic recovery [27]. Unlike species-specific and transplantation antigens no T or other differentiation antigens are expressed on stem cells in mice. We are not therefore dependent on leukemia-specific antibodies (which may not exist at all) for the purging of leukemic marrow. For leukemias that express differentiation antigens the corresponding complement-fixing antibodies can be assumed to lyse them while sparing the stem cells necessary for hematopoietic and immunological reconstitution.

How many leukemic cells can be inhibited by antibodies in this mouse model? We inhibited 10^5 cells of a lethal leukemia with a cell dose 1/100 th of this number [27]. Bernstein et al. studied the antileukemic effects of monoclonal anti-Th-1 injected in to mice bearing a transplantable T leukemia [1]. They found that 3×10^5 leukemic cells injected SC could be inhibited provided the antibody was injected early (1–2 h) after the tumor cells had been inoculated. It was concluded from these studies that the in vivo therapy was limited because host mechanisms failed to eliminate larger numbers of subcutaneous cells coated with the

Table 2. Survival of irradiated AKR/J mice following grafts of syngeneic marrow mixed with 10^5 lymphocytes of an AKR/J T cell leukemia and incubated with anti-T cell globulin

Group no.	Incubation of donor cells	No. of recipients	Individual survival times (days)
1	Buffer	12	8, 8, 11, 11, 11, 11, 11, 11, 11, 11, 12, 13
2	Complement	12	8, 8, 8, 8, 8, 11, 11, 11, 11, 11, 11, 11
3	Complement + ATCG	12	9, 16, 18, 19, 19, 21, 22, > 100, > 100, > 100, > 100, > 100[a]

[a] No leukemia was detected in group 3, in contrast to the mice in the other groups

Table 3. Recovery of cellular immunity after transplantation of syngeneic bone marrow incubated with ATCG into normal or thymectomized CBA mice

Group no.	Thymectomy[a]	Incubation with ATCG	No. of recipients	Survival of skin grafts[b] (days)
1	+	+	15	84, > 100, > 100, > 100, > 100, > 100, > 100,
2	+	–	9	28, 29, 30, 35, 35, 35, 70, 77, 84
3	–	+	9	11, 12, 14, 14, 15, 16, 16, 16, 16

[a] Thymectomy was performed 2 weeks before bone marrow transplantation
[b] H-2-incompatible C57BL/6 skin was grafted 1 month after bone marrow transplantation

infused antibody, partly due to the emergence of deviant leukemic cells lacking the target antigen. A large number of earlier studies with polyclonal antibodies all seem to show that tumors and leukemias can only be inhibited if unrealistically high amounts of antibodies are injected within 24 h after tumor cell inoculation. Later injections did not eradicate transplanted T leukemias even under ideal conditions in congenic hosts, where the leukemia and the host T antigen were different so that the applied antibody could not be absorbed by host tissue but only by the leukemic cell [15].

Our approach of lysing leukemic cells in vitro before bone marrow transplantation was conceived to avoid dependence on host mechanisms for the elimination of tumor cells coated with antibodies. Suppression of opsonizing functions has to be considered in patients after maximal cytoreductive treatment.

Much lower amounts of antibodies are required for the in vitro approach. However, its limits in tumor cell inhibition are not yet well defined. Antibodies coupled to the A chain of the plant toxin were demonstrated to effectively kill neoplastic B cells [31, 32] or normal T cells [12, 21] in vitro and in vivo. Further experiments are needed to find out whether such immunotoxins clearly kill more T leukemic cells than cytotoxic antibodies while sparing hematopoietic stem cells.

Clinical Considerations

Since leukemia may relapse after months or years of remission, autologous bone marrow transplantation requires a bone marrow bank allowing long-term storage of bone marrow cells preserved in liquid nitrogen. Long-term studies of cryopreserved bone marrow have demonstrated that bone marrow cells can indeed be stored in liquid nitrogen for over 6 years without significant loss of stem cell function [19]. As autologous bone marrow transplantation in remission will probably lead to better clinical results the answer to the question as to whether to harvest marrow during the first or the second remission will depend on the logistics of collection and storage. So far patients with acute lymphoblastic leukemia of the common type have made up the largest group treated with autologous bone marrow transplantation and antibodies [5, 20, 22, 23]. Several patients with acute nonlymphoblastic leukemia received autologous marrow pretreated by chemoseparation [13, 26] with 4-hydroperoxycyclophosphamide in a phase I study, with an observation time up to 15 months of complete remission. Various physical methods have been tested to separate leukemic cells from normal hematopoietic cells on the basis of cell differences such as density, size, or varying heat sensitivity; there have been no clear results. The use of a discontinuous albumin gradient for separating residual leukemic cells did not affect the relapse rate, as was shown by comparison with patients who had received unfractionated bone marrow cells [6].

Although the antibody approach appears quite promising in autologous bone marrow transplantation, there is still no definite ruling on what type of antibody should be used. Polyclonal antibodies require purification from stem cell toxicity. They are preferably rabbit antibodies, which bind complement better than monoclonal mouse antibodies usually do. Monoclonal antibodies are restricted to one epitope of an antigen, while polyclonal antibodies represent a mixture of antibody subclasses directed against several epitopes of a given antigen. Monoclonal antibodies, of course, have the great advantage of standardization.

The type of leukemia that can be treated depends on the antibodies available. With antibodies against T or cALL more than 90% of childhood lymphatic leukemias would be candidates for autologous bone marrow transplantation [17]. But acute myeloid leukemia should also be considered for treatment with autologous bone marrow transplantation if antibodies against myeloid or Ia antigens are available. Whether acute B lymphoblast leukemia cells can be more effectively inhibited by anti-idiotype antibodies than by antibodies reacting with Ia or other B cells antigens remains to be shown. Clearly autologous bone marrow transplantation for the treatment of leukemias is still in an early experimental phase, where results are preliminary and experience has still to be drawn from every single case.

Patients, Materials, and Methods

Bone marrow was obtained from patients in remission by multiple aspirations from the anterior and posterior iliac crest under general anesthesia, and was suspended in a preservative-free heparin medium mixture. The bone marrow (800–1,700 ml) was filtered through fine screens; after fractionation in a cell separator the red cell suspension depleted of mononuclear cells was washed and immediately reinfused to the donor. The marrow cell suspension was mixed at 4° C to a final concentration of 10% DMSO, transferred to polyolefine bags, sandwiched into metal sleeves and frozen to −30° C at a rate of 1 deg

C/min with automatic compensation of the phase transition time, then to −100° C at a rate of 5−7 deg C/min, followed by storage in liquid nitrogen at −196° C. Thawing was performed in a 45° C water bath within 2 minutes.

After an ACDA plasma correction of pH to 6.9, the cryopreserved bone marrow was directly infused to the patient without clearing the cryopreservation medium from the marrow. Antisera against human T- antigen and cALL antigen were developed in rabbits. Immunization, absorption, and fractionation methods are described in detail elsewhere [24]. For the clinical use of incubation with antisera, which was performed before storage of the marrow, the following requirements have to be satisfied: sterility, pyrogen-free technique, negative hemagglutination titer; no cross-reactions against glomerular basement membrane, hematopoietic stem cells, plasma proteins, or complement. Cross-reactions of antisera with normal hematopoietic stem cells were studied in inhibition tests using the CFU-C assay and the diffusion chamber test [18]. The final dilution of the antiserum in the bone marrow suspension was 1 : 200 of a 10 mg/ml antibody preparation. Standard methods were applied for microcytotoxicity testing. Patients were conditioned with the following antileukemic therapeutic regimen: BCNU (200 mg/m^2 on days −13 and −12), cytosine arabinoside (200 mg/m^2 on days −12 to −8), cyclosphosphamide (1.8 g/m^2 on days −7 and −6), and total-body irradiation with 10 Gy from two opposing ^{60}Co sources at a dosage of 5.5 cGy/min 24 h before transplantation. During hospitalization the patients were kept in a laminar flow unit.

Results and Discussion

In various clinical centers different treatment protocols have been used to eradicate leukemia in the recipient before autografting. We combine the Seattle regimen [28] with BCNU and cytosine arabinoside. Tolerance in allogeneic bone marrow transplantation has so far been good [25].

Figure 1 shows the cytotoxic activity of specific anti-cALL globulin against leukemic cells and normal hematopoietic cells. All blasts of three typical cALL cases at diagnosis (99% blasts in the bone marrow) and one case in relapse (48% blasts in the bone marrow) were lysed to a dilution of 1 : 256. No cytotoxic effect was observed in T-ALL leukemic cells, normal bone marrow cells, or normal peripheral blood lymphocytes.

The cytotoxic activity of anti-cALL globulin against normal hematopoietic stem cells was investigated in frozen marrow cells from patient 1 (Table 4). Short-term incubation of marrow cells with nonabsorbed anti-cALL antiserum and complement completely inhibited the growth of stem cells committed to granulocytic-myeloid differentiation (CFU-C). The absorption of cross-reacting antibodies produced a cleared globulin fraction with no cytotoxic activity against normal progenitor cells but a high cytotoxic activity against cALL-type leukemic cells.

Figure 2 illustrates the clinical course of patient 1, a 7-year-old girl in her third relapse of cALL. At 24 h after total body irradiation, 1.9 × 10^8 nucleated marrow cells/kg (86,000 CFU-C/kg) were infused. The marrow cells had been harvested during her first remission, cryopreserved in liquid nitrogen for 30 months, and prepared with anti-cALL globulin before grafting. The clinical course was uneventful and the patient achieved complete hematopoietic recovery with a WBC count of 1,000/mm^3 on day 21, a platelet count of 20,000/mm^3 on day 50, and a remission period of 6 months.

The second patient, an 8-year-old boy in his third cALL relapse, received 3.7 × 10^8 nucleated bone marrow cells/kg that had been cryopreserved at −196° C for 12 months.

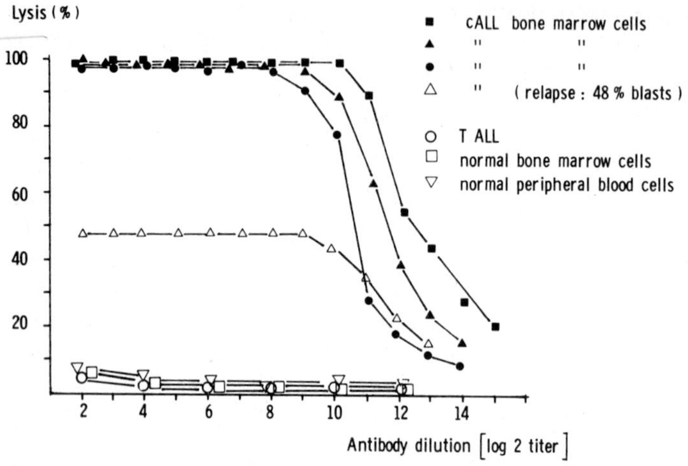

Fig. 1. Cytotoxic activity of anti-cALL globulin in three cases of cALL at diagnosis, one case in relapse, and one case of T-ALL as well as cytotoxic activity against normal bone marrow and peripheral blood cells

Table 4. Cytotoxicity of nonabsorbed and absorbed anti-cALL globulin in committed progenitor cells (CFU-C)

	Antibody dilution[b]	CFU-C/2 $\times$ 10^5 nucleated marrow cells[c]
Anti-cALL globulin[a]		
Nonabsorbed	1: 4 + C	0
	1:16 + C	0
Absorbed	1: 4 + C	102 ± 6
	1:16 + C	92 ± 8
Normal rabbit globulin	1: 4 + C	89 ± 5

[a] All preparations were adjusted to a protein concentration of 10 mg/ml
[b] *C*, complement
[c] Mean CFU-C ± SEM

The patient died of cardiac failure 7 days after bone marrow transplantation. The bone marrow was characterized by incipient normal myelopoietic and erythropoietic differentiation, but no leukemic cells could be detected. Autografting (3.3 × 10^8/kg marrow cells, preservation at −196° C for 15 months) was also performed in an 8-year-old girl in her third relapse. On day 23 the patient died of septicemia. Histopathology showed the onset of remission in bone marrow and peripheral blood, but no leukemic cells.
In spite of the clinical outcome in the three patients this phase 1 study demonstrated that bone marrow cells harvested during the first remission and prepared with antileukemic antisera have the capacity to repopulate the recipient's bone marrow and produce hematopoietic recovery.

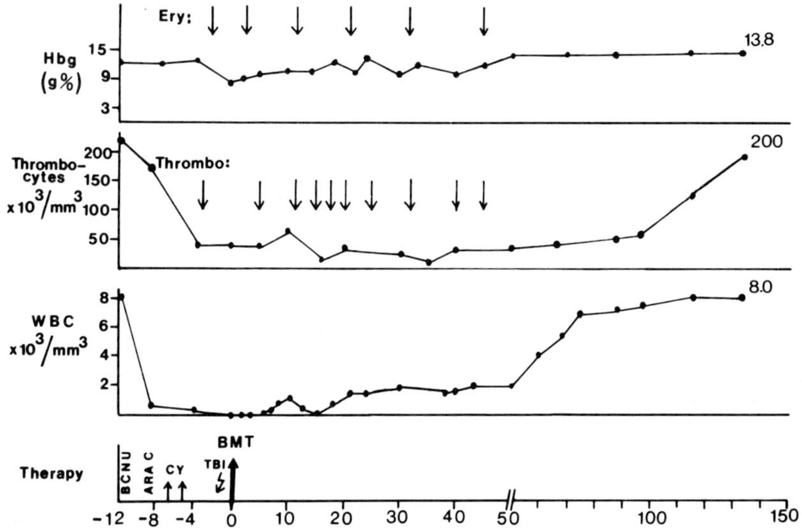

Fig. 2. Clinical course of patient 1 after transplantation of autologous bone marrow cells prepared with anti-cALL globulin. *TBI,* total body irradiation; *BMT,* bone marrow transplantation; ↓, transfusion

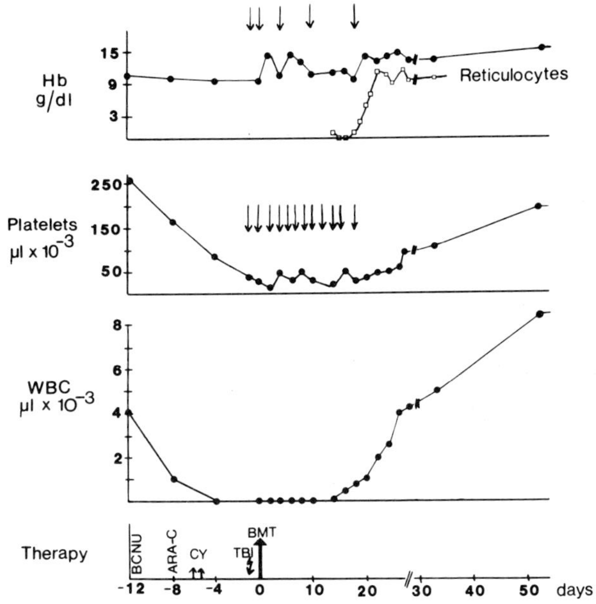

Fig. 3. Clinical course in patient 4 after transplantation of nucleated marrow cells in his third remission. ↓, transfusion

The analysis of patient data after allogeneic bone marrow transplantation showed that leukemic relapse ranked second in the causes of death. There is clear evidence that relapse occurs predominantly in patients in whom grafting is performed in late relapse [29, 30, 33]. This was also observed in patient 1, who relapsed 6 months after bone marrow transplantation.

Our present phase 2 study is designed to investigate improvement in survival rates after bone marrow transplantation in the second or at latest third remission. Patient 4, an

$8^1/_2$-year-old boy, had a graft of 2.5×10^8 nucleated marrow cells/kg, which had been preserved for 51 months at −196° C, in his third remission (Fig. 3). The clinical course after transplantation was uneventful and the patient is in complete remission 10 months after the bone marrow transplantation. Patient 5, a 9-year-old girl, had an autograft (2.2×18^8/kg nucleated marrow cells preserved for 50 months at −196° C) in her third remission and is in complete remission 2 months after bone marrow transplantation.
Whether these observations will translate into an improved cure rate remains to be determined by long-term follow-up studies.

References

1. Badger CC, Bernstein ID (1983) Therapy of murine leukemia with monoclonal antibody against a normal differentiation antigen. J Exp Med 157,3: 828
2. Baumgartner C, Bleher EA, Brun del Re U, Bucher KA, Deubelbeiss R, Greiner A, Hirt P, Imbach R, Odavic R, Wagner HP (1981) Transplantation of cryopreserved autologous bone marrow after intensive chemotherapy and total body irradiation in children and adolescents with advanced cancer. Exp Hematol 9,9: 139
3. Boranic M, Tonkovic I (1971) Time pattern of the antileukemic effect of graft-versus-host reaction in mice. Cancer Res 31: 1140
4. Chertkov JL, Sukyasyan GV, Novikova MN, Nemenova NM, Kotlyarov AM, Malanina VN, Samoylina NL, Udalov GA, Semenov LF (1971) Autologous bone marrow transplantation in irradiated baboons. Radiat Res 46: 129–143
5. Deisseroth A, Mangalik A, Robinson W, Weiner R (eds) (1979) Keystone conference on autologous bone marrow transplantation. Exp Hematol [Suppl 5] 7
6. Dicke KA, Zander A, Spitzer G, Verma DS, Peters LJ, Vellekoop L, McCredie JB, Hester J (1979) Autologous bone marrow transplantation in relapsed adult acute leukemia. Lancet 1: 514
7. Fay JW, Silberman HR, Moore JO, Noell KT, Huang AT (1979) Autologous marrow transplantation for patients with acute myelogenous leukemia – a preliminary report. Exp Hematol 7,5: 303
8. Fefer A, Cheever MA, Thomas ED et al. (1981) Bone marrow transplantations for refractory acute leukemia in 34 patients with identical twins. Blood 57,3: 421
9. Goldman JM (1980) Haemopoietic stem cell autografts for leukaemia. Blut 41: 71
10. Gorin NC, Najman A, Salmon C, Muller JY, Petit JC, David R, Stachowiak J, Hirsch Marie F, Parlier Y, Duhamel G (1979) High dose combination chemotherapy (TACC) with and without autologous bone marrow transplantation for the treatment of acute leukemia and other malignant diseases. Kinetics of recovery of haemopoesis. A preliminary study of 12 cases. Eur J Cancer 15: 1113
11. Jacobson LO, Simmons EL, Marks EK, Eldredge JH (1951) Recovery from radiation injury. Science 113: 510–511
12. Jansen FK, Blythman HE, Carriere D, Casellas P, Diaz J, Gros P, Henequin JR, Paolucci F, Pau B, Poncelet P, Richter G, Salhi SL, Vidal H, Voisin GA (1980) High specific cytotoxicity of antibody-toxin hybrid molecules (immunotoxins) for target cells. Immunol Lett 2: 97–102
13. Kaizer H, Tutschka P, Stuart R, Körbling M, Braine H, Saral R, Colvin M, Santos G (1982) Autologous bone marrow transplantation in acute leukemia and non-hodgkin's lymphoma: a phase I study of 4-hydroperoxycyclophosphamide (4HC) incubation of marrow prior to cryopreservation. In: Neth R, Gallo RC, Greaves M, Moore R, Winkler K (eds) Modern trends in human leukemia 5. Springer, Berlin Heidelberg New York, pp 90–91 (Hämatologie und Bluttransfusion, vol 28)
14. Kaizer H, Wharam MD, Johnson RJ, Economou JG, Shin HS, Santos GW, Elfenbein GJ, Tutschka PJ, Braine HG, Munoz LL, Leventhal BG (1980) Requirements of the successful

application of autologous bone marrow transplantation in the treatment of selected malignancies. Haematol Bluttransfus 25: 285
15. Kirch ME, Hämmerling U (1981) Immunotherapy of murine leukemias by monoclonal antibody. I. Effect of passively administered antibody on growth of transplanted tumor cells. J Immunol 127,2: 805
16. Mannick JA, Lochte HL, Thomas ED, Ferrebee JW (1960) In vitro and in vivo assessment of the viability of dog marrow after storage. Blood 15: 517–524
17. Netzel B, Rodt H, Thiel E, Haas RJ, Thierfelder S (1979) Neuere Aspekte zur Anwendung spezifischer Antiseren bei der Diagnose und Therapie der akuten lymphatischen Leukämie im Kindesalter. Klin Pädiat 191: 175
18. Netzel B, Rodt H, Lau B, Thiel E, Haas RJ, Dörmer P, Thierfelder S (1978) Transplantation of syngeneic bone marrow incubated with leukocyte antibodies. II. Cytotoxic activity of anti-cALL globulin on leukemic cells in man. Transplantation 26: 157
19. Netzel B, Rodt H, Haas RJ, Janka G, Thierfelder S (1980) The concept of antileukemic, autologous bone marrow transplantation in acute lymphoblastic leukemia. Haematol Bluttransfus 25: 297
20. Netzel B, Haas RJ, Rodt H, Kolb HJ, Thierfelder S (1980) Immunological conditioning of bone marrow for autotransplantation in childhood acute lymphoblastic leukemia. Lancet 1: 1332
21. Neville DM, Youle RJ (1981) Monoclonal antibody-ricin or ricin a chain hybrids: kinetic analysis of cell killing for tumor therapy. Immunol Rev 62: 135
22. Ritz J, Bast RC, Clavell LA, Hercend T, Sallan SE, Liton JM, Feeney M, Nathan DG, Schlossman SF (1982) Autologous bone marrow transplantation in cALLA-positive acute lymphoblastic leukemia after in vitro treatment with J5 monoclonal antibody and complement. Lancet 2: 8289
23. Ritz J, Sallan SE, Bast RC, Lipton JM, Nathan DG, Schlossman SF (1982) In vitro treatment with monoclonal antibody prior to autologous bone marrow transplantation in acute lymphoblastic leukemia. In: Neth R, Gallo RC, Greaves M, Moore R, Winkler K (eds) Modern trends in human leukemia 5. Springer, Berlin Heidelberg New York, p 117 (Haematologie und Bluttransfusion, vol 28)
24. Rodt H, Netzel B, Thiel E, Jäger G, Huhn D, Haas RJ, Götze D, Thierfelder S (1977) Classification of leukemic cells with T and 0-ALL specific antisera. Haematol Bluttransfus 20: 87
25. Rodt H, Netzel B, Kolb HJ, Janka G, Rieder I, Belohradsky B, Haas RJ, Thierfelder S (1979) Antibody treatment of marrow grafts in vitro: a principle for prevention of GvH disease. In: Baum SJ, Ledney GD (eds) Experimental haematology today. Springer, Berlin Heidelberg New York, p 197
26. Sharkis SJ, Santos GW, Colvin M (1980) Elimination of acute myelogenous leukemic cells from marrow and tumor suspensions in the rat with 4-hydroperoxycyclophasphamide. Blood 55: 521
27. Thierfelder S, Rodt H, Netzel B (1977) Transplantation of syngeneic bone marrow incubated with leucocyte antibodies. I. Suppression of lymphatic leukemia of syngeneic donor mice. Transplantation 26: 460
28. Thomas ED, Storb R, Clift RA, Fefer A, Johnson FL, Neiman PE, Lerner KG, Glucksberg H, Buckner CD (1975) Bone marrow transplantation. N Engl J Med 292: 832
29. Thomas ED, Buckner CD, Clift RA, Fefer A, Johnson FL, Neiman PE, Sale GE, Sanders JE, Singer JW, Shulman H, Storb R, Weiden PL (1979) Marrow transplantation for acute non-lymphoblastic leukemia in first remission. N Engl J Med 302: 597
30. Thomas ED, Sanders JE, Johnson FL, Buckner CD, Clift RA, Fefer A, Goodell BW, Storb R, Weiden PL (1979) Marrow transplantation for patients with acute lymphoblastic leukemia in remission. Blood 54: 468
31. Thorpe PE, Detre SI, Mason DW, Cumber AJ, Ross WC (1982) Monoclonal antibody therapy: "model" experiments with toxin-conjugated antibodies in mice and rats. In: Neth R, Gallo RC, Greaves M, Moore R, Winkler K (eds) Modern trends in human leukemia 5. Springer, Berlin Heidelberg New York, pp 107–111 (Haematologie und Bluttransfusion, vol 28)

32. Vitetta ES, Krolik KA, Uhr JW (1982) The use of antibody-ricin A chain immunotoxins for the therapy of a B cell leukemia (BCL_1) in mice. Academic Press, New York, pp 473–480 (UCLA symposium vol XIV.)
33. Weiden PL, Flurnoy N, Thomas ED, Prentice R, Fefer A, Buckner CD, Storb R (1979) Antileukemic effect of graft-versus-host disease in human recipients of allogeneic-marrow graft. N Engl J Med 300: 1068

Subject Index